Pain Management

made **Incredibly Easy!**®

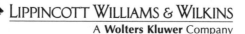

LIPPINCOTT WILLIAMS & WILKINS
A **Wolters Kluwer** Company

Philadelphia • Baltimore • New York • London
Buenos Aires • Hong Kong • Sydney • Tokyo

Staff

Publisher
Judith A. Schilling McCann, RN, MSN

Editorial Director
David Moreau

Clinical Director
Joan M. Robinson, RN, MSN

Senior Art Director
Arlene Putterman

Art Director
Mary Ludwicki

Clinical Editors
Bonnie L. McGonigle, RN, MSN, CCRN, CRNP;
Marcy Caplin, RN, MSN, CS; Pamela Kovach, RN, BSN

Editors
Julie Munden (senior editor), Ty Eggenberger,
Kathy E. Goldberg, Judd Howard, Brenna H. Mayer,
Carol Munson

Copy Editors
Kimberly Bilotta (supervisor), Amy Furman,
Shana Harrington, Dona Hightower Perkins,
Pamela Wingrod

Designer
Lynn Foulk

Illustrators
Bot Roda, Jackie Facciolo

Electronic Production Services
Diane Paluba (manager), Joyce Rossi Biletz (senior
desktop assistant), Richard Eng (desktop assistant)

Manufacturing
Patricia K. Dorshaw (senior manager),
Beth Janae Orr (book production coordinator)

Editorial Assistants
Danielle J. Barsky, Beverly Lane, Linda Ruhf

Indexer
Karen C. Comerford

Printed in the United States of America. For information, write Lippincott Williams & Wilkins, 1111 Bethlehem Pike, P.O. Box 908, Springhouse, PA 19477-0908.

PMMIE – D N O S A J J M A
05 04 03   10 9 8 7 6 5 4 3 2 1

Library of Congress Cataloging-in-Publication Data
Pain management made incredibly easy.
    p. ; cm.
    Includes index.
    1. Pain — Treatment. 2. Analgesia.
    [DNLM: 1. Pain — therapy. 2. Palliative Care. WL 704 P46595
    2003] I. Lippincott Williams & Wilkins.

RB127.P33238 2003
616'.0472 — dc21
ISBN 1-58255-227-4 (pbk. : alk. paper)   2003000868

Contents

Contributors and consultants

Paul M. Arnstein, PhD, APRN-BC, FNP-C
Assistant Professor
Boston College
Chestnut Hill, Mass.

Patricia A. Brandon, RN
Nurse Clinician Anesthesia Pain Service
Ochsner Foundation Hospital
New Orleans

Mary Milano Carter, RN, MS, ANP, BC
Director of Clinical Services
North Shore Pain Services
Syossett, N.Y.

Mark A. Chamberlain, PharmD
Drug Information Specialist
Clinical Assistant Professor
University of Maryland
Baltimore

Patricia Manda Collins, RN, MSN, AONC
Clinical Nurse Specialist
Baptist Health (Education Services)
Miami

Laura K. Crooks, RN, BSN, MEd
Independent Pain Management Educator
Pittsburgh

Linda M. Dean, MSN, CRNP, ACRN
Director of Clinical Education
HIV/AIDS Medicine Division
Drexel University College of Medicine
Philadelphia

Annabel D. Edwards, RN, MSN, ANP
Clinical Nurse Specialist
Massachusetts General Hospital
Boston

Una M. Edwardson, RN,C, ANP
Adult Nurse Practitioner
United Hospital (Allina Health System) Pain
  Clinic
St. Paul

Judith M. Fouladbakhsh, RN, MSN, APRN, BC
Faculty Member
Wayne State University College of Nursing
Detroit

Cynthia L. Frozena, RN, MSN
Medical Education & Communication
Enzymatic Therapy
Green Bay, Wis.

Nyla R. Gardner, RN,C, MSN
Nurse Manager
Dr. O'Connell's PainCare Centers, Inc.
Somersworth, N.H.

Monica S. Haley, RN, MHA
Administrator, Clinical Nurse
Dr. O'Connell's PainCare Centers, Inc.
Somersworth, N.H.

Eleftheria Karapas, RN, MS
Pain Management Coordinator
Silver Cross Hospital
Joliet, Ill.

Anne Marie Kelly, RN,C, BSN
Director of Staff Development and Pain
  Management
Catholic Memorial Home
Fall River, Mass.

Nancy R. Kowal, RN,C, MS, ANP
Pain Consultant
Past President ASPMN
President Sigma Theta Tau
Adjunct Professor
University of Massachusetts
Worcester

Kathleen Lowinger, ARNP, MSN, BC
Pain Management Clinical Nurse Specialist
Baptist Hospital of Miami

Erin McMenamin, MSN, CRNP, AOCN
Pain Medicine Nurse Practitioner/Program
  Manager
University of Pennsylvania
Philadelphia

Debbie Miller-Saultz, RN, MS, FNP
Nurse Practitioner – Department of Pain
  Medicine and Palliative Care
Beth Israel Medical Center
New York

Rhonda Nichols, RN, MS, CNS
Pain Management Consultant
San Francisco

June E. Oliver, RN, MSN, CCNS, CCRN
Clinical Nurse Specialist
Advocate Illinois Masonic Medical Center
Chicago

Lourdes "Cindy" Santoni-Reddy, MSN, MEd, NP-C, FAAPM
Faculty
Hahnemann University
Philadelphia
Nurse Practitioner
American Academy of Pain Management
Sonora, Calif.

Barbara St. Marie, MA, CS, ANP, GNP
Nurse Practitioner – Pain Management
Fairview University Medical Center
Minneapolis

Lisa Salamon, RN,C, MSN, CNS, ET
Clinical Nurse Specialist
Cleveland Clinic Foundation

Helen N. Turner, RN, MSN, CNS
Pediatric Pain Management Clinical Nurse
  Specialist
Doernbecher Children's Hospital
Oregon Health & Science University
Portland

Foreword

Every day, health care professionals in all settings encounter patients who are experiencing pain. Uncontrolled pain slows healing, contributes to the development of complications, and causes needless suffering. For this reason, you're required by the Joint Commission on Accreditation of Healthcare Organizations and by your own facility's policies and procedures to meet standards for assessing and managing your patients' pain.

Despite the ever-increasing importance of pain management in your practice, you'd be hard pressed to find an authoritative resource on pain management that presents reliable clinical information in such an easy-to-understand format. *Pain Management Made Incredibly Easy* is a much-needed breath of fresh air in pain-management literature because it combines concise information on pain principles from noted experts with practical, hands-on solutions that will enable you to provide quality care for your patients who experience pain.

This innovative book explores all the major topics associated with pain management, including:
• the fundamentals of pain—anatomy and physiology, theories of pain transmission, psychosocial aspects of pain, and barriers to effective pain management
• pain assessment—history and physical examination, pain assessment tools, nonverbal pain clues, psychological evaluation, and documentation of pain assessment findings
• pharmacologic pain management, from NSAIDs and opioids to adjuvant analgesics, local anesthetics, and patient-controlled analgesia
• nonpharmacologic pain management approaches, ranging from acupuncture, biofeedback, and homeopathy to music therapy, traction, and yoga
• management of acute pain, chronic nonmalignant pain, cancer, and HIV-AIDS–related pain
• pain management in pediatric and geriatric patients, including age-appropriate pain assessment guidelines, intervention techniques, and medications
• pain management in patients with addictive disease
• patient teaching and lifestyle management issues.

Throughout the book, you'll find plenty of features to aid your understanding of pain-management principles and practices, such as:
• clear, simple explanations and definitions of key terms
• illustrations that clarify technical concepts
• checklists that identify key points
• quick quizzes to help you assess what you've learned.

To make the content both useful and user-friendly, *Pain Management Made Incredibly Easy* offers these remarkably unique features:

Peak technique — tells you how to perform specific pain management procedures

Now I get it! — clarifies the pathophysiology of pain and the mechanisms underlying various pain management techniques

Rein in the pain — offers pointers on how to manage pain

Myth busters — clears the air about stereotypes and prejudices related to pain and its perception.

With its light-hearted approach and get-right-to-the-point presentation, *Pain Management Made Incredibly Easy* takes the incredibly complex experience of pain and explains it in clear-cut ways that will help you manage your patients' pain more quickly and more effectively than ever before. How many of your high-priced medical references can do that?

Paul M. Arnstein, PhD, APRN-BC, FNP-C
Member, Board of Directors
American Society of Pain Management Nurses
Assistant Professor
Boston College
Chestnut Hill, Mass.

Understanding pain

Just the facts

In this chapter, you'll learn:

♦ the nociceptive and psychological responses to pain

♦ definitions of acute, chronic nonmalignant, and cancer pain

♦ current models of pain theory

♦ beliefs about pain that affect pain behaviors.

A look at the physiology of pain

Pain has existed since the beginning of time— and so have attempts to understand and treat it. Pain alerts us to injury or illness and serves as a protective mechanism.

Reactions to pain vary among individuals. In fact, they even vary within the same person at different times.

Not so simple

Although pain may seem like a simple sensation, it's actually a complex experience influenced by:
• a person's cultural background
• the anticipation of pain
• previous experience with pain
• the context in which pain occurs
• emotional and cognitive responses.

The process of pain involves complex physiologic and psychological responses that vary from person to person and even from day to day. To understand pain fully, you must be familiar with its physiologic aspects, called nociception, and its psychological aspects.

> My pain is producing complex physiologic and psychological responses, including the need to say !@#$%!

Understanding nociception

The word sounds complicated, but *nociception* simply means the sensation of pain. Nociception results from the stimulation of *nociceptors* — special injury-sensing receptors embedded in the skin or in the walls of internal organs. Injury may come from a physical source (mechanical, thermal, or electrical) or a chemical source (such as a toxin).

The body contains millions of nociceptors — roughly 1,300 for every square inch of skin. Some nociceptors detect burns while others detect cuts, chemical changes, pressure, infection, and other sensations.

Just can't help reacting that way

Nociceptors use nerve impulses to send messages to other nerves, which in turn forward the messages to the spinal cord and brain at lightning speed. This process activates involuntary (autonomic and reflexive) responses. Involuntary responses caused by painful stimuli include:
- elevated blood pressure
- an increasing pulse rate
- an increased respiratory rate or breath holding
- muscle flexion (withdrawal) of the affected part of the body.

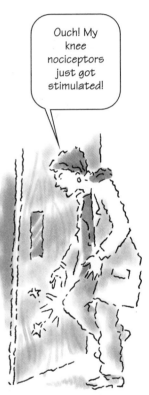

Ouch! My knee nociceptors just got stimulated!

Is it pain — or nociception?

Nociception and the pain experience aren't identical. Nociception refers to the neurologic events and reflex responses caused by an event that damages, or threatens to damage, tissue.

Pain, on the other hand, is an unpleasant sensory and emotional experience associated with actual or potential tissue injury, or described in terms of such injury. Pain is subjective; nociception isn't.

Nociception doesn't necessarily cause the perception of pain — and pain can occur even without nociception. That explains why patients with certain pain syndromes may have no obvious pathology yet still experience debilitating pain.

Stages of nociception

Nociception has four stages:
- transduction
- transmission
- perception
- modulation.

Transduction

Transduction—the first stage of nociception—refers to the conversion of mechanical, chemical, or thermal information into electrical activity in the nervous system. When a sensory (afferent) neuron receives a nociceptive stimulus, its leglike extension, or axon, conveys electrical information toward the spinal cord or to cells leading to the cranial nerves.

Special sensory nerve endings in the skin, deep tissue, and viscera (soft internal organs) change mechanical, thermal, and chemical energy into electrical energy. These sensory receptors are excited only by stimuli in the area they innervate, called their receptive fields.

> Transduction converts mechanical, chemical, and thermal information into electrical impulses.

Don't touch my transducer molecules!

Transduction works differently for thermal, mechanical, and chemical stimuli. But in all cases, the stimulus interacts with highly specialized molecules, called transducer molecules, embedded in the receptor membrane. (See *Transduction: First stage of nociception and pain*, page 4.)

With excitation, the transducer molecule changes in a way that causes sodium channels in the receptor membrane to open. Extracellular sodium flows into the cell, causing the receptor to depolarize (lose its electrical charge). This, in turn, causes an action potential—a momentary change in electrical potential on the cell surface.

Let's get specific

Transducer molecules vary with the type of stimulus to which they're sensitive.
- Those sensitive to chemicals have binding sites that accept only one type of chemical.
- Those sensitive to mechanical stimulation have ion channels that are opened by mechanical distortion of a cell membrane.
- Those sensitive to temperature have molecular "gates" that open when heated or cooled.

Different receptors have varying degrees of specificity for different types of stimuli. Receptors that respond to only one type of stimulus—heat, for example—are called *unimodal* receptors. In contrast, *polymodal* receptors respond to two or more types of stimuli.

Receptors also differ in their sensitivity—the number of action potentials that result from a given stimulus.

> I'm Uni Modal, and I respond to just one type of stimulus.

> And I'm Poly Modal, and I respond to a whole lot more.

Transduction: First stage of nociception and pain

In transduction, a mechanical, thermal, or chemical stimulus interacts with receptor molecules at the tips of nociceptive primary afferent neurons (commonly called free nerve endings). As a result, sodium channels open and extracellular sodium flows in, causing the receptor molecule to depolarize, which creates an action potential. Electrical energy then travels to the spinal cord and on to the brain, signaling pain.

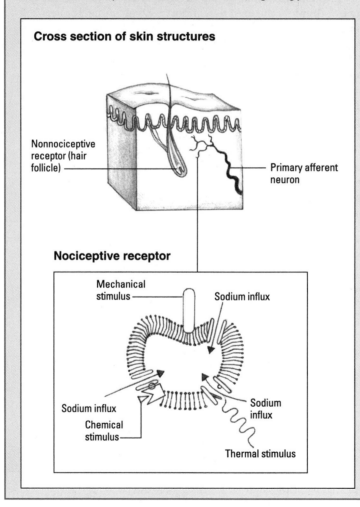

Cross section of skin structures

Nonnociceptive receptor (hair follicle)

Primary afferent neuron

Nociceptive receptor

Mechanical stimulus

Sodium influx

Sodium influx

Chemical stimulus

Sodium influx

Thermal stimulus

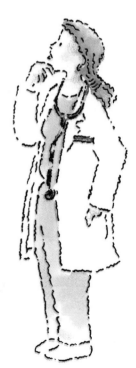

You seem hypersensitive today

Receptors that respond to stimuli in the viscera and the body wall, called *somatovisceral* receptors, vary greatly in specificity and sensitivity. Somatovisceral receptors fall into three groups:
• *nonnociceptive* (innocuous, or harmless) receptors. These receptors are activated by stimuli that don't cause damage or produce pain (such as touch and hair movement).
• *nociceptive-specific* receptors (nociceptors). These receptors respond only to stimuli that damage (or could damage) tissue.
• *silent nociceptors*. These receptors only become active in instances of chemical sensitization or inflammation. They can amplify and spread pain, or change nonpainful stimuli into nociceptive signals.

Nociceptors, nonnociceptive receptors, and silent nociceptors are distributed throughout the body, but their densities vary. For example, the fingertips contain many nonnociceptive receptors but relatively few nociceptors. This is probably because pain sensations could interfere with the sense of touch, for which the fingers are specially adapted. In contrast, the cornea and teeth abound in nociceptors, making them especially responsive to painful stimuli.

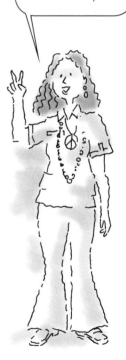

My fingertips have relatively few nociceptors, so they're less sensitive to pain.

Nonnociceptive receptors

Although somatovisceral nonnociceptive receptors rarely signal pain directly, they can affect pain perception in several ways:
• In some disorders, innocuous stimuli can become painful. This condition is called *allodynia*.
• Innocuous sensory input can amplify pain perception. This is called *hyperalgesia*.
• When nociceptive pathways are absent, excessive activity in nonnociceptive (and perhaps silent nociceptors) neurons alerts the nervous system to noxious (pain-producing) stimuli.

Several types of nonnociceptive sensory receptors exist. Each type has a distinctive structure, function, location in the body, depth under the skin, and conduction speed. Also, each type responds to different stimuli.

All nonnociceptive receptors are unimodal, specialized, and highly sensitive, responding to extremely slight stimulation. This low activation threshold differentiates them from nociceptors.

Nociceptive receptors

Specialized for pain, nociceptors appear throughout the skin, deep tissue, and viscera. Types of nociceptors include:
• superficial somatic nociceptors
• deep somatic nociceptors
• visceral nociceptors. (See *How visceral nociception works*, page 6.)

> **Now I get it!**
>
> # How visceral nociception works
>
> Years ago, most experts thought the soft internal organs, or viscera, lacked nociceptors because direct organ manipulation didn't cause pain during light surgical anesthesia.
>
> But such disorders as appendicitis and angina—in which internal organs give rise to pain—contradict this notion. Such pain probably results from slow-conducting, unencapsulated nerve endings of certain nerve fibers found throughout the viscera and somatic structures.
>
> **Name your stimuli**
>
> Stimuli that cause pain when applied to the viscera differ from those that cause pain when applied to the skin. Also, such stimuli may differ from organ to organ.
> • In the colon, stomach, and other hollow organs, distention stimulates nociceptors.
> • In the testes and other solid organs, compression most effectively stimulates nociceptors.

Somatovisceral nociceptors respond *only* to mechanical, thermal, or chemical stimuli that damage, or threaten to damage, tissue. For example, they respond when you touch a hot frying pan but not when you touch a cool one.

Nociceptors differ from nonnociceptive receptors in several ways:
• They have a highly complex structure and function, reflecting their highly specialized transduction properties.
• Some are polymodal, whereas all nonnociceptive receptors are unimodal.
• They can be activated by chemicals that originate either from within tissues (such as inflammatory mediators) or externally.

Stimulation of nociceptors creates the physiologic response that we recognize as pain. But pain doesn't result from a single stimulation of a single nociceptor. For a person to perceive pain, either the action potential must occur repeatedly in a single nociceptor, or it must occur in many nociceptors at once.

Superficial somatic nociceptors

Somatic nociceptors respond mainly to mechanical and thermal stimuli. Superficial (cutaneous) somatic nociceptors come in two types:

• Unimodal receptors give rise to myelinated sensory (afferent) nerve fibers with conduction speeds of up to 40 miles per hour. Called A-delta fibers, these fibers have a large diameter. When activated, they evoke sharp localized pain or pricking pain.

• Polymodal nociceptors give rise to unmyelinated afferent nerve fibers with conduction speeds of 3 miles per hour. Called C fibers, they account for roughly 75% of all nociceptors. C fibers have a smaller diameter than A-delta fibers. When activated, they typically evoke long-lasting dull, aching, or burning pain.

Polymodal nociceptors respond to mechanical, thermal, and chemical stimuli—especially chemicals released during inflammation, exercise, or disease.

When A-delta and C fibers are activated—for example, you stick your toe in scalding bath water—you feel an immediate, sharp, localized pain followed by long-lasting, burning pain. That's because the painful stimulus evokes fast (A-delta) and slow (C) pain fibers.

In too deep

Deep somatic nociceptors occur in muscle, fascia, connective tissue, and joints. Although they resemble cutaneous nociceptors, they respond to somewhat different stimuli.

Deep somatic nociceptors commonly respond to stimuli that evoke deep pain—such as the excessive force that can occur in traumatic injury or the chemicals (such as prostaglandins, substance P, acids, and potassium) that cause muscle pain. Most people would describe the pain evoked by these nociceptors as throbbing or aching.

Transmission

In the second phase of nociception, called transmission, depolarized neurons transfer electrical impulses to the central nervous system (CNS), which processes nociceptive signals to extract relevant information.

The whole (ob)noxious picture

To understand this process, think of the information provided by nociceptors as a "picture" of noxious stimulation.

For instance, consider a newspaper photograph. Although the photo consists of many tiny dots, your brain doesn't just recognize the dots. It also recognizes the overall image.

The brain does the same thing with a picture of incoming noxious stimuli. It abstracts the important features—the meaning—of the overall picture.

Unimodal receptors give rise to myelinated A-delta fibers. I can identify them by their large diameters.

I need a drink. I just got bombarded with noxious stimuli.

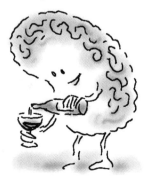

Movin' on up

The action potential created by this process moves from the injury site to the spinal cord and then climbs to higher neurologic centers. Transmission refers to the processing and extraction of relevant features of sensory input. (See *Transmission: Second stage of nociception and pain.*)

Perception

The third stage of nociception, perception of pain, and other sensory stimuli is dynamic, changing in response to a person's development, environment, disease, or injury. Pain perception can be brief (seconds to hours), prolonged (hours to weeks), or even permanent.

Transmission: Second stage of nociception and pain

In the second stage of nociception, the action potential progresses from the injury site to the spinal cord. This stage, called transmission, occurs in the spinal cord's dorsal horn (the central gray matter at the back of the cord). Substance P and other neurotransmitters transfer the impulse from the nociceptor to the spinothalamic tract. The thalamus then acts as a relay station that sends the pain impulses to different areas of the brain for processing.

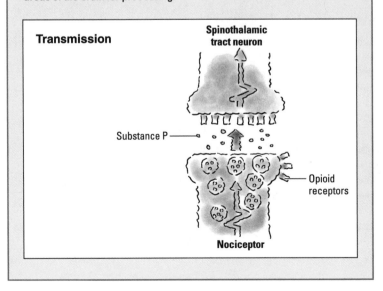

The CNS response to nociceptive stimuli can result from inflammatory tissue damage, peripheral nerve injury, or damage to parts of the CNS that mediate pain sensations. The response also can result from a past or present experience of pain or current attitudes toward pain.

Perceiving a whole lot of pain

One example of pain perception is *allodynia*—the feeling of pain in response to a stimulus that normally isn't painful. For instance, a patient may perceive that a bedsheet touching a wounded limb is painful.

Another example is *hyperalgesia*—the perception that a normally painful stimulus is more painful than usual.

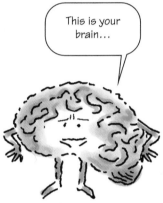

This is your brain...

Modulation

The fourth stage of nociception, modulation (also called adjustment) refers to internal and external ways of reducing or increasing pain. The gelatinous substance that bathes the interneurons can be disposed to excite or inhibit pain signals. One obvious external way to reduce pain is to use analgesic drugs. Other types of modulation involve cognitive influences, which can either reduce pain (distraction) or increase it (anticipation). Many other physical and psychological influences can modulate pain as well. (See *Modulation: Fourth stage of nociception and pain,* page 10.)

Midbrain mechanism

The body itself can modulate nociceptive inputs and pain perception through a pain control mechanism in the midbrain. Here, external opioids (such as morphine) and endogenous opioid peptides (endorphins, the body's natural painkillers) trigger inhibitory influences that flow down to the spinal cord.

Descending pain modulation

Neurotransmitters—mainly serotonin and norepinephrine—mediate this descending inhibition. Terminals, or endpoints, of neurons descending from the medulla (the part of the brainstem that attaches to the spinal cord) contain serotonin. Terminals of neurons descending from the pons (located just above the medulla) contain norepinephrine.

That's why drugs that prevent the removal of serotonin or norepinephrine can have analgesic properties. For example, clonidine and tricyclic antidepressants may be useful adjuvants when pain medicines alone prove ineffective.

Stress, anxiety, and fear typically contribute to the amplification of pain. However, in some circumstances (major trauma, for

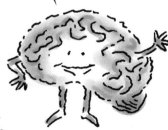

...This is your brain on endorphins (thanks to inhibitory influences that decrease pain).

Modulation: Fourth stage of nociception and pain

In modulation, nociceptive impulses may be restrained in response to the stimulus. Impulses from the brain travel down the spinal cord, triggering release of such substances as serotonin, norepinephrine, and endogenous opioids. These substances bind to the opioid receptors and prevent the release of neurotransmitters, such as substance P, thereby inhibiting the transmission of pain impulses.

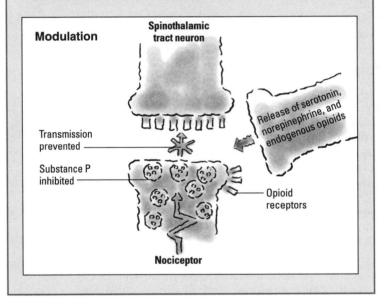

Modulation

Spinothalamic tract neuron

Release of serotonin, norepinephrine, and endogenous opioids

Transmission prevented

Substance P inhibited

Opioid receptors

Nociceptor

I don't mean to brag, but my terminals are brimming with neurotransmitters.

example), excessive adrenaline (norepinephrine) or substance P related to sudden, intense stress or pain can activate descending modulation to inhibit pain perception.

A world of pain

Descending pain modulation may play a key role in unusual chronic pain states. In these disorders, the pain-facilitating system may be activated but not turned off. This may promote rather than inhibit spinal neuron activity.

In certain circumstances, enhanced nociceptive information has a protective effect such as during tissue repair. But if pain facilitation persists after tissue repair is complete, typical nonnociceptive stimulation could be perceived as pain.

Types of pain

Pain falls into three broad categories—acute pain, chronic non-malignant pain (also called chronic persistent pain), and cancer pain.

Acute pain

Acute pain comes on suddenly—for instance, after trauma, surgery, or an acute disease—and lasts from a few days to a few weeks. It causes a withdrawal reflex and may trigger involuntary bodily reactions, such as sweating, fast heart and respiratory rates, and elevated blood pressure. (See *Acute pain: A sympathetic response.*)

Acute pain may be constant (as in a burn), intermittent (as in a muscle strain that hurts only with activity), or both (as in an abdominal incision that hurts a little at rest and a lot with movement or coughing).

Treating acute pain

The cause of acute pain can be diagnosed and treated, and the pain resolves when the cause is treated or analgesics are given. Drug regimens and invasive procedures that aren't reasonable for extended periods can be used more freely in acute pain.

> Ow! That really hurts! Acute pain causes a withdrawal reflex.

Now I get it!

Acute pain: A sympathetic response

In acute pain, certain involuntary (autonomic) reflexes may occur. Acute pain causes the sympathetic branch of the autonomic nervous system (ANS) to trigger the release of epinephrine and other catecholamines. These substances, in turn, cause physiologic reactions such as those seen in the fight-or-flight response.

It'll get your attention
Sympathetic activation directs immediate attention to the injury site. This promotes reflexive withdrawal and fosters other actions that prevent further damage and enhance healing. For example, if you place your hand on a hot stove, the ANS immediately generates a reflex withdrawal that jerks your hand away and minimizes tissue damage.

Chronic nonmalignant pain

Pain is considered chronic when it lasts beyond the normal time expected for an injury to heal or an illness to resolve. Many experts define chronic nonmalignant pain as pain lasting 6 months or longer and may continue during the patient's lifetime.

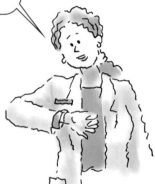

> This could be a long wait. Chronic nonmalignant pain can last as long as a patient's lifetime.

Chronic nonmalignant pain is unrelated to cancer. This type of pain affects more people — roughly 100 million Americans — than any other type. It can cause serious disability (as in arthritis or avascular necrosis), or it may be related to poorly understood disorders such as fibromyalgia and complex regional pain syndrome. Neuropathic pain is one type of chronic pain. (See *Understanding neuropathic pain.*)

Treating chronic nonmalignant pain

Medical treatment for chronic nonmalignant pain must be based on the patient's long-term benefit, not just the current complaint of pain. Drug therapy and surgery, which typically provide only partial and temporary relief, should be individualized.

Drug treatment alone almost never effectively relieves chronic nonmalignant pain. The patient must receive a combination of treatments. These may include drugs, nondrug therapies, temporary or permanent invasive therapies (such as nerve blocks or surgery), cognitive-behavioral therapy, alternative and complementary therapies, and self-management techniques.

> To control chronic pain, the patient might need to combine drugs with yoga, meditation, biofeedback — whatever rocks her boat.

It pains me to say this, but...

Even with medical management, chronic nonmalignant pain can be lifelong. For this reason, treatments that carry significant risks or aren't likely to prove effective over the long term may be inappropriate.

Rewards of rehab

In many cases, treatment of chronic nonmalignant pain must focus on rehabilitation rather than a cure. Rehabilitation aims to:
• maximize physical and psychological functional abilities
• minimize pain experienced during rehabilitation and for the rest of the patient's life
• teach the patient how to manage residual pain and handle pain exacerbation caused by increased activity or unexplained reasons.

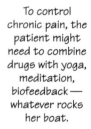

Now I get it!

Understanding neuropathic pain

Commonly described as tingling, burning, or shooting, neuropathic pain is a puzzling type of chronic pain generated by the nerves. It often has no apparent cause and responds poorly to standard pain treatment.

We don't know the precise mechanism of neuropathic pain. Possibly, the peripheral nervous system has experienced damage that injures sensory neurons, causing continuous depolarization and pain transmission. Or perhaps repeated noxious stimuli cause hypersensitivity and excitement in the spinal cord. The result: chronic neuropathy in which a normally harmless stimuli causes pain.

The limb is gone, but the pain remains

Phantom pain syndrome is one example of neuropathic pain. This condition occurs when an arm or a leg has been removed but the brain still gets pain messages from the nerves that originally carried the limb's impulses. The nerves seem to misfire, causing pain.

Types of neuropathic pain

Neuropathic pain can involve either peripheral or central pain.

Peripheral pain can occur as:
• polyneuropathy—pain felt along the peripheral nerves, as in diabetic neuropathy
• mononeuropathy—pain associated with an established injury and felt along the nerve, as in trigeminal neuralgia.

Central neuropathic pain also comes in two varieties:
• sympathetic pain, which results from dysfunction of the autonomic nervous system
• deafferentation pain, marked by elimination of sensory (afferent) impulses, as from damage to the central or peripheral nervous system (as in phantom limb pain).

> I'm puzzled because I don't know why I'm in pain.

Cancer pain

Cancer pain is a complex problem. It may result from the disease itself or from treatment. About 70% to 90% of patients with advanced cancer experience pain. Although cancer pain can be treated with oral medications, only one-third of patients with cancer pain achieve satisfactory relief.

Sometimes pain results from the pressure of a tumor impinging on organs, bones, nerves, or blood vessels. In other cases, limitations in activities of daily living may lead to muscle aches.

Don't treat me like that!

These cancer treatments may cause pain:
• chemotherapy, radiation, or drugs used to offset the impact of these therapies on blood counts and the infection risk (such as

mouth sores, peripheral neuropathy, and abdominal, bone, or joint pain from chemotherapy agents)
• surgery
• biopsies
• blood withdrawal
• lumbar punctures.

Treating cancer pain

Whether pain results from cancer or its treatment, it may cause the patient to lose hope — especially if he thinks the pain means his illness is progressing. He's then likely to suffer additional feelings of helplessness, anxiety, and depression.

However, most types of cancer pain can be managed effectively, diminishing physical and mental suffering.

Unwise to undertreat

Unfortunately, however, cancer pain commonly goes undertreated because of:
• inadequate knowledge of — or attention to — pain control by health care professionals
• failure of health care professionals to properly assess pain
• the reluctance of patients to report their pain
• the reluctance of patients and doctors to use morphine and other opioids for fear of addiction.

Undertreated cancer pain diminishes the patient's activity level, appetite, and sleep. It may prevent the patient from working productively, enjoying leisure activities, or participating in family or social situations.

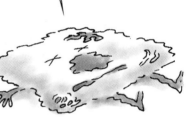

Untreated cancer pain can make your patient feel utterly hopeless.

Psychological responses to pain

Although the pain experience and nociception are related, they aren't the same thing. Nociception refers only to the body's physiologic reactions to certain stimuli. The pain experience also includes a crucial psychological component.

Can you feel my pain?

The experience of pain is influenced by a person's cultural and religious background, anticipation of pain, previous experiences with pain, various emotional and cognitive factors, and the context in which the pain occurs. That's why something that causes considerable pain in one person may cause little or no pain in another. In fact, the things that cause pain can vary even for the same person at different times.

Sometimes pain is so subjective that it has nothing to do with nociception—and vice versa. In the patient with a spinal cord injury, for instance, noxious stimuli below the injury level may cause nociceptive withdrawal reflexes because the peripheral nociceptors and spinal reflex circuitry are intact. But the cord injury prevents transmission of this information past the injury to the brain, so the patient doesn't perceive pain.

> Oh no—not this again! I'll be in pain for days, just like last time.

Interpreting pain

When a person touches an unexpectedly hot surface, his body responds in two ways:
• the part of the body that touched the hot surface withdraws reflexively
• the person becomes consciously aware that a burn has occurred.

An experience like no other

To become consciously aware of pain, the brain must integrate the information in several regions—and then interpret the event consciously. The combination of integrating the information and interpreting it consciously makes pain a unique experience.

Two aspects of pain

The two aspects of pain that people experience are called the sensory-discriminative and motivational-affective aspects.

Sensory-discriminative aspect

In the sensory-discriminative aspect of pain, neural processes converge so the person can quickly pinpoint the location, intensity, and duration of the painful stimulus.

Burned again!

Using the previous example, let's say you touch a hot surface. You know instantly which hand and finger are involved and which area of your finger touched the heat. The ability to quickly characterize and locate the pain site is best developed in the skin and relatively poorly developed in deeper tissues, such as the viscera.

Motivational-affective aspect

The motivational-affective aspect of pain refers to the emotional responses that make pain personal and unique for everyone. These responses don't occur in the same brain regions as sensory-discriminative activities.

What color is your pain?

Motivational-affective activities are accomplished by more basic, relatively indirect neural pathways that emotionally color a person's response to nociceptive input.

> Would you like to talk about the painful information you've been integrating and receiving?

Cognitive and evaluative issues

Overlying the sensory-discriminative and motivational-affective components of pain are cultural and cognitive issues (called the cognitive-evaluative phase) that influence interpretation of and concerns about pain. Cognitive contributions include attention, anxiety, anticipation, and other experiences with pain.

Not-so-great expectations

Let's say the patient has had a traumatic experience with a painful medical procedure. The next time he faces that procedure, he's likely to be anxious because he'll expect to feel that pain again. The patient's anxiety will color his interpretation of and response to any pain he'll feel from the procedure.

Theories about pain

Over the years, the prevailing medical view of pain evolved from a completely sensory model to an almost completely psychogenic one. Today, the prevailing view of pain encompasses physical and emotional components.

According to the sensory model, pain results entirely from physical factors. In contrast, the psychogenic model sees the origin of pain as mental or emotional rather than physiologic. Even today, a report of pain that can't be confirmed by observed pathology is viewed as pain with a psychological component.

These models come up a bit short

The pain models described share a basic shortcoming: They rely solely on either physical or psychological factors to explain the pain response (especially in chronic pain). In reality, the model that best explains the pain experience is probably the one that best integrates physical and psychological factors.

Motivational model

The motivational model (apparently favored by many insurance companies) holds that pain unsubstantiated by observed physical problems must stem from:

- malingering—conscious faking of symptoms for financial or other gain
- exaggeration of symptoms.

You think I'm faking?

However, no studies have shown dramatic improvement in pain reports after a person receives a disability award. And according to the Institute of Medicine, malingering is extremely rare in patients who complain of chronic pain.

Operant conditioning model

The operant conditioning model holds that behavioral signs of acute pain—withdrawal, avoiding activities thought to worsen pain, and attempts to escape from noxious sensations—are subject to the principles of positive reinforcement, negative reinforcement, and avoidance learning. (See *Principles of operant conditioning.*)

In the operant view, acute pain behaviors may be controlled by external reinforcements, or secondary gain. These behaviors may be appropriate and helpful in the short term, but may become problematic over time. For example, when back pain flares up, a

---

Principles of operant conditioning

Operant conditioning encompasses three major concepts: positive reinforcement, negative reinforcement, and avoidance learning.

Positive reinforcement

Positive reinforcement occurs when a behavior elicits positive consequences or a reward of some type. As a result, the person is motivated to repeat the behavior.

Pain behaviors may be positively reinforced, for example, when a person receives attention from others for limping or grimacing.

Negative reinforcement

Negative reinforcement occurs when *stopping* a behavior elicits positive consequences or a reward. Pain behaviors may be negatively reinforced, for example, when a person gets attention from others when he stops complaining about minor aches and pains.

Avoidance learning

Avoidance learning occurs when performing a behavior helps the person avoid a negative consequence or loss of a reward. For example, a patient with a back injury may undergo avoidance learning when he understands that exercise, although possibly painful, ultimately will help him avoid increased disability through loss of muscle strength, flexibility, and endurance.

The three major concepts of operant conditioning are positive reinforcement, negative reinforcement, and avoidance learning.

woman may lie down on the floor and hold her back. Unwittingly, her husband may reinforce her pain behaviors by spending extra time with her, rubbing her back, or letting her avoid undesirable activities during pain flare-ups.

The operant model doesn't suggest conscious deception or malingering. The pain sufferer isn't consciously trying to get attention or avoid undesirable activities. Instead, reinforcement of pain behaviors more likely results from a gradual, unintended process.

In the operant model, the pain sufferer isn't trying to deceive or to get attention.

Stop being so nice

The operant conditioning model may provide the basis for effective treatment of selected patients with chronic pain. Treatment based on this model aims to eliminate pain behaviors by withdrawing attention from them and positively reinforcing well behaviors instead.

Like other pain models, the operant conditioning model has flaws. For instance, it uses overt behaviors as the sole basis for understanding pain, distress, and suffering. In truth, we have no way of knowing whether an observed behavior results from pain, a structural abnormality, or a coping response.

Respondent conditioning model

The respondent (or classic) conditioning model proposes that if a nociceptive stimulus is frequently paired with a neutral stimulus, the neutral stimulus eventually will come to elicit a pain response.

Some experts believe chronic or recurrent acute pain fits the respondent conditioning model of pain perception.

Let's get physical

Consider, for example, the patient who gets painful treatments from a physical therapist. Eventually, he may become conditioned to having a negative emotional response to the therapist, the treatment room, or another stimulus linked to the original nociceptive stimulus. This negative reaction may cause his muscles to tense and his pain to worsen—reinforcing the link between the physical therapist and pain.

Over time, a patient may associate a growing number of stimuli with pain production—a process called stimulus generalization. Sitting, walking, engaging in demanding work or social interaction, having sex, or even thinking about these activities may worsen anticipatory anxiety and cause physiologic and biochemical changes. The patient then may show maladaptive responses to many activities other than those that initially caused pain.

Cycle of pain

Physical abnormalities thought to result from chronic pain—such as a distorted gait, decreased range of motion, and muscle fatigue—actually may be secondary to maladaptive behavior changes adopted through learned responses to pain.

As pain becomes linked to a growing list of situations and activities, the patient avoids them. The likely result is greater physical deconditioning, isolation, physical and emotional disability and, ultimately, more pain.

Social learning model

The social learning model holds that people can acquire pain behaviors through observation and modeling. People (especially children) acquire new behaviors by observing others. From their parents and society, they acquire attitudes about health, health care, symptoms, and physiologic processes as well as appropriate responses to injury and disease. Depending on their social learning experiences, they may ignore or overreact to symptoms.

> I predict the patient will have pain caused by stimulus generalization.

Teach me about pain

Ample experimental evidence points to the role of social learning in pain. Physiologic responses to pain stimuli may be conditioned by observing others in pain. For example, patients on a burn unit have ample opportunity to observe other burn patients' responses.

Similarly, children of parents with chronic pain tend to display more illness behaviors, make more visits to the school nurse, and choose more pain-related responses to defined scenarios compared to children of parents who rarely exhibit pain behaviors. Differences in social learning may be one reason why people with similar physical problems have highly variable behavioral responses.

> Children learn new behaviors and attitudes about health from their parents and society.

Gate control model

Now more than three decades old, the gate control model integrates physiologic and psychological responses in its definition of pain. It holds that the spinal cord has a "gating" mechanism that inhibits or promotes transmission of peripheral nerve impulses to the brain.

According to this theory, spinal cord cells that transmit nociceptive information to sites above the cord function as a spinal "gate." Activity in small-diameter afferent nerve fibers (A-d and C fibers) opens the gate to nociception.

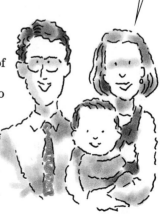

Close the gate — please!

In contrast, activity in large-diameter, myelinated nonnociceptive afferent fibers (A-a and A-b fibers) closes the gate to nociception. The balance of activity between nociceptive and nonnociceptive fibers can affect gate position. A relatively open gate means more pain; a relatively closed gate means less pain.

Gateway to grief

Whether pain is inhibited or transmitted depends on the diameters of active peripheral fibers and the influence of certain brain processes. In short, the spinal "gate" is influenced by the relative amount of activity in afferent large-diameter (myelinated) and small-diameter (unmyelinated) nociceptive fibers that converge in the spinal cord's dorsal horn.

The gate control model rejects the notion that pain is either somatic or psychogenic. Instead, it holds that somatic and psychogenic factors enhance or moderate pain perception. Fear, anger, anxiety, and stress originate in the brain and can open the gates, increasing the intensity of pain. Conversely, laughter, exercise, sexual orgasm, and self-efficacious beliefs, which also originate in the brain, release endorphins and, in turn, close the gate on pain.

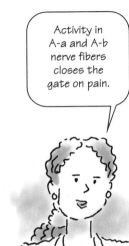

Activity in A-a and A-b nerve fibers closes the gate on pain.

Cognitive-behavioral model

The cognitive-behavioral model incorporates many of the psychological variables of operant and respondent learning—namely anticipation, avoidance, and reinforcement. But it places central importance on cognitive factors (particularly expectations) rather than conditioning.

Self-fulfilling prophecy?

Pain management strategies based on the cognitive-behavioral model stem from certain central assumptions about people and the conditions that influence pain perception. (See *Understanding the cognitive-behavioral model.*)

The cognitive-behavioral model suggests that so-called conditioned reactions, such as feeling anxiety and pain when thinking about exercise, are largely self-activated. These reactions aren't evoked automatically by conditioned stimuli but are based on learned expectations. In other words, people learn to predict painful events and then engage in anticipatory anxiety and avoidance behaviors.

I prefer my pain with filters

In the cognitive-behavioral view, behavior and emotions are influenced by personal interpretation—not just by an event's objective

Now I get it!

Understanding the cognitive-behavioral model

The cognitive-behavioral model of pain perception stems from five basic beliefs.

Active processing

An individual actively processes information rather than simply reacting to the environment. To make sense of stimuli, a person filters and organizes information based on previous learning, information-processing strategies, and more.

Reciprocal influence of thinking on physiology and behavior

Thinking influences a person's affect (outward manifestation of emotions) and physiologic arousal—both of which may influence behavior. Conversely, affect, physiology, and behavior can influence thinking.

Reciprocal influence of behavior and environment

Behavior is determined reciprocally by the environment and the person. An individual doesn't simply respond passively to the environment—he creates his own environment. A patient who seeks medical attention for symptoms creates an environment different from one created by someone who self-medicates.

Ability to change maladaptive responses

Because people develop and maintain maladaptive thoughts, feelings, and behaviors, they can also change those maladaptive modes of responding.

Three-pronged approach

Successful interventions to alter maladaptive behavior focus on maladaptive thoughts and feelings as well as on behaviors. Changing only thoughts, only feelings, or only behaviors doesn't necessarily change the other two.

characteristics. Thus, the pain experience is shaped by personal attitudes and beliefs that filter and interact reciprocally with sensory experience, emotions, social influences, and behavioral responses. These behaviors may elicit responses from the patient's family and friends that reinforce adaptive and maladaptive ways of thinking, feeling, and behaving.

Beliefs about pain

Patients' attitudes, beliefs, expectations of themselves, coping resources, and beliefs about the health care system affect the entire spectrum of their pain behaviors.

Behavior and emotions are influenced by the interpretation as well as the facts of an event. This partly explains why patients may differ greatly in their beliefs about pain.

> People have widely varying beliefs about pain — and these beliefs affect their pain behavior and recovery prospects.

Bob and Carol and Ted and Alice — in pain

Take Carol and Alice, for instance. Both have lower back pain. Carol thinks her pain indicates a progressive disease, while Alice thinks her pain results from a stable, manageable problem. Who's likely to experience more suffering and behavioral dysfunction? You guessed it — Carol.

Let's peek in on their significant others, Bob and Ted. Both awaken with a headache. Bob assumes the headache is from a hangover, while Ted thinks he might have a brain tumor. Like Carol, Ted is setting himself up for more suffering than Bob.

Because of their beliefs, Bob and Alice will respond to their pain in markedly different ways than Ted and Carol. In essence, they're likely to experience less suffering and disability.

Coping

Patients' beliefs, judgments, and expectations about an event's consequences — and belief in their ability to influence the outcome — can affect their ability to function. That's because such beliefs, judgments, and expectations can influence mood directly and alter coping ability.

Patients with low back pain offer a good example. Many fail to comply with prescribed exercises. Their previous pain experience may foster a negative view of their abilities and an expectation of increased pain during exercise. These beliefs form a rationale for avoiding exercise.

> Get the patient into the fighting spirit. Active ways of coping with pain lead to adaptive functioning and decreased pain.

Helpless without feedback

The expectation of exercise-related pain reinforces patients' beliefs that their disability is pervasive. Patients who see disability as a necessary reaction to pain and view activity as dangerous are more likely to experience continued disability. Their failure to perform prescribed activities has negative effects:
• It robs them of the corrective feedback that could help counteract their beliefs.
• It reinforces the perception of helplessness and incapacity.

In contrast, developing positive coping strategies may alter the perception of pain intensity and promote the patient's ability to manage or tolerate pain and continue activities of daily living.

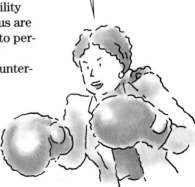

Can you cope with these concepts?

Coping can be overt or covert; active or passive. *Overt* coping strategies include rest, drug therapy, and use of relaxation techniques. *Covert* coping strategies include distraction, reassuring oneself that the pain will diminish, seeking information, and solving problems.

Active coping strategies — efforts to function despite pain or to distract oneself from pain — lead to adaptive functioning. *Passive* coping strategies — restricting one's activities and depending on others for help in pain control — lead to greater pain and depression. (See *Encouraging active pain-coping strategies.*)

Attention

Pain can change the way the patient processes pain-related and other information by focusing attention on bodily signals. As these signals change, he may assume these changes mean that the un-

---

Rein in the pain

Encouraging active pain-coping strategies

The patient's strategy for coping with pain may be active or passive. *Active* strategies include attempts to function despite pain. *Passive* strategies include relying on others for help in pain control.

If possible, steer the patient toward active coping strategies. A patient who uses adaptive coping strategies tends to experience less pain and increased pain tolerance than one who uses maladaptive strategies.

One strategy doesn't fit all
However, keep in mind that one particular active coping strategy isn't necessarily better than another. What's more, a given strategy may be helpful in one situation or for one patient, but not helpful in a different situation or for another patient.

Likewise, certain strategies may help at one time but prove maladaptive or ineffective in other situations.

Out-of-control thoughts
The most important feature of poor coping seems to be "catastrophizing" — thinking extremely negative thoughts about one's plight rather than choosing poorly among adaptive coping strategies.

If the patient falls into this trap, teach him that imagining more positive outcomes may help reduce his pain.

By encouraging active pain-coping strategies, I foresee a positive outcome in the patient's future.

derlying disease is getting worse and, as a result, may report increased pain.

In contrast, a patient who doesn't attribute symptoms to worsening disease tends to report less pain, even if his disease actually is progressing.

Too little feedback

Beliefs and expectations about a disease are hard to change. Patients tend to avoid experiences that might invalidate their beliefs and guide their behavior in keeping with their beliefs. Too often, health professionals refrain from challenging patients about irrational beliefs and excessively restrictive activities. Because of this, the patient may receive little or no corrective feedback.

Successful rehabilitation

Beliefs about pain can influence the patient's disability level, response to treatment, and compliance with prescribed activities. For rehabilitation to succeed, the patient must change from believing he's helpless and passive to believing in his ability to function regardless of pain.

A patient with chronic nonmalignant pain must learn to minimize the role of pain in determining his functioning level. Those patients who find successful ways to cope with pain tend to establish a balance between trying new activities despite persistent pain and respecting the physical limitations imposed by their condition.

Efficacy has its advantages

Being able to minimize the role of pain may stem in part from a personal conviction that one can successfully follow a course of action to produce a desired outcome. Known as *self-efficacy*, this concept is crucial to coping and successful rehabilitation.

A belief in self-efficacy grows from the patient's conviction that the demands of his situation won't exceed his ability to cope. A patient can build a sense of self-efficacy by performing increasingly difficult tasks to learn what physical sensations mean, and by using the relaxation and learning strategies that have helped others with similar conditions.

Pain beyond control?

What about pain that's hard to control? Commonly, patients with chronic pain—and limited success in controlling it—think of the pain as outside their control. They're unlikely to try new pain-management strategies.

Instead, they grow frustrated and demoralized by pain that interferes with their recreational, occupational, and social activities.

I feel so self-efficacious! I'm sure I'll get rid of this pain in no time.

They may resort to passive coping strategies—inactivity, self-medication, or alcohol abuse—to reduce emotional distress and pain.

It seems catastrophic

Patients who feel little control over pain also are more likely to "catastrophize" the impact of a pain episode and any situations that tend to worsen pain. Depression and anxiety—common among patients with chronic pain—can influence pain perception.

In fact, anxiety about pain can change a person's pain threshold and tolerance level. Likewise, depression symptoms can reduce the capacity for successful coping.

> Don't turn every ache and pain into a catastrophe. It will only make your pain worse.

Physical links to pain

Just as physical factors can affect a patient's psychological condition, psychological factors can affect his mood, coping ability, and nociception.

Cognitive interpretations and affective arousal may influence physiology by increasing autonomic sympathetic nervous system (SNS) arousal and promoting endogenous opioid (endorphin) production.

Autonomic arousal

Thinking about pain and stress can increase muscle tension, especially in already painful areas. Chronic and excessive SNS arousal is a precursor to increased skeletal muscle tone. It may set the stage for hyperactive and persistent muscle contractions, which promote muscle spasms and pain.

Arousing sympathy

Patients who exaggerate the significance of their problems or focus on them too closely may influence sympathetic arousal. This predisposes them to further injury and can complicate recovery in other ways.

> There, there! Try to think positive thoughts. It may improve your pain tolerance.

How thoughts affect endorphins

Studies show that thoughts can influence the concentration of endorphins available to control pain. Research results indicate that:
• a patient's feelings of self-efficacy predicted their pain tolerance; those with high self-

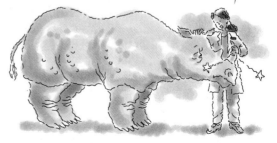

Self-efficacy and arthritis pain

Research suggests that feelings of self-efficacy can directly affect the physiology of pain. In one study, researchers provided stress management treatment to patients with rheumatoid arthritis. This autoimmune disorder, which may result from impaired suppressor T-cell functioning, causes inflammation of synovial membranes. Among the symptoms are joint pain and stiffness.

A boost to T cells
The study found that patients with increased feelings of self-efficacy had greater levels of suppressor T cells. Self-efficacy levels also related directly to the degree of pain and joint impairment the patients experienced.

---

efficacy had greater levels of endorphins. (See *Self-efficacy and arthritis pain.*)
• naloxone, an opioid antagonist, blocked the pain-relieving effects of cognitive coping.
• lower concentrations of endorphins were associated with learned helplessness.

The second finding shows how thoughts can directly affect endorphins. Self-efficacy may influence pain perception at least partially through endogenous opioids.

Treating pain successfully

When caring for a patient experiencing pain, you have three overall goals:
• reduce pain intensity
• improve the patient's ability to function
• improve the patient's quality of life.

To accomplish these goals, you must work with the patient to agree upon goals that are mutually desirable, realistic, measurable, and achievable. In addition, you'll need to focus on the nociceptive and emotional aspects of pain. A patient responds to a painful physical condition based, in part, on his subjective interpretation of illness and symptoms. His beliefs about the meaning of pain and his ability to function despite discomfort are important aspects of coping ability.

Harmful beliefs

Maladaptive responses to pain are more likely in a patient who believes that:
- he has a serious debilitating condition
- disability is a necessary aspect of pain
- activity is dangerous
- pain is an acceptable reason to reduce one's responsibilities.

Sometimes it pays to be a control freak

Many factors can promote or disrupt a patient's sense of control over the pain experience. They include:
- personal beliefs and expectations about pain
- coping ability
- social supports
- the specific disorder that's causing the pain
- response of employers.

These factors also influence a patient's investment in treatment, acceptance of responsibility, perceptions of disability, adherence to treatment, and support from significant others.

To start the patient on the road to successful pain management, consider physical, psychosocial, and behavioral factors —and the changes that occur in these relationships over time.

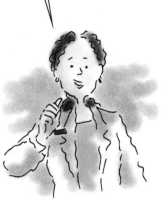

Help a patient with chronic pain gain control over the pain. She'll find she's more capable than she thought.

Making the effort

Treatment that increases perceived control over pain and reduces "catastrophizing" can decrease pain severity ratings and functional disability. Maintaining this sense of control—and the behavioral changes it fosters—depends on the patient's belief that successful pain control stems from one's own efforts.

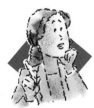

Quick quiz

1. Which of the following stimulates the pain response?
   A. Nociceptors
   B. Nonnociceptive receptors
   C. Dendrites
   D. Axons

Answer: A. Nociceptors create the physiologic response to a painful stimulus.

2.   What's the first step in the nociceptive process?
A.   Perception of pain
B.   Exposure to noxious stimuli
C.   Transmission and central processing
D.   Descending modulation

Answer: B. Exposure to noxious stimuli triggers the process of nociception.

3.   Which time frame do many experts use when defining chronic nonmalignant pain?
A.   Several weeks
B.   6 months or longer
C.   12 months
D.   More than 12 months

Answer: B. Many experts define chronic nonmalignant pain as pain that lasts 6 months or longer. However, it can be permanent.

4.   Which pain model may prove effective when treating a patient with chronic nonmalignant pain?
A   Motivational model
B.   Change model
C.   Pain prone model
D.   Operant conditioning model

Answer: D. The operant conditioning model aims to eliminate pain behaviors by withdrawing attention from the patient and providing positive reinforcement.

Scoring

☆☆☆   If you answered all four questions correctly, perfect! You've reached the pinnacle of pain understanding!

☆☆   If you answered three questions correctly, congrats! You're about to turn the corner on pain!

☆   If you answered fewer than three questions correctly, don't catastrophize! A little extra studying will make the pain go away!

Assessing pain

Just the facts

In this chapter, you'll learn:

♦ the new JCAHO standards for pain assessment

♦ rating scales you can see to quantify the patient's pain

♦ effective ways to document pain assessment findings

♦ the history and examination techniques for the patient with pain

♦ methods to recognize psychogenic pain and emotional distress.

A look at pain assessment

To ensure that the patient receives effective pain relief, you must conduct a thorough and accurate pain assessment. That's a tall order, because pain is so subjective.

Pain is influenced not just by physical pathology but by cultural and social factors, expectations, mood, and perceptions of control. What's more, you and the patient may have dramatically different pain thresholds and tolerances, expectations about pain, and ways of expressing pain.

You may even doubt the patient's complaints of pain—particularly if you think his behavior doesn't match his report of pain. For instance, he may tell you he has moderate pain yet continue to chat and laugh with visitors. If no pathologic cause for pain is found, you may even question the patient's report of pain. (See *Debunking myths about pain*, page 30.)

> How about that! Pain can be influenced by social and cultural factors.

Myth busters

Debunking myths about pain

Even today, myths about pain and its management abound among both patients and health care providers. Below we expose some of these myths.

Myth: The goal of pain management is to use as little pain medication as possible.

Fact: The goal of pain management is to keep the patient as comfortable as possible. Help the patient choose a target pain rating that will reduce his discomfort to a tolerable level and let him participate comfortably in self-care. Regularly assess and document his pain intensity using an appropriate pain rating scale.

Myth: If the patient doesn't seem to be in pain, he isn't in pain.

Fact: Pain is subjective—it's whatever the patient says it is, occurring whenever he says it does. Don't expect to find physiologic markers of pain, such as vital sign changes, grimacing, or diaphoresis, in a patient with chronic pain. Chances are his body has adapted to the pain.

Myth: A patient who's sleeping isn't in severe pain.

Fact: Patients can fall asleep despite severe pain. Some patients even use sleep as a way to control pain.

Myth: If the patient jokes with visitors, he can't be in severe pain.

Fact: Joking with visitors can be a form of distraction that the patient uses to cope with pain. The best indicator of pain is the patient's own report of pain.

Pain is whatever the patient says it is, occurring whenever he says it does.

The patient knows best

To keep your pain assessment on track, keep in mind the first principle of pain assessment: Pain is whatever the patient says it is, occurring whenever he says it does.

The patient's self-report of the presence and severity of pain is the most accurate, reliable means of pain assessment. If the patient reports pain, respect what he says and act promptly to assess and control it.

Pain threshold and tolerance

Pain threshold refers to the intensity of the stimulus a person needs to sense pain. *Pain tolerance* is the duration and intensity of pain that a person tolerates before openly expressing pain. Tolerance has a strong psychological component. Identifying pain threshold and tolerance are crucial to pain assessment and the development of a pain management plan.

But remember—pain threshold and tolerance vary widely among patients. They may even fluctuate in the same patient as circumstances change.

Interdisciplinary pain management team

An interdisciplinary team approach promotes effective pain control. Team members typically include a doctor, a nurse, a pharmacist, a social worker, a spiritual advisor, a psychologist, physical and occupational therapists, an anesthesiologist or a certified registered nurse anesthetist, a pain management specialist and, of course, the patient and his family.

Go for the goal

The success of a pain management plan hinges on having the patient choose an appropriate goal—a pain intensity rating that will reduce his discomfort to a tolerable level and let him engage comfortably in self-care activities. Team members should work together to choose a rating scale for measuring the patient's pain intensity and to develop appropriate pain management goals.

Thorough documentation and pain assessment tools communicate vital patient information to all team members. If the patient has chronic pain, periodic team meetings also may be crucial.

All members of the pain management team must be on the same page.

Differentiating acute and chronic pain

Pain can be classified in several ways. One simple classification is based on its duration—acute or chronic.

Acute pain

Acute pain comes on abruptly after a sudden physical crisis. Typically, it's sharp, intense, and easily localized. Acute pain activates the sympathetic branch of the autonomic nervous system (ANS), causing such responses as heavy perspiration, increasing blood pressure, and rapid heart and respiratory rates.

Acute pain can be prolonged or recurrent. (See *Differentiating acute and chronic pain*, page 32.)

Differentiating acute and chronic pain

Acute pain may cause certain physiologic and behavioral changes that you won't observe in a patient with chronic pain.

Type of pain	Physiologic evidence	Behavioral evidence
Acute	• Increased respirations • Increased pulse • Increased blood pressure • Dilated pupils • Diaphoresis	• Restlessness • Distraction • Worry • Distress
Chronic	• Normal respirations, pulse, blood pressure, and pupil size • No diaphoresis	• Reduced or absent physical activity • Despair, depression • Hopelessness

Prolonged acute pain

Prolonged acute pain can last days to weeks. Usually it results from tissue injury and inflammation (as from a sprain or surgery) and subsides gradually.

At the injury site, release or synthesis of chemicals heightens sensitivity in nearby tissues. This hypersensitivity, called *hyperalgesia*, is normal. In fact, tenderness and tissue hypersensitivity help protect the injury site and prevent further damage.

Good grief! Prolonged acute pain can last for weeks.

Recurrent acute pain

Recurrent acute pain refers to brief painful episodes that recur at variable intervals. Examples include sickle cell vaso-occlusive crisis and migraine headache.

Pain with a purpose

In migraine and some other recurrent conditions, pain serves no apparent useful purpose—no protective action can be taken and tissue damage can't be prevented. But in others, such as sickle cell disease, acute pain encourages the person to seek medical treatment.

Chronic pain

Chronic pain is commonly defined as pain lasting 6 months or longer and may continue during the patient's lifetime. Although it sometimes begins as acute pain, more typically it starts slowly and builds gradually. Unlike acute pain, chronic pain isn't protective and doesn't warn of significant tissue damage.

Causes of chronic pain include nerve damage, such as in brain injury, tumor growth, or unexplained and abnormal responses to tissue injury by the central nervous system.

High cost of chronic pain

Chronic pain may be severe enough to limit a patient's ability and desire to participate in career, family life, and even activities of daily living. If it's severe or intractable, the patient may experience decreased function, pain behaviors, depression, opioid dependence, "doctor shopping," and suicide.

Challenges in assessing chronic pain

You may find pain assessment especially difficult in a patient with chronic pain. Over time, the ANS adapts to pain, so the patient may lack typical autonomic responses — dilated pupils, increased blood pressure, and fast heart and respiratory rates. Also, his facial expression may not suggest he's in pain. He may sleep periodically and shift his attention away from his pain. But don't let the lack of outward signs lead you to conclude that he isn't in pain.

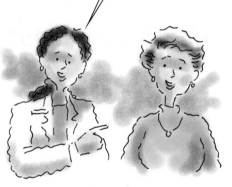

It may not look like it, but she's in chronic pain. She doesn't exhibit classic signs of pain because her body has adapted to it.

JCAHO pain management standards

In 2000, the Joint Commission on Accreditation of Healthcare Organizations (JCAHO) issued new standards for pain assessment, management, and documentation. These standards require that patients be asked about pain when admitted to a JCAHO-accredited facility. Any patient who reports pain must be assessed further by licensed personnel. Facility policies must identify a standard pain screening tool to be used for all patients able to use it.

If you work in a JCAHO-accredited facility, check policies and procedures for information on which screening tool to use, how often to assess pain, and which pain level warrants further assessment and action. (In many facilities, this level is 4 or higher on a scale of 0 to 10.)

The fifth vital sign

Pain is commonly called the fifth vital sign because pain assessment scores must be monitored and recorded regularly—and at least as vigilantly as you monitor and record vital signs. To meet JCAHO standards, you must record pain assessment data in a way that promotes reassessment.

JCAHO standards also mandate that health care facilities plan and support activities and resources that assure pain recognition and use of appropriate interventions. These activities include:
• initial pain assessment
• regular reassessment of pain
• education of health care workers about pain assessment and management
• development of quality improvement plans that address pain assessment and reassessment.

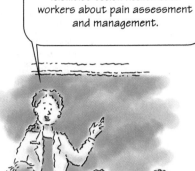

JCAHO requires that facilities teach health care workers about pain assessment and management.

Pain assessment tools

When the patient is admitted, ask him if he's currently in pain or has ongoing problems with pain. If he has ongoing pain, find out if he has an effective treatment plan. If so, continue with this plan if possible. If he doesn't have such a plan, use an assessment tool, such as a pain rating scale, to further assess his pain.

Pain rating scales

Pain rating scales quantify pain intensity—one of pain's most subjective aspects. These scales offer several advantages over semistructured and unstructured patient interviews:
• They're easier to administer.
• They take less time.
• They can uncover concerns that warrant a more thorough investigation.
• When used before and after a pain control intervention, they can help determine if the intervention was effective.

Pain rating scales come in many varieties. When choosing an appropriate scale for your patient, consider his visual acuity, age, reading ability, and level of understanding.

Even a beast like this gets sad when he's in pain.

Pain intensity rating scale

You can evaluate pain in a nonverbal manner for pediatric patients ages 3 and older or for adult patients with language difficulties. One common pain rating scale consists of six faces with expressions ranging from happy and smiling to sad and teary.

Putting a face on pain

To use a pain intensity rating scale, tell the patient that each face represents a person with progressively worse pain. Ask him to choose the face that best represents how he feels. Explain that although the last face has tears, he can choose this face even if he isn't crying. (See *Using a pain intensity rating scale.*)

Visual analog scale

The visual analog scale is a horizontal line, 10 cm long, with word descriptors at each end — "no pain" on one end, "pain as bad as it can be" on the other. The scale also may be used vertically.

Drawing the line on pain

Ask the patient to place a mark along the line to indicate the intensity of his pain. Then measure the line in millimeters up to his mark. This measurement represents the patient's pain rating. Be aware that this scale may be too abstract for some patients to use. (See *Visual analog scale*, page 36.)

Numerical rating scale

The numerical rating scale is perhaps the most commonly used pain rating scale. Simply ask the patient to rate his pain on a scale from 0 to 10, with 0 representing no pain and 10 representing the worst pain imaginable. Instead of giving a verbal rating, the patient can use a horizontal or vertical line consisting of descriptive words and numbers.

Although most patients find the numerical rating scale quick and easy to use, it may be too abstract for some patients. (See *Using the numerical rating scale*, page 37.)

Verbal descriptor scale

With the verbal descriptor scale, the patient chooses a description of his pain from a list of adjectives, such as "none," "annoying," "uncomfortable," "dreadful," "horrible," and "agonizing."

Like the numerical rating scale, the verbal descriptor scale is quick and easy, but it does have drawbacks:
• It limits the patient's choices.

Using a pain intensity rating scale

A pediatric patient or an adult patient with language difficulties may not be able to express the pain he's feeling. In such instances, use the pain intensity scale below. Ask your patient to choose the face that best represents the severity of his pain, on a scale from 0 to 5.

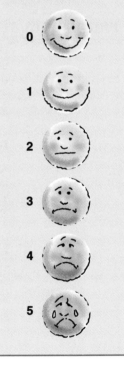

0
1
2
3
4
5

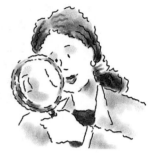

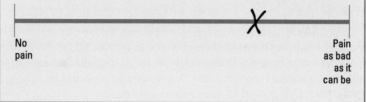

Visual analog scale

To use the visual analog scale, ask the patient to place a line across the scale to indicate his current level of pain. The pain rating is determined by measuring the distance, in millimeters, from "no pain" to his marking.

No pain

Pain as bad as it can be

- Patients tend to choose moderate rather than extreme descriptors.
- Some patients may not understand all the adjectives.

Overall pain assessment tools

Overall pain assessment tools evaluate pain in multiple dimensions, providing a wider range of information. These tools are time-consuming and may be more practical for outpatient use. Still, you might want to use one for a hospitalized patient with hard-to-control chronic pain.

Pain assessment guide

Although lengthy, a pain assessment guide can help you collect important information about the patient's overall pain experience. These guides may vary from one facility to the next. (See *Pain assessment guide,* pages 38 and 39.)

Brief pain inventory

The brief pain inventory (BPI) focuses on the patient's pain during the past 24 hours. Either the patient or health care provider can complete it in about 15 minutes. It comes in several languages besides English, including Chinese, French, and Vietnamese.

Point to the pain, please

To use the BPI, have the patient rate the least and worst pain he's experienced over the past 24 hours and at the present time. Have him point to the location of his pain on a body map.

The BPI also asks questions that focus on:
- whether the patient has had pain other than common types (such as a headache or toothache)

Using the numerical rating scale

A numerical rating scale (NRS) can help the patient quantify his pain. Have him choose a number from 0 (indicating no pain) to 10 (indicating the worst pain imaginable) to reflect his current pain level. He can either circle the number on the scale itself or verbally state the number that best describes his pain.

No pain | 0 | 1 | 2 | 3 | 4 | 5 | 6 | 7 | 8 | 9 | 10 | Pain as bad as it can be

Not as simple as it sounds
To be on the safe side, don't assume that your patient knows how to use the scale. Provide teaching and then verify that he understands what you've taught him. Be sure to document your teaching and your method of evaluating his understanding.

Work toward a comfort goal
Help the patient establish a comfort goal—a numerical pain level that will enable him to perform self-care activities, such as ambulation, coughing, and deep breathing. Usually, a level of 3 or less on a 0-to-10 scale is an adequate comfort level.

   If the patient chooses a comfort goal of 4 or higher, teach him that unrelieved pain can damage his health. Discuss concerns he may have about using analgesics and clear up misconceptions such as those related to addiction.

When to evaluate the pain management plan
If the patient rates his pain as 10, he's experiencing severe pain—a sign that his pain management plan is ineffective. Consult with the doctor about increasing the analgesic dose or adding another analgesic.

When to use a vertical scale instead
Like some children, many adults who speak languages that are read from right to left (or vertically) may have trouble with the NRS because it's horizontal. They may find a vertical scale easier to use. When using a vertical scale, place 0 at the bottom of the scale and 10 at the top.

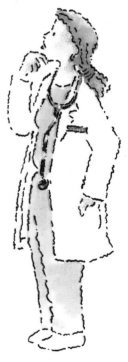

• whether pain has interfered with his activities (such as walking, work, and sleep) in the past 24 hours, and if so, to what extent
• whether the patient's current pain management plan is effective. (See *Brief pain inventory,* pages 40 and 41.)

McGill pain questionnaire

The McGill pain questionnaire assesses the multiple dimensions of neuropathic pain (a tingling, burning, or shooting pain generated

(Text continues on page 42.)

Pain assessment guide

A pain assessment guide like the one below can help you conduct a thorough assessment of the patient's pain status on admission. Although lengthy, this guide provides more information than a simple rating scale. It may be especially appropriate for a patient with chronic pain.

Patient name: _Marie Koller_

Patient goal: _Pain rating of 3 or less_

Past medical conditions: _Arthritis, Cataracts_

Past surgeries and hospitalization: _None_

Past tests and results: _N/A_

Drug allergies and reactions: _NKA_

Do you drink alcohol? (Specify substance and amount.) _NO_

Do you smoke? (Specify substance and amount.) _NO_

Do you use drugs? (Specify substance and amount.) _NO_

When did your pain begin? _6 months ago_

Are you aware of something that started it? _NO_

Where is your pain?

How severe is your pain right now?

No pain 0 1 2 3 4 5 6 7 8 9 10 Worst possible pain

(6 is circled)

How would you describe your pain? (Circle all that apply.)

(Shooting)   Stabbing   Gnawing   (Sharp)

Dull   Aching   Numb   (Throbbing)

Radiating   Burning   Unbearable

Is your pain intermittent, occasional, or continuous? (Circle one.)

What makes your pain better? _Rest and heat_

What makes your pain worse? _Activity_

Pain assessment guide *(continued)*

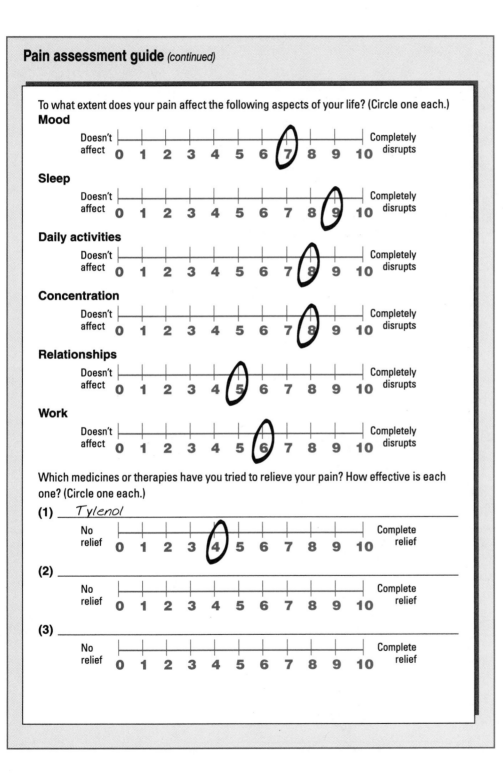

To what extent does your pain affect the following aspects of your life? (Circle one each.)

Mood

Doesn't affect · 0 1 2 3 4 5 6 **7** 8 9 10 · Completely disrupts

Sleep

Doesn't affect · 0 1 2 3 4 5 6 7 8 **9** 10 · Completely disrupts

Daily activities

Doesn't affect · 0 1 2 3 4 5 6 7 **8** 9 10 · Completely disrupts

Concentration

Doesn't affect · 0 1 2 3 4 5 6 7 **8** 9 10 · Completely disrupts

Relationships

Doesn't affect · 0 1 2 3 4 **5** 6 7 8 9 10 · Completely disrupts

Work

Doesn't affect · 0 1 2 3 4 5 **6** 7 8 9 10 · Completely disrupts

Which medicines or therapies have you tried to relieve your pain? How effective is each one? (Circle one each.)

(1) _Tylenol_

No relief · 0 1 2 3 **4** 5 6 7 8 9 10 · Complete relief

(2) _____

No relief · 0 1 2 3 4 5 6 7 8 9 10 · Complete relief

(3) _____

No relief · 0 1 2 3 4 5 6 7 8 9 10 · Complete relief

Brief pain inventory

The pain inventory below can help you assess your patient's pain in the past 24 hours.

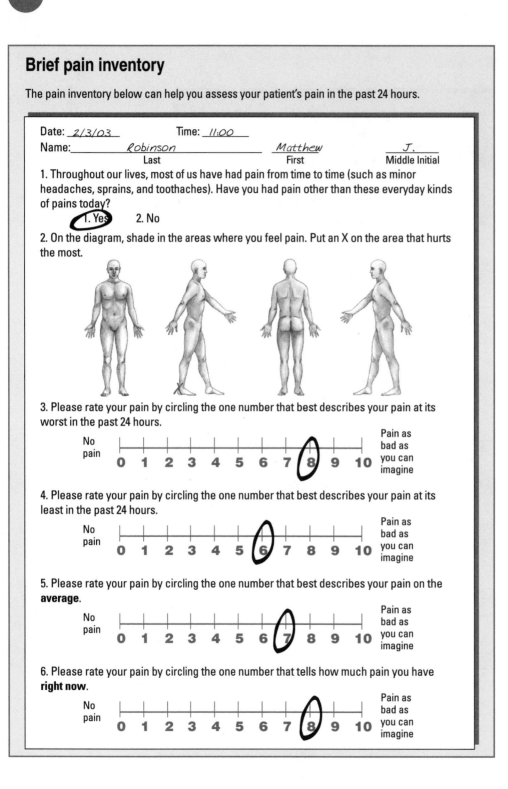

Date: _2/3/03_   Time: _11:00_

Name: _____Robinson_____   _____Matthew_____   ____J.____
          Last   First   Middle Initial

1. Throughout our lives, most of us have had pain from time to time (such as minor headaches, sprains, and toothaches). Have you had pain other than these everyday kinds of pains today?

    (1. Yes)   2. No

2. On the diagram, shade in the areas where you feel pain. Put an X on the area that hurts the most.

3. Please rate your pain by circling the one number that best describes your pain at its worst in the past 24 hours.

No pain   0 1 2 3 4 5 6 7 (8) 9 10   Pain as bad as you can imagine

4. Please rate your pain by circling the one number that best describes your pain at its least in the past 24 hours.

No pain   0 1 2 3 4 5 (6) 7 8 9 10   Pain as bad as you can imagine

5. Please rate your pain by circling the one number that best describes your pain on the **average**.

No pain   0 1 2 3 4 5 6 (7) 8 9 10   Pain as bad as you can imagine

6. Please rate your pain by circling the one number that tells how much pain you have **right now**.

No pain   0 1 2 3 4 5 6 7 (8) 9 10   Pain as bad as you can imagine

Brief pain inventory *(continued)*

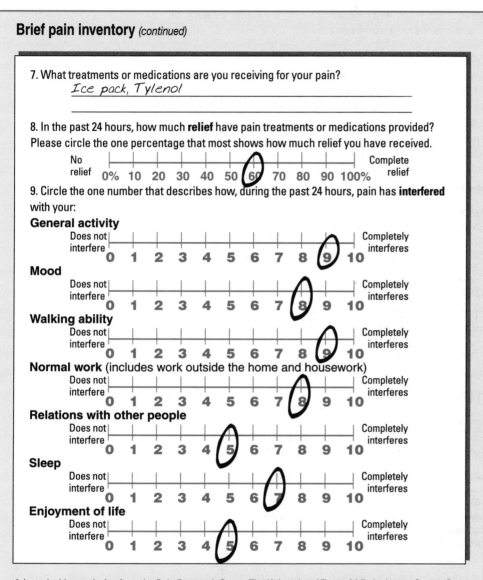

7. What treatments or medications are you receiving for your pain?

Ice pack, Tylenol

8. In the past 24 hours, how much **relief** have pain treatments or medications provided? Please circle the one percentage that most shows how much relief you have received.

No relief   0%   10   20   30   40   50   **60**   70   80   90   100%   Complete relief

9. Circle the one number that describes how, during the past 24 hours, pain has **interfered** with your:

General activity

Does not interfere   0   1   2   3   4   5   6   7   8   **9**   10   Completely interferes

Mood

Does not interfere   0   1   2   3   4   5   6   7   **8**   9   10   Completely interferes

Walking ability

Does not interfere   0   1   2   3   4   5   6   7   8   **9**   10   Completely interferes

Normal work (includes work outside the home and housework)

Does not interfere   0   1   2   3   4   5   6   7   **8**   9   10   Completely interferes

Relations with other people

Does not interfere   0   1   2   3   4   **5**   6   7   8   9   10   Completely interferes

Sleep

Does not interfere   0   1   2   3   4   5   6   **7**   8   9   10   Completely interferes

Enjoyment of life

Does not interfere   0   1   2   3   4   **5**   6   7   8   9   10   Completely interferes

Adapted with permission from the Pain Research Group, The University of Texas, M.D. Anderson Cancer Center, 1991.

by nerves). It provides word descriptors to measure sensory, affective, and evaluative pain domains.

The long and the short of it

This tool is available in a short and long form. The short form has 15 word descriptors and takes less than 5 minutes. The long form consists of 78 word descriptors and takes about 20 minutes.

The McGill questionnaire can be used for baseline and periodic assessments. However, it doesn't quantify the patient's pain and isn't useful for frequent assessments.

Minnesota Multiphasic Personality Inventory

Used particularly for patients with chronic pain, the Minnesota Multiphasic Personality Inventory consists of 566 true-or-false questions that help assess personality characteristics in patients. Its main value lies in predicting responses to pain interventions.

Self-monitoring record

If your patient has chronic or recurrent pain, consider giving him a self-monitoring record to help him accurately describe pain occurrence and severity. (See *Pain self-monitoring record.*)

Pain self-monitoring record

A self-monitoring record (sometimes called a pain diary) like the one shown below helps you better understand the patient's symptoms, their timing and severity, and his ways of responding to them. It also helps him understand the active role he must play in managing his pain. Consider asking him to keep such a diary before his first interview with a pain specialist.

Name: _Robert Waters_

Date Time	Symptoms (How bad on a scale of 0 to 10?)	Situation (What were you doing?)	What were you thinking?	What did you do?	With what result?
1/6 8 a.m.	Low back pain shooting down my leg. (8)	Lying in bed	Why is this hurting now?	Got up; took 500 mg. Naproxen	Minimal relief
1/6 6 p.m.	Low back pain (7)	Sitting in chair, watching TV.	————	Applied a heating pad; took 500 mg Naproxen	Some relief

Documenting pain assessment findings

Be sure to document baseline pain assessment findings so that you and other team members can use them for later comparison. You may want to use a standardized documentation form such as the pain assessment guide mentioned earlier.

If the patient has unrelieved pain, you'll need to conduct frequent assessments. To make pain assessment findings more visible, consider using a graphic sheet that lets you document pain severity next to vital signs.

Using pain assessment flow sheets

A pain assessment flow sheet provides a convenient way to track the patient's pain level and response to interventions over time. On a typical flow sheet, you record information about the patient's pain severity rating, therapeutic interventions, effects of each intervention, and adverse effects of treatments (such as nausea or sedation).

Dear Pain Diary

A pain assessment flow sheet is useful inside and outside the hospital. After discharge, the patient and his family may want to use the flow sheet along with a pain diary, in which the patient records his activities, pain intensity, and pain interventions. The diary can reveal the extent to which pain management measures and activities affect his pain level.

Analgesic infusion flow sheet

If the patient is receiving an analgesic infusion, you may use an analgesic infusion flow sheet to speed documentation and track his progress. Information to record on the flow sheet includes the:
• medication name and dosage
• date and time of each dose
• concentration and dose
• volume infused and volume remaining. (See *Pain management flow sheet*, page 44.)

Oral medication flow sheet

An oral medication flow sheet can be a valuable tool for:
• patients who will receive analgesics after discharge
• home-care patients with pain caused by progressive illness
• patients with chronic nonmalignant pain.

These flow sheets should be brief and simple to use. (See *Monitoring analgesic effectiveness*, page 45.)

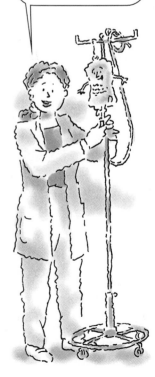

Giving analgesics by I.V. infusion? Using a flow sheet can speed up your documentation.

Pain management flow sheet

The flow sheet below helps ensure that all pain management team members have the information they need to monitor medication use in patients receiving analgesic infusions. If you work in a facility accredited by the Joint Commission on Accreditation of Healthcare Organizations (JCAHO), be sure to follow JCAHO guidelines when administering and documenting pain medications.

Pain Management Flow Sheet

Date 1/14/03   Epidural ☐   I.V. ☑

Mary Smith
12 Christmas Lane
Doylestown PA 18901

Stamp of patient's name

Pain scale (0 to 10)

Other measures
1. Back rub
2. Massage
3. Heat
4. Relaxation
5. Other

Sedation scale
1. Awake
2. Drowsy
3. Awake, only
   when aroused
4. Not arousable

Time	Pain before / Sedation level	Medication & strength	Basal rate	PCA dose	Delay time	Bolus	4-hr limit	Other measures	Pain after / Sedation	Comments	Initials
0800	8 / 1	Morphine 30 mg	1 mg/ml	5 ml/dose	10 minutes	0	25 mg	None	3 / 1	None	M.S.

Monitoring analgesic effectiveness

If your patient is receiving oral analgesics, you can help ensure effective pain control by teaching him to record his pain rating before and after each dose. In the space provided on the form below, enter the patient's target pain rating (the pain level he thinks would be acceptable). Below that rating, list the activities he wishes to perform comfortably.

Instruct him to rate his pain before each analgesic dose and then 1 to 2 hours after the dose. Explain that keeping this record will help him and the health care team find the right drug, dose, and frequency to provide adequate pain relief. He can also list any adverse effects on the form.

Date: _2/24/03_

Target pain rating: _2_

Target activities: _Walking, household activities_

No pain | 0 1 2 3 4 5 6 7 8 9 10 | Worst pain imaginable

Instructions: Rate your pain before you take pain medicine and 1 to 2 hours later. Record any side effects and other notes (if needed).

Time	Pain rating before dose	Medicine I took	Pain rating 1 to 2 hours after dose	Side effects	Other
9 a.m.	6	2 400 mg Ibuprofen	2	NONE	
2 p.m.	7	2 400 mg Ibuprofen	2	NONE	

If your pain is greater than _8_ or if you have other problems with your pain medicine, call:
Name/phone _Dr. Smith, 215-555-6531_

Have your patient rate his pain before and after each analgesic dose.

History and physical examination

Accurate pain assessment yields information that serves as the basis for an individualized pain management plan. For a patient with acute pain, a brief assessment may be adequate to formulate an appropriate plan.

However, a patient with chronic pain may require a thorough assessment that evaluates physical and psychosocial factors. Still, even the best history and examination techniques may not produce the definitive findings needed to make a precise diagnosis and clearly identify the origin of chronic pain. Usually, history and physical findings help the doctor interpret the results of diagnostic tests.

Patient history

Assessment begins with the patient interview. If he has acute pain from a traumatic injury, the interview may last for mere seconds. If he has chronic pain, it may be lengthy.

When interviewing a patient with chronic pain, try to elicit information that sheds light on his thoughts, feelings, behaviors, and physiologic responses to pain. Also find out about the environmental stimuli that can alter his response to pain.

Play the match game

During the interview, assess the cognitive, affective, and behavioral components of the patient's pain experience. This can help you later when working with the patient to develop pain management goals. Also ask questions to determine how his pain affects his mental state, relationships, and work performance.

Find out how long your patient's pain lasts.

Pain characteristics

Question the patient about these characteristics of his pain:
• **Onset and duration.** When did the pain begin? Did it come on suddenly or gradually? Is it intermittent or continuous? How often does it occur? How long does it last? Is it prolonged or recurrent?
• **Location.** Ask the patient to point to the painful parts of his body or to mark these areas on a diagram. Be sure to assess each pain site separately.
• **Intensity.** Using a pain rating scale, ask the patient to quantify the intensity of his pain at its worst and at its best.
• **Quality.** Ask the patient what the pain feels like, in his own words. Does it have a burning quality? Is it knifelike? Does he feel pressure? Throbbing? Soreness?

- **Relieving factors.** Does anything help relieve the pain, such as a certain position or heat or cold applications? Besides helping to pinpoint the cause of the pain, his answers may aid in developing a pain management plan.
- **Aggravating factors.** What seems to trigger the pain? What makes it worse? Does it get worse when the patient moves or changes position?

You may find the PQRST technique valuable when assessing pain. Each letter stands for a crucial aspect of pain to explore. (See *PQRST: The alphabet of pain*, page 48.)

Medical and surgical history

The patient's medical history may offer clues to the source of pain or a condition that may exacerbate it. Ask him to list all of his past medical conditions, even those that have been resolved. Also question him about previous surgeries.

Past experience with pain

Explore the patient's experiences with pain. If he experienced significant pain in the past, he may have anticipatory fear of future pain—especially if he received inadequate pain relief.

Play "20 Questions"

Ask the patient which previous treatments—pharmacologic and otherwise—he tried, and find out which treatments helped and which didn't. Keep in mind that nonpharmacologic treatments include physical and occupational therapy, acupuncture, hypnosis, meditation, biofeedback, heat and cold therapy, transcutaneous nerve stimulation, and psychological counseling.

Drug history

Obtain a complete list of the patient's medications. (Many medications can alter the effectiveness of analgesics.) Besides prescribed drugs, ask if he takes over-the-counter preparations, vitamins, nutritional supplements, or herbal or homemade remedies. Record the name, dose, frequency, administration route, and adverse effects of each agent he has used. Also ask him about drug allergies.

Find out if the patient currently takes or has previously taken medications to control pain and whether these were effective. If he currently receives analgesics, have him describe exactly how he takes them. If he hasn't been taking them according to instructions, he may need additional teaching on proper administration. If a particular analgesic agent or regimen didn't work for him in the past, you may be able to teach him how to use it effectively by tailoring the dosage or regimen to his needs.

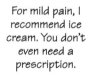

I provide my own music therapy. I don't know about you, but it sure eases my pain.

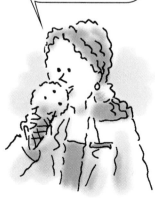

For mild pain, I recommend ice cream. You don't even need a prescription.

PQRST: The alphabet of pain

Use the PQRST mnemonic device to obtain more information about the patient's pain. Asking the questions below elicits important details about his pain.

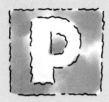 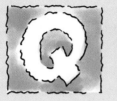 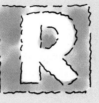 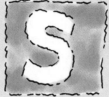 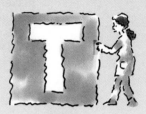

P: Provocative or palliative
Ask the patient:
• What provokes or worsens your pain?
• What relieves or causes the pain to subside?

Q: Quality or quantity
Ask the patient:
• What does the pain feel like? Is it aching, intense, knifelike, burning, or cramping?
• Are you having pain right now? If so, is it more or less severe than usual?
• To what degree does the pain affect your normal activities?
• Do you have other symptoms along with the pain, such as nausea or vomiting?

R: Region and radiation
Ask the patient:
• Where is your pain?
• Does the pain radiate to other parts of your body?

S: Severity
Ask the patient:
• How severe is your pain? How would you rate it on a 0-to-10 scale, with 0 being no pain and 10 being the worst pain imaginable?
• How would you describe the intensity of your pain at its best? At its worst? Right now?

T: Timing
Ask the patient:
• When did your pain begin?
• At what time of day is your pain best? What time is it worst?
• Is the onset sudden or gradual?
• Is the pain constant or intermittent?

Satisfaction survey

Ask the patient if he's satisfied with the level of pain relief his current medications bring. Find out how long these drugs take to work and whether the pain returns before the next dose is due.

Question the patient about adverse effects, such as nausea, constipation, or drowsiness. If he's taking opioids for pain relief, note any worries he has about becoming drug dependent. Listen carefully for concerns he may have about any medication.

Social history

Thorough pain assessment includes a social history. Many social factors can influence the patient's perception and reports of pain and vice versa. This information also helps guide interventions.

Find out how the patient feels about himself, his place in society, and his relationships with others. Ask about his marital status, occupation, support systems, financial status, hobbies, exercise and sleep patterns, responsibilities, and religious, spiritual, and cultural beliefs. Determine his patterns of alcohol use, smoking, and illicit drug use.

Chronic pain can have wide-ranging effects on a person's life. If your patient has chronic pain, explore the impact it has on his moods, emotions, expectations, coping efforts, and resources. Also ask how his family responds to his condition.

Stoics don't say much

To provide culturally sensitive care, you must determine the meaning of pain for each patient — particularly in the context of his culture and religion. Determine how his cultural background and religious beliefs may affect his pain experience. In some cultures, pain is openly expressed. Other cultures value stoicism and denial of pain. A patient who comes from a stoic culture may lead you to believe that he isn't in pain.

But be sure not to stereotype your patient. Keep in mind that within each culture, the response to pain may vary from person to person. Also recognize your own cultural values and biases. Otherwise, you may end up evaluating the patient's response to pain according to your own beliefs instead of his.

Physical examination

Start the physical examination by observing the patient. He may display a broad range of behaviors to convey pain, distress, and suffering. Some behaviors are controllable. Others, such as heavy perspiring or pupil dilation, are involuntary.

As you observe the patient before or during the physical examination, note and document his behaviors. (See *Pain behavior checklist*, page 50.) Use your observations to help quantify his pain.

Overt means observable

These overt behaviors may indicate that the patient is experiencing pain:
- verbal reports of pain
- vocalizations, such as sighs and moans
- altered motor activities (frequent position changes, guarded positioning, slow movements, rigidity)
- limping
- grimacing and other expressions
- functional limitations, including reclining for long periods
- actions to reduce pain such as taking medication.

Heavy sweating is an involuntary behavior that may indicate pain.

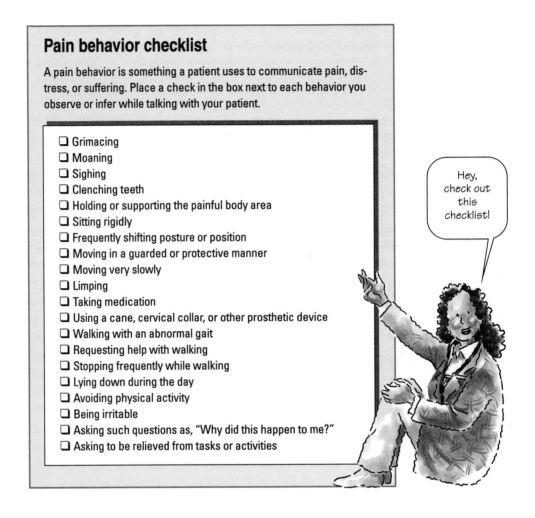

Pain behavior checklist

A pain behavior is something a patient uses to communicate pain, distress, or suffering. Place a check in the box next to each behavior you observe or infer while talking with your patient.

❑ Grimacing
❑ Moaning
❑ Sighing
❑ Clenching teeth
❑ Holding or supporting the painful body area
❑ Sitting rigidly
❑ Frequently shifting posture or position
❑ Moving in a guarded or protective manner
❑ Moving very slowly
❑ Limping
❑ Taking medication
❑ Using a cane, cervical collar, or other prosthetic device
❑ Walking with an abnormal gait
❑ Requesting help with walking
❑ Stopping frequently while walking
❑ Lying down during the day
❑ Avoiding physical activity
❑ Being irritable
❑ Asking such questions as, "Why did this happen to me?"
❑ Asking to be relieved from tasks or activities

Hey, check out this checklist!

If it's acute, think "autonomic"

Next, measure the patient's blood pressure, heart and respiratory rates, and pupil size. Acute pain may raise blood pressure, speed the heart and respiratory rates, and dilate pupils.

Remember, however, that these autonomic responses may be absent in a patient with chronic pain because the body gradually adapts to pain. Don't assume lack of autonomic responses means lack of pain.

To complete the examination, use a systematic technique to perform palpation, percussion, and auscultation. If the patient is in severe pain, you may need to shorten the examination, completing it later when his pain has decreased.

Psychological characteristics of pain

If diagnostic tests don't find a physical basis for the patient's pain, some health care providers may label the pain *psychogenic*. Psychogenic pain refers to pain associated with psychological factors. A patient with psychogenic pain may have organic pathology, or a psychological disorder may be the predominant influence on pain intensity.

Common psychogenic pain syndromes include chronic headache, muscle pain, back pain, and stomach or pelvic pain of unknown cause.

Keepin' it real

Keep in mind that psychogenic pain is *real* pain and doesn't mean the patient is malingering. Remember, too, that although pain can cause emotional distress, such distress isn't necessarily the cause of the psychogenic pain.

If objective physical findings don't substantiate the patient's complaints or if his pain severity rating seems excessive in light of physical findings, consider referring him to a psychologist or psychiatrist who specializes in evaluating chronic pain.

Emotional by-products of pain

A patient with chronic pain may suffer significant emotional distress. Because pain is subjective, his suffering and disability are hard to prove, disprove, or even quantify. So others may suspect he's faking or imagining the pain. (In fact, over time, he himself — rather than his pain — may become the subject of evaluation.)

If the patient is concerned that his pain may stem from an undiagnosed, possibly life-threatening condition, this obviously will add to his stress.

Shopping around

Many patients with chronic pain go from doctor to doctor and undergo exhausting procedures seeking a diagnosis and effective treatment. If their pain doesn't respond to treatment, they may feel health care providers, employers, and family are blaming — or doubting — them. In time, pain may become the central focus of their lives. They may withdraw from society, lose their jobs, and alienate family and friends.

Not surprisingly, many patients with chronic pain feel anxious, depressed, demoralized, helpless, hopeless, frustrated, an-

> Some patients with chronic pain go "doctor shopping" in search of relief.

gry, and isolated. They may suffer from insomnia, disruption of usual activities, drug abuse and dependence, anger, and violence. Some even attempt suicide.

Road to success

For health care providers, assessment and management of patients with pain—especially chronic pain—can be equally frustrating. But that doesn't mean you should lose heart or blame the patient. Through careful assessment and regular reevaluation, you can increase the odds for successful pain management—even in patients with seemingly intractable or chronic pain.

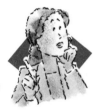

Quick quiz

1.   A patient who has been chatting with visitors tells you that his pain intensity rates a 5 on a 0-to-10 scale. How should you document this report?

    A.   By recording a lower pain rating than that reported by the patient

    B.   By recording a pain rating of 5

    C.   By recording that the patient doesn't appear to be in pain

    D.   By recording that the patient doesn't understand how to use the pain rating scale

Answer: B. Pain is whatever the patient says it is, occurring whenever he says it occurs. A patient who chats with visitors may simply be using distraction as a way to cope with pain.

2.   Which of the following statements accurately reflects JCAHO pain standards?

    A.   Only patients with certain diagnoses need to be assessed for pain on admission.

    B.   A pain level of 3 doesn't warrant reassessment.

    C.   The nurse may delegate pain assessment to unlicensed personnel.

    D.   Facility policies must identify a standard pain screening tool.

Answer: D. JCAHO standards require that all JCAHO-accredited facilities determine a standardized screening tool for use with all patients who are able to use that tool.

3. Because the ANS can adapt to pain, a patient with chronic pain may show which of the following?

    A.   Increased respirations

    B.   Dilated pupils

    C.   Diaphoresis

    D.   Hopelessness

Answer: D. The ANS adapts to pain over time. A patient with chronic pain is more likely to experience hopelessness (along with anxiety and anger) than to exhibit the autonomic responses listed.

4. On which pain rating scale does the patient place a line to indicate his current pain level?

    A.   Numerical rating scale

    B.   Visual analog scale

    C.   Pain intensity rating scale

    D.   Verbal descriptor scale

Answer: B. In the visual analog scale, the patient places a line on the scale to show his current pain level.

5. Which statement accurately describes the effects of culture on pain experience and expression?

    A.   People from all cultures respond to pain the same way.

    B.   All individuals within a given culture respond to pain the same way.

    C.   Cultural values can significantly influence a patient's response to pain.

    D.   A patient's cultural values have little importance in pain assessment.

Answer: C. The patient's cultural values play an important role in his response to pain. Remember, don't assess the patient's response to pain based on *your* cultural values.

6. When choosing an appropriate pain scale to use for your patient, consider his:

    A.   Visual acuity, age, reading ability, and level of understanding.

    B.   Past experiences with pain, age, and reading ability.

    C.   Level of education, visual acuity, and past experience with pain.

    D.   Visual acuity, culture, and ability to speak.

Answer: A. Factors to consider when choosing an appropriate pain scale for your patient include visual acuity, age, reading ability, and level of understanding.

Scoring

☆☆☆ If you answered all six questions correctly, awesome! You're an
        ace at assessing pain!

☆☆   If you answered four or five questions correctly, terrific! That
        didn't hurt so much, did it?

☆   If you answered fewer than four questions correctly, don't assess
        your condition as hopeless. Another dose of studying will lift
        you out of the doldrums.

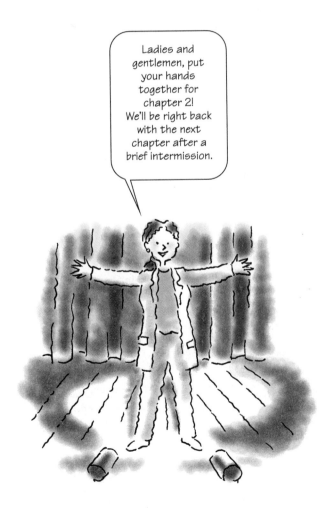

Pharmacologic pain management

Just the facts

In this chapter, you'll learn:

♦ the classes of drugs used to control pain

♦ specific uses of pain medications

♦ the pharmacokinetics (drug circulation) and pharmacodynamics (drug action) of pain medications

♦ drug interactions and adverse reactions caused by pain
medications.

A look at pain medications

Uncontrolled or poorly controlled pain diminishes a patient's
physical and mental health. Because pain can be so difficult to
treat, many drug and nondrug treatments have been developed for
all types of pain.

Pick your potency

This chapter reviews drugs used to manage pain, ranging from
mild to potent. Types of drugs used to control pain include:
• nonopioid analgesics
• opioid agonist and opioid antagonist agents
• local anesthetics
• anticonvulsants, antidepressants, muscle relaxants, and other types of drugs used adjunctively (additionally) for pain management.

> My friends
> here can help
> relieve all kinds
> of pain.

Nonopioid analgesics

Nonopioid (nonnarcotic) analgesics are used to treat pain that's either nociceptive (caused by stimulation of injury-sensing receptors) or neuropathic (arising from nerves). These agents are particularly effective against the somatic component of nociceptive pain such as joint and muscle pain. Besides controlling pain, nonopioid analgesics reduce inflammation and fever.

Drug types in this category include:

- acetaminophen
- nonsteroidal anti-inflammatory drugs (NSAIDs)
- salicylates.

Combination package

When used alone, acetaminophen and NSAIDs provide relief from mild pain. NSAIDs also can relieve moderate pain; in high doses, they may help relieve severe pain.

Given in combination with opioids, nonopioid analgesics provide additional analgesia, allowing a lower opioid dose and thus a lower risk of adverse opioid effects.

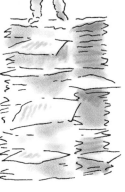

Pass the NSAIDs! This paperwork is giving me a nasty headache.

Acetaminophen

A para-aminophenol derivative, acetaminophen relieves mild pain and reduces fever. It's commonly the drug of choice for patients who need a mild analgesic, especially when aspirin and NSAIDs are contraindicated. Unlike those drugs, acetaminophen has no anti-inflammatory effect. It doesn't alter platelet function and rarely causes GI problems.

Pharmacokinetics

When taken orally, acetaminophen is absorbed quickly and entirely from the GI tract. About 60% to 98% of a dose is absorbed. It's widely distributed in body fluids and metabolized almost completely by the liver. The drug is excreted through the kidneys and in breast milk.

With rectal administration, only about 30% to 40% of the dose is absorbed. Also, absorption is slower.

Pharmacodynamics

Acetaminophen's pain control mechanism isn't well understood, but the drug is thought to inhibit prostaglandin synthesis in the central nervous system (CNS). Fever reduction comes from direct

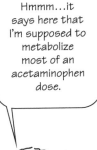

Hmmm...it says here that I'm supposed to metabolize most of an acetaminophen dose.

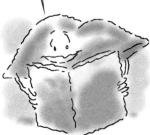

action on the body's "thermostat"—the temperature-regulating center in the brain's hypothalamus.

Pharmacotherapeutics

Acetaminophen is used to relieve headache, muscle aches, and general pain as well as to reduce fever. It's the first-choice drug for treating fever and flulike symptoms in children. According to the American Arthritis Association, acetaminophen also effectively relieves pain in some forms of arthritis.

Drug interactions

Acetaminophen may slightly increase the effects of oral anticoagulants and thrombolytics when taken in combination. It may increase the risk of liver toxicity when combined with phenytoin, barbiturates, carbamazepine, isoniazid, or chronic alcohol abuse. (See *Adverse reactions to acetaminophen.*)

> ### Adverse reactions to acetaminophen
>
> Well tolerated, acetaminophen is one of the safest nonopioid analgesics. The main concern, liver toxicity, can be prevented by carefully monitoring the patient and ensuring that the total daily dosage doesn't exceed 4,000 mg (2,400 mg for patients who have three or more alcoholic drinks daily).

NSAIDs

NSAIDs provide temporary relief from mild to moderate pain. They're also used adjunctively to manage cancer pain—especially in patients with bone metastasis. For long-term treatment, NSAIDs may be prescribed for osteoarthritis or rheumatoid arthritis.

NSAIDs have several advantages:
- They can be taken orally.
- They don't cause CNS or respiratory depression when used in therapeutic doses.
- They're generally available without a prescription.

No dearth of NSAIDs

Many NSAIDs are available. They include:
- celecoxib
- diclofenac
- fenoprofen
- flurbiprofen
- ibuprofen
- indomethacin
- ketoprofen
- ketorolac
- meclofenamate
- mefenamic acid
- nabumetone
- naproxen
- oxaprozin
- piroxicam

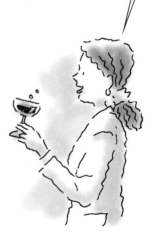

Acetaminophen may damage the liver when taken by a chronic alcohol abuser.

- rofecoxib
- sulindac
- tolmetin sodium
- valdecoxib.

Pharmacokinetics

Most NSAIDs are absorbed rapidly with limited tissue distribution (because of high protein binding) and are metabolized by the liver. Duration of action varies among specific agents.

The half-life is dose-dependent and ranges from 2 to 4 hours (ibuprofen) to 40 to 60 hours (oxaprozin). The kidneys eliminate a small amount of unchanged drug.

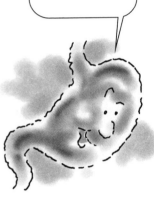

> I feel a lot better since I started taking COX-2 inhibitors.

Pharmacodynamics

NSAIDs work by interfering with prostaglandin production. Prostaglandins are hormonelike substances that promote inflammation, pain, and fever; support platelet function; and protect the stomach lining.

Prostaglandins are produced by the enzyme cyclooxygenase (COX). Actually, COX comes in two types—COX-1 and COX-2. Both types produce prostaglandins that promote inflammation, pain, and fever. But only COX-1 produces prostaglandins that protect the stomach lining and support platelet function.

Traditional NSAIDs inhibit COX-1 and COX-2. By blocking COX-2, they may damage the stomach lining, causing GI distress, stomach bleeding and ulcers, and altered platelet function.

News about NSAIDs

A new class of NSAIDs, COX-2 inhibitors, suppresses only COX-2. Because they spare COX-1, these agents reduce the risk of GI toxicity and altered platelet function. (See *NSAID innovation: COX-2 inhibitors.*)

> Thanks to NSAIDs, we can dance even though we have arthritis!

Pharmacotherapeutics

NSAIDs are used mainly to treat inflammation.
Secondary uses include menstrual cramps and mild to moderate pain after certain types of surgery.

NSAIDs typically bring favorable results in patients with:
- moderate to severe rheumatoid arthritis (an inflammatory disease of peripheral joints)
- osteoarthritis (a degenerative joint disease)
- acute gouty arthritis (urate deposits in the joints)
- dysmenorrhea (painful menstruation).

Rein in the pain

NSAID innovation: COX-2 inhibitors

A new type of nonsteroidal anti-inflammatory drug (NSAID) may improve arthritis treatment for millions. Called COX-2 inhibitors, these agents block only the COX-2 enzyme, a subtype of the enzyme cyclooxygenase (COX). COX-2 plays an important role in pain — and pain relief — because it stimulates the inflammatory response.

COX-2 inhibitors are used mainly to treat pain and inflammation associated with osteoarthritis and rheumatoid arthritis. They're also used to treat episodes of acute pain of mild to moderate intensity. Currently approved COX-2 inhibitors include celecoxib, rofecoxib, and valdecoxib.

A break with tradition

Traditional NSAIDs block the COX-1 and COX-2 enzymes. COX-1 protects the stomach lining and affects kidney function and blood clotting. That explains why traditional agents can alter platelet or kidney function and cause GI distress, bleeding, and ulcers.

Because COX-2 inhibitors don't affect COX-1 enzymes, they're less likely to cause serious GI, kidney, or platelet problems.

Pharmacokinetics

COX-2 inhibitors reach peak concentration 2 to 3 hours after ingestion. Food, especially a high-fat meal, delays this peak for another 1 to 2 hours (except for celecoxib, which is absorbed better with a high-fat meal). The half-life ranges from 11 to 17 hours, making once-daily dosing possible.

COX-2 inhibitors are metabolized extensively in the liver and may require dosage adjustment. Celecoxib and valdecoxib are extensively bound to albumin. Most elimination occurs in the urine as metabolites. Studies on breast-milk excretion haven't been conducted.

Pharmacodynamics

COX-2 is produced after tissue injury caused by an inflammatory stimulus. Because COX-2 inhibitors selectively decrease inflammation at the tissue site, they lack the systemic effects of other NSAIDs. But they still share some adverse effects with traditional NSAIDs.

Pharmacotherapeutics

COX-2 inhibitors are indicated for rheumatoid arthritis, osteoarthritis, acute pain, and dysmenorrhea. But they aren't superior to traditional NSAIDs in treating these conditions. Unless a patient has a compelling reason to use them, their relatively high cost doesn't warrant their use in treating acute pain or inflammation.

Drug interactions

COX-2 inhibitors may:
- decrease the effectiveness of some antihypertensives
- worsen peripheral edema when combined with other drugs that can cause such swelling (for instance, calcium channel blockers)
- increase bleeding time when given with warfarin
- increase the risk of GI bleeding when combined with low-dose aspirin
- raise lithium concentrations when therapy starts
- cause bone marrow suppression and GI toxicity when given with methotrexate.

Adverse reactions

COX-2 inhibitors may cause photosensitivity, peripheral edema, hypertension, and stomach upset (although they usually cause fewer GI adverse effects than other NSAIDs). They must be used cautiously in patients with renal or hepatic impairment.

They're contraindicated in patients with sulfonamide sensitivity and in those who've had allergic reactions to aspirin or other NSAIDs.

Adverse reactions to NSAIDs

All nonsteroidal anti-inflammatory drugs (NSAIDs) can cause similar adverse reactions. These include:
• abdominal pain, bleeding, anorexia, diarrhea, nausea, and stomach ulcers
• liver toxicity
• drowsiness, headache, dizziness, confusion, tinnitus, vertigo, and depression
• bladder infection, blood in the urine, and kidney necrosis.
    The risk of adverse reactions decreases with short-term, low-dose, and single-dose use.

Generally speaking
Adverse reactions follow several patterns:
• The longer the drug's half-life, the greater the risk of liver toxicity.
• Buffered or coated NSAIDs may reduce GI toxicity.
• The risk of GI bleeding rises with the patient's age, alcohol use, and multiple NSAID use.
• Patients with heart failure, renal insufficiency, or liver disease typically have more adverse reactions.

Risky business
Phenylbutazone has an unusually high incidence of adverse reactions. It commonly causes nausea, vomiting, abdominal discomfort, stomach discomfort after eating, diarrhea, and rashes.

Drug interactions

NSAIDs can interact with many drugs—especially indomethacin, mefenamic acid, phenylbutazone, piroxicam, and sulindac. Because NSAIDs are highly protein-bound, they're likely to interact with other protein-bound drugs such as oral anticoagulants. Some NSAIDs can also interact with antihypertensive drugs. (See *Adverse reactions to NSAIDs*.)

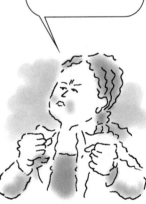

Salicylates are commonly prescribed to eliminate pain. Oooh, I sure could use one now!

Salicylates

Salicylates, such as aspirin, are among the most commonly used pain medications. A single salicylate dose of 650 mg brings maximum pain relief and fever-reducing effects. Doses of up to 5 g/day confer maximum anti-inflammatory effects.

Pharmacokinetics

Taken orally, salicylates are absorbed partly in the stomach but mainly in the upper part of the small intestine. Pure and buffered aspirin forms are absorbed readily. With sustained-release and enteric-coated aspirin, absorption is delayed. Toxicity rarely is life-threatening, and symptoms are mild.

Pharmacodynamics

Salicylates relieve pain by inhibiting prostaglandin synthesis.

Pharmacotherapeutics

Salicylates are used mainly to relieve pain and inflammation and reduce fever. They aren't effective against visceral pain (pain arising from the organs or smooth muscle) or severe pain related to trauma.

Drug interactions

Salicylates are highly protein-bound and may displace other protein-bound drugs from binding sites. This raises the serum level of the unbound active drug, leading to increased drug effects.

For example, when taken with NSAIDs, salicylates may have a reduced therapeutic effect and may heighten the risk of adverse GI effects. (See *Adverse reactions to salicylates.*)

Bleeding problems also can occur. One 650-mg dose of aspirin can prolong bleeding time for 4 to 7 days.

Adverse reactions to salicylates

The most common adverse reactions to salicylates include:
• gastric distress, diarrhea, nausea, and vomiting
• confusion
• dizziness
• hyperventilation
• thirst
• sweating
• hearing loss (with prolonged use)
• tinnitus
• impaired vision
• Reye's syndrome (in children with chickenpox and flulike symptoms).

Opioids

Opioids (narcotics) include derivatives of the opium (poppy) plant and synthetic drugs that imitate natural narcotics. Unlike NSAIDs, which act peripherally, opioids produce their primary effects in the CNS.

Agonist vs. antagonist

Opioids include opioid agonists, opioid antagonists, and mixed agonist-antagonists. Opioid agonists are used to treat moderate to severe pain without causing loss of consciousness.

Actually, opioid antagonists aren't pain medications, but block the effects of opioid agonists. They're used to re-

Opioid agonists cause analgesic effects.

Opioid antagonists reverse them.

verse adverse drug reactions, such as respiratory and CNS depression produced by opioid agonists. Unfortunately, by reversing analgesic effects, they may cause the patient's pain to recur.

Mixin' and matchin'

As their name implies, mixed opioid agonist-antagonists have agonist and antagonist properties. The agonist component relieves pain, while the antagonist component reduces the risk of toxicity and drug dependence. These agents also decrease the risk of respiratory depression and drug abuse.

Opioid agonists

Opioid agonists include:
- codeine
- fentanyl citrate
- hydromorphone hydrochloride
- levorphanol tartrate
- meperidine hydrochloride
- methadone hydrochloride
- morphine sulfate (including sustained-release tablets and intensified oral solution)
- oxycodone hydrochloride.

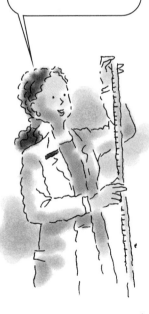

Morphine is the gold standard of pain relief. Every other pain medication is measured against it.

Go for the gold

Morphine is the "gold standard" against which the effectiveness and adverse reactions of other pain medications are measured.

Pharmacokinetics

Opioid agonists can be given by any route, although inhalation administration is rare. Oral doses are absorbed readily from the GI tract.

I.V. agents provide the most reliable and fastest pain relief (almost immediate). With the subcutaneous (S.C.) and intramuscular (I.M.) routes, absorption may be delayed, especially in patients with poor circulation.

Distribution deal

Opioid agonists are widely distributed to the muscles, kidneys, liver, intestines, lungs, spleen, and brain. They're metabolized in the liver. Meperidine, for instance, is metabolized to normeperidine — a toxic metabolite with a longer half-life than meperidine.

The kidneys excrete the metabolites. A small amount is excreted in the stool. Opioid agonists also are excreted in breast milk.

Pharmacodynamics

Opioid agonists reduce pain by binding to opiate receptor sites in the CNS. When these drugs stimulate opiate receptors, they mimic the effects of endorphins—naturally occurring opiates that are part of the body's pain relief system.

This receptor-site binding causes analgesic effects and cough suppression as well as adverse reactions, such as respiratory depression and constipation. (See *How opioid agonists control pain*, page 64.)

> I'm feeling no pain! The opioid agonist I took is mimicking my natural endorphins.

Pharmacotherapeutics

Opioid agonists are used to relieve severe pain in acute, chronic, and terminal conditions. Morphine also relieves shortness of breath in patients with pulmonary edema and left-sided heart failure.

Drug interactions

Opiate agonists may cause additive CNS depression in patients who are also receiving general anesthesia, phenothiazines, tranquilizers, sedative-hypnotics, or other CNS depressants. For such combined therapy, the dosage of one or both drugs should be reduced. (See *Adverse reactions to opioid agonists*, page 65.)

Mixed opioid agonist-antagonists

Mixed opioid agonist-antagonists relieve pain while carrying a lower risk of toxic effects and drug dependency. These agents include:
- buprenorphine hydrochloride
- butorphanol tartrate
- dezocine
- nalbuphine hydrochloride
- pentazocine hydrochloride (combined with pentazocine lactate, naloxone hydrochloride, aspirin, or acetaminophen).

> Opiate agonists may cause additive CNS depression in patients receiving other drugs that depress the CNS.

Potent potential

Originally, mixed agonist-antagonists seemed to have less addiction potential than pure opioid agonists as well as a lower risk of drug dependence. However, butorphanol and pentazocine reportedly have caused dependence.

CAUTION!

Now I get it!

How opioid agonists control pain

Opioid agonists, such as meperidine, inhibit pain transmission by mimicking the body's natural pain-control mechanisms.

Where neurons meet

In the dorsal horn of the spinal cord, peripheral pain neurons meet central nervous system (CNS) neurons. At the synapse, the pain neuron releases substance P (a pain neurotransmitter). This agent helps transfer pain impulses to the CNS neurons that carry the impulses to the brain.

Taking up space

In theory, spinal interneurons respond to stimulation from descending CNS neurons by releasing endogenous opiates. These opiates bind to the peripheral pain neuron to inhibit release of substance P and retard the transmission of pain impulses.

Stopping substance P

Synthetic opiates supplement this pain-blocking effect by binding with free opiate receptors to inhibit the release of substance P. Opiates also alter consciousness of pain, but how this mechanism works remains unknown.

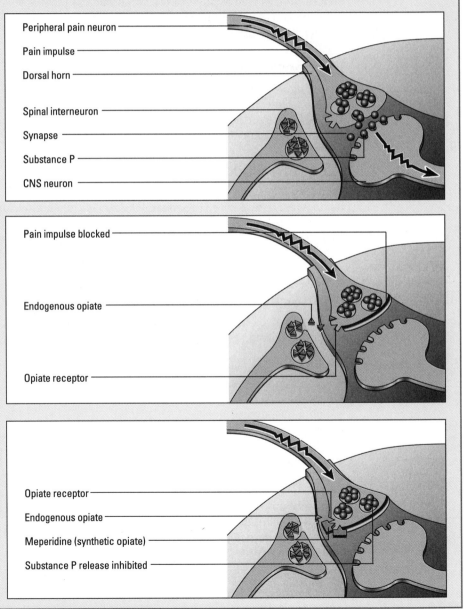

Peripheral pain neuron
Pain impulse
Dorsal horn
Spinal interneuron
Synapse
Substance P
CNS neuron

Pain impulse blocked
Endogenous opiate
Opiate receptor

Opiate receptor
Endogenous opiate
Meperidine (synthetic opiate)
Substance P release inhibited

Adverse reactions to opioid agonists

Respiratory depression (decreased breathing rate and depth) is one of the most common adverse reactions to opioid agonists. The higher the dose, the worse the respiratory depression. Some patients may experience periodic, irregular breathing or even asthma attacks.

Other adverse reactions to opioid agonists include:
- flushing
- decreased blood pressure when rising (orthostatic hypotension)
- pupil constriction (miosis)
- constipation
- light-headedness
- dizziness
- sedation
- nausea
- vomiting.

Too tolerant

With repeated opioid use, psychological or physical dependence and tolerance may develop. Abrupt cessation may lead to withdrawal syndrome—fever, chills, nausea, vomiting, and insomnia.

More with meperidine

Meperidine commonly produces tremors, palpitations, tachycardia, and delirium.

Added risk

Opioid agonists should be used with particular caution in elderly patients or those who have impaired hepatic or renal function, hypothyroidism, Addison's disease, prostatic hypertrophy, or urethral stricture.

Pharmacokinetics

Absorption of opioid agonist-antagonists occurs rapidly from parenteral administration sites. These drugs are distributed to most body tissues and cross the placenta.

Metabolized in the liver, they're excreted mainly by the kidneys. However, more than 10% of a butorphanol dose and a small amount of dezocine and pentazocine doses are excreted in the stool.

Pharmacodynamics

The exact mechanism of action isn't known. However, buprenophine binds with CNS receptors, altering the perception of pain and the emotional response to it. The drug releases slowly from binding sites, producing a longer duration than other drugs in this class.

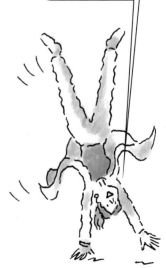

Opioid agonist-antagonists don't just alter pain perception. They also change the emotional response to pain.

Pharmacotherapeutics

Mixed opioid agonist-antagonists are used mainly to:
- relieve moderate to severe pain
- reduce preoperative anxiety and pain
- provide analgesia during childbirth.

Breathing a little easier

Mixed agents may be preferred over opioid agonists because they may carry a lower risk of drug dependence and respiratory depression. However, they can produce other adverse reactions.

Drug interactions

Increased CNS depression and an additive decrease in respiratory rate and depth may occur when mixed opioid agonist-antagonists are used along with CNS depressants, such as barbiturates or alcohol.

These drugs shouldn't be given to patients with a history of opioid abuse because they can cause withdrawal symptoms. (See *Adverse reactions to mixed opioid agonist-antagonists.*)

Opioid antagonists

Opioid antagonists attach to opiate receptors but don't stimulate them. As a result, they prevent other opioids, enkephalins, and endorphins from producing their effects.

Opioid antagonists include naloxone hydrochloride and naltrexone hydrochloride.

Pharmacokinetics

Naloxone is given I.M., S.C., or I.V. Naltrexone is given orally in tablet or liquid form. Both drugs are metabolized by the liver and excreted by the kidneys.

Pharmacodynamics

Opioid antagonists block opioid effects by occupying opioid receptor sites, displacing other drugs that attach to opiate receptors, and blocking further binding at these sites.

Pharmacotherapeutics

Naloxone is the preferred drug for managing opioid overdose. It reverses respiratory depression and sedation and helps stabilize vital signs within seconds.

Adverse reactions to mixed opioid agonist-antagonists

The most common adverse reactions to mixed opioid agonist-antagonists include:
- nausea
- vomiting
- light-headedness
- sedation
- euphoria.

Pain makes an encore

Because naloxone reverses opioids' analgesic effects, a patient who receives an opioid for pain relief may complain of pain or even experience withdrawal symptoms after receiving an opioid antagonist.

Detoxify first

Naltrexone is used to treat drug abuse — typically in combination with psychotherapy. It's given only to patients who've gone through a detoxification program to eliminate all opioids from the body. When given to someone who still has opioids in the body, acute withdrawal symptoms may occur.

Drug interactions

Naloxone doesn't produce significant drug interactions. Naltrexone may cause withdrawal symptoms in patients who are receiving opioid agonists or are opioid-dependent. (See *Adverse reactions to opioid antagonists.*)

Adjuvant analgesics

Adjuvant analgesics are drugs that have other primary indications but are used as analgesics in some circumstances. Adjuvants may be given in combination with opioids or used alone to treat chronic pain. Patients receiving adjuvant analgesics should be reevaluated periodically to monitor their pain level and check for adverse reactions.

A real potpourri

Drugs used as adjuvant analgesics include certain anticonvulsants, local and topical anesthetics, muscle relaxants, tricyclic antidepressants (TCAs), serotonin 5-HT1 agonists, selective serotonin reuptake inhibitors (SSRIs), ergotamine alkaloids, benzodiazepines, psychostimulants, cholinergic blockers, and corticosteroids.

Anticonvulsants

Anticonvulsants may be used to treat neuropathic pain (pain generated by peripheral nerves). These agents include:
- carbamazepine
- clonazepam
- divalproex sodium

Adverse reactions to opioid antagonists

The opioid antagonists naloxone and naltrexone cause different adverse reactions.

Naloxone: Scary wake-up call
Naloxone may cause nausea and vomiting. Occasionally, adverse reactions include hypertension and tachycardia.

Also, an unconscious patient who regains consciousness abruptly after naloxone administration may hyperventilate and experience tremors.

Naltrexone: A list of its own
Naltrexone may cause:
- edema, hypertension, palpitations, phlebitis (vein inflammation), and shortness of breath
- anxiety, depression, disorientation, dizziness, headache, and nervousness
- anorexia, diarrhea or constipation, nausea, thirst, and vomiting
- urinary frequency
- liver toxicity.

- gabapentin
- lamotrigine
- oxcarbazepine
- phenytoin
- tiagabine
- topiramate
- valproic acid
- zonisamide.

Carbamazepine and gabapentin are the anticonvulsants most commonly used as adjuvant analgesics.

Pharmacokinetics

Anticonvulsants are absorbed slowly from the GI tract. The half-life ranges from 5 to 25 hours, depending on the specific drug and dose. These drugs are distributed widely throughout the body.

> Some anticonvulsants are excreted in exhaled air.

Head straight for the protein

Roughly 75% to 95% of a dose is protein bound. Anticonvulsants are metabolized by the liver and excreted in urine, feces, breast milk and, in some cases, exhaled air.

Pharmacodynamics

Anticonvulsants help prevent excessive nerve impulses, which may be perceived as pain. Gabapentin and valproic acid, for instance, suppress excessive nerve impulses by blocking the calcium channel and boosting production of gamma-aminobutyric acid (GABA), an inhibitory neurotransmitter. Carbamazepine and phenytoin act on the sodium channel.

Pharmacotherapeutics

Carbamazepine and gabapentin may be prescribed adjunctively to help relieve neuropathic pain in adults. Carbamazepine is the drug of choice for treating trigeminal neuralgia (shooting pains of the facial area around one or more branches of the trigeminal nerve).

Drug interactions

Anticonvulsants can interact with many drugs. For example, carbamazepine and phenytoin may reduce the effectiveness of many other drugs — and, in turn, certain drugs can reduce their effectiveness.

Valproic acid may worsen bleeding in patients receiving anticoagulants. It also may increase serum phenobarbital levels. Gener-

---

Adverse reactions to anticonvulsants

Anticonvulsants that block the sodium channel — carbamazepine, lamotrigine, and phenytoin — may cause adverse reactions involving most body systems.

Use with caution
Because anticonvulsants may undergo altered absorption and metabolism, they should be used cautiously in elderly patients and those with cardiac, renal, or hepatic dysfunction.

ally, alcohol decreases the effectiveness of anticonvulsants. Anticonvulsants also have the potential to adversely affect many body systems. (See *Adverse reactions to anticonvulsants.*)

Local anesthetics

Local anesthetics may be used to help manage neuropathic pain or as an alternative to general anesthesia. These agents include:
• amide drugs, such as bupivacaine, etidocaine, lidocaine, mepivacaine, prilocaine, and ropivacaine
• ester drugs, such as benzocaine, cocaine, chloroprocaine, procaine, and tetracaine. (See *Pain-numbing cousins.*)

Pharmacokinetics

Absorption time varies with the specific drug, dose, administration route, lipid solubility, and protein binding. The half-life ranges from 1 to 10 hours.

Here, there, and everywhere

Local anesthetics are distributed widely throughout the body. Duration of action ranges from 30 to 60 minutes for the esters and 1 to 5 hours for the amides.

Metabolism varies with the specific drug. Local anesthetics are excreted by the kidneys in varying degrees.

Pharmacodynamics

Local anesthetics selectively block sodium channel permeability, thereby disrupting ectopic nerve impulses centrally and peripherally. They don't affect normal nerve conduction.

Pharmacotherapeutics

Local anesthetics are used to prevent and relieve pain from medical procedures, disease, or injury. They're also prescribed for severe pain not relieved by topical anesthetics or analgesics.

Drug interactions

Local anesthetics don't cause significant interactions with other drugs. When given in combination with clonidine, epinephrine, or opioids, their anesthetic activity increases. (See *Adverse reactions to local anesthetics.*)

Pain-numbing cousins

Local anesthetics include two main groups. *Amides* (which include lidocaine and prilocaine) contain nitrogen in their molecular makeup.

Give them oxygen

In contrast, *esters* (such as cocaine and procaine) contain oxygen, not nitrogen.

Adverse reactions to local anesthetics

Major adverse reactions to local anesthetics are dose- and drug-dependent. Lidocaine is a Class IB antiarrhythmic. Besides its pain-numbing effects on the central nervous system, it may cause:
• hypotension
• cardiac arrhythmias and depression
• cardiac arrest.

Topical anesthetics

Topical anesthetics are applied directly to the skin or mucous membranes to prevent or relieve minor pain. These agents include:
- amide drugs, such as dibucaine and lidocaine
- ester drugs, such as benzocaine, cocaine, dyclonine, pramoxine hydrochloride, and tetracaine.

Mixin' it up

This drug category also includes topical combinations of local anesthetics, such as:
- Aerocaine—a mixture of benzocaine and benzethonium
- Cetacaine—a mixture of benzocaine, butamben, dyclonine, lidocaine hydrochloride, and tetracaine hydrochloride
- EMLA (eutetic mixture of local anesthetics), which contains lidocaine and prilocaine.

Pharmacokinetics

Although topical anesthetics cause little systemic absorption, such absorption may occur with frequent or high-dose applications to the eye or large areas of burned or injured skin.

Discreet excretion

Tetracaine and other esters are metabolized in the blood and, to a lesser extent, the liver. Amides are metabolized by the liver. Both types of topical anesthetics are excreted in the urine.

Pharmacodynamics

Topical anesthetics relieve pain by preventing nerve impulse transmission. These drugs accumulate in the nerve membrane, causing it to expand and lose its ability to depolarize, thus blocking impulse transmission.

Pharmacotherapeutics

Topical anesthetics are used to:
- relieve or prevent pain, especially from minor burns
- relieve itching and irritation
- numb a selected area before an injection
- numb mucosal surfaces before tube insertion
- relieve sore throat or mouth pain (when used as a spray or solution).

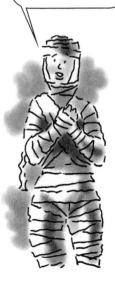

Aren't you going a bit overboard? Topical anesthetics cause little systemic absorption.

Drug interactions

Topical anesthetics cause few interactions with other drugs because they aren't well-absorbed into the systemic circulation. (See *Adverse reactions to topical anesthetics.*)

Muscle relaxants

Muscle relaxants can be classified as:
• neuromuscular agents (such as metocurine and tubocurarine), used primarily as adjuncts to general anesthesia (and secondarily to induce muscle relaxation and promote relaxation in patients on mechanical ventilation)
• antispasmodic agents, used to relieve spasticity associated with CNS disorders
• agents used for short-term pain relief and muscle spasms.
   We'll discuss only the latter two categories in detail.

Spasm stoppers

Antispasmodic agents include:
• baclofen
• dantrolene
• diazepam
• tizanidine.

Good for a brief respite

Agents used for short-term pain relief and muscle spasms include:
• carisoprodol
• chlorzoxazone
• cyclobenzaprine
• methocarbamol
• tizanidine.

Pharmacokinetics

Antispasmodic drugs are absorbed rapidly from the GI system — except for dantrolene, whose absorption is slow and incomplete. The half-life ranges from 2.5 to 100 hours. These drugs are distributed widely, metabolized by the liver, and excreted mainly in urine.

Get a half-life

Agents used for short-term relief from pain or muscle spasms are absorbed, metabolized, and distributed in similar ways. The half-life varies from 1 hour (chlorzoxazone) to 3 days (cyclobenzaprine).

> **Adverse reactions to topical anesthetics**
>
> All topical anesthetics can cause hypersensitivity reactions, such as rash, hives, itching, mouth and throat swelling, and respiratory difficulty.
>
> Those also used as local anesthetics (such as benzocaine, cocaine, lidocaine, and tetracaine) may cause central nervous system and cardiovascular reactions.

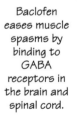

Baclofen eases muscle spasms by binding to GABA receptors in the brain and spinal cord.

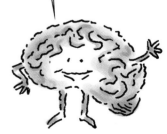

Pharmacodynamics

Antispasmodic effects of baclofen and diazepam are similar. Baclofen suppresses release of excitatory neurotransmitters by binding to GABA-B receptors in the dorsal horn of the spinal cord, brain stem, and other CNS sites. Diazepam acts on GABA-A receptors.

Agents used for short-term relief from pain and muscle spasms act centrally in various ways, helping to minimize pain through sedation. Tizanidine has the effects of both muscle relaxant categories and can be used for both spasticity and painful muscle conditions.

Pharmacotherapeutics

Muscle relaxants are used to relieve common musculoskeletal pain or acute traumatic sprains or strains.

Agents used for short-term relief of pain and muscle spasms are prescribed to relax skeletal muscles.

Drug interactions

Concomitant use of muscle relaxants with other anticonvulsants or CNS depressants may intensify CNS depression. Cyclobenzaprine may interact with monoamine oxidase inhibitors (MAOIs), exacerbating CNS depression or causing anticholinergic effects — such as reduction of smooth muscle spasms and decreased secretions and sweating. (See *Adverse reactions to muscle relaxants.*)

Tricyclic antidepressants

Of the various types of antidepressants, TCAs have the longest history in managing pain — particularly neuropathic pain.

TCAs include:
- amitriptyline
- amoxapine
- clomipramine
- desipramine
- doxepin
- imipramine
- maprotiline
- nortriptyline
- protriptyline.

Adverse reactions to muscle relaxants

Most muscle relaxants can cause drowsiness, dizziness, weakness, and light-headedness. Baclofen also may cause nausea, fatigue, vertigo, depression, and headache. Carisoprodol can cause light-headedness when standing. Tizanadine can cause:
- sleepiness
- sedation
- hypotension
- slow heartbeat
- dry mouth
- urinary tract infections.

Let's get serious

More serious adverse reactions also may occur.
- Dantrolene can cause fatigue, malaise, and seizures.
- Methocarbamol may cause seizures when given I.V.
- Cyclobenzaprine can cause seizures and arrhythmias.
- Diazepam may cause cardiovascular collapse, slow heart rate, and respiratory depression.

Pharmacokinetics

TCAs are absorbed rapidly from the GI tract and metabolized by the liver. The half-life ranges from 12 to 89 hours. Steady state occurs between 4 and 10 days.

The sooner, the better

Although the full antidepressant effect may take up to 4 weeks, pain relief may occur as early as 5 to 10 days after TCA therapy begins. TCAs are widely distributed in the CNS and excreted in urine and breast milk.

Pharmacodynamics

The mechanism of action varies with the specific drug. Generally, TCAs inhibit reuptake of brain neurotransmitters (norepinephrine, serotonin, or dopamine) at nerve terminals. Also, they may block noradrenergic neuronal firing, providing analgesia to damaged nerve fibers.

Pharmacotherapeutics

TCAs are helpful in treating neuropathic pain.

Drug interactions

TCAs may interact with cimetidine, certain antiarrhythmics and neuroleptics, barbiturates, direct-acting sympathomimetics (such as phenylephrine), warfarin, MAOIs, and centrally acting antihypertensives (such as clonidine and methyldopa). (See *Adverse reactions to tricyclic antidepressants.*)

Serotonin 5-HT1 receptor agonists

Serotonin 5-HT1 receptor agonists (commonly called triptans) prevent or relieve migraine. These drugs include:
- almotriptan
- frovatriptan
- naratriptan
- rizatriptan
- sumatriptan
- zolmitriptan.

Pharmacokinetics

Absorption and distribution vary with the administration route. Generally, suppositories have a faster onset than oral agents and

---

Adverse reactions to tricyclic antidepressants

Tricyclic antidepressants (TCAs) may cause:
- dry mouth, blurred vision, and constipation
- irritation, dizziness, drowsiness, and sedation
- difficulty urinating
- postural hypotension
- poor libido and erectile dysfunction
- weight gain
- increased sensitivity to the sun
- increased sweating
- hand tremors
- unusual energy
- difficulty falling or staying asleep
- weakness
- increased heart rate.

Rare events
Rarely, TCAs cause cardiac changes and should be used with caution in patients with cardiac conduction disorders. Other serious adverse effects include:
- liver inflammation
- myocardial infarction
- cardiovascular accident
- seizures.

are absorbed more rapidly and consistently. With injection, onset occurs within 10 minutes; with nasal sprays, within 15 minutes.

Through the kidneys or liver

The half-life ranges from 2.5 to 6 hours. Elimination is predominantly renal. With some exceptions, these agents are metabolized in the liver.

Pharmacodynamics

Serotonin 5-HT1 receptor agonists bind to serotonin receptors on the trigeminal nerve. This inhibits serotoninergic neuron firing and reduces serotonin synthesis and release. Dural blood vessels then constrict.

Drug interactions

These agents may interact with ergot-containing drugs, prolonging vasospastic effects. Some agents also may interact with cimetidine, SSRIs, and MAOIs. (See *Adverse reactions to serotonin 5-HT1 receptor agonists.*)

SSRIs

A well-known class of antidepressants, SSRIs are being investigated for pain relief as well. These agents include:
- fluoxetine
- paroxetine
- sertraline hydrochloride.

Pharmacokinetics

SSRIs are absorbed almost completely after oral administration and are highly protein-bound. Primarily metabolized in the liver, they're excreted in the urine.

Pharmacodynamics

SSRIs inhibit neuronal reuptake of serotonin.

Pharmacotherapeutics

Used mainly to treat depression, SSRIs are currently being studied in the management of neuropathic pain. They've also shown potential in treating chronic nonmalignant pain syndromes. However, evidence doesn't support their role in managing acute pain. As analgesics, SSRIs perform best when used as adjuncts to opioids.

Adverse reactions to serotonin 5-HT1 receptor agonists

Serotonin 5-HT1 receptor agonists may cause such effects as:
- dry mouth
- nausea
- dizziness
- muscle weakness
- tingling
- sensations of warmth, heaviness, pressure, or tightness
- ear, nose, and throat discomfort.

It gets worse

More serious problems include:
- coronary vasospasm, possibly leading to myocardial infarction or cardiovascular accident
- serotonin syndrome, in patients who also take antidepressants that increase serotonin levels. Serotonin syndrome involves mental changes, restlessness, tremor, chills, sweating, and colitis.

Drug interactions

SSRIs may competitively inhibit a liver enzyme responsible for oxidizing numerous other drugs—including TCAs, certain antipsychotics, carbamazepine, metoprolol, flecainide, and encainide.

Fatal interaction

When used with MAOIs, potentially fatal reactions may occur. Individual SSRIs also have their own particular interactions. (See *Adverse reactions to SSRIs*.)

Ergotamine alkaloids

Ergotamine alkaloids are used to prevent or abort migraine and cluster headaches. They include ergotamine tartrate and dihydroergotamine mesylate.

Pharmacokinetics

When given orally, ergotamine alkaloids have variable GI absorption. Peak blood levels occur in roughly 2 hours. When given by inhalation, absorption is rapid and complete. With buccal administration, absorption is poor. (Giving caffeine simultaneously aids drug absorption.)

The half-life is 2 hours. However, these drugs have long-lasting effects because they're stored in the tissues.

Where does it all go?

Ergotamine alkaloids are metabolized in the liver, with 90% of metabolites excreted in the bile. Unmetabolized drug is secreted erratically in saliva, and trace amounts are excreted in the stool and urine.

Pharmacodynamics

Ergotamine alkaloids exhibit partial agonist or antagonist activities on certain receptors. They constrict cranial and peripheral blood vessels, act as potent emetics, and affect uterine tone.

Pharmacotherapeutics

These agents are used to prevent migraine or cluster headaches. Dihydroergotamine mesylate may be for acute migraine treatment.

Drug interactions

Ergotamine alkaloids may interact with:
• antacids

> Adverse
> reactions to
> SSRIs
>
> Selective serotonin reuptake inhibitors (SSRIs) may cause many adverse reactions. These include:
> • dry mouth, blurred vision, and constipation
> • urinary retention
> • drowsiness and sedation
> • irritability, agitation, and anxiety
> • difficulty sleeping
> • diminished or increased appetite
> • weight gain or loss
> • headache
> • nausea, diarrhea, and other GI disturbances
> • headache.
>
> **Sexual adverse effects**
> Many patients who take SSRIs experience such sexual problems as:
> • poor libido
> • erectile dysfunction
> • inability to achieve orgasm.

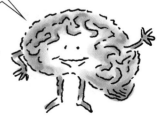

No migraine today, thanks to that ergot drug I just took.

- anticoagulants
- anticholinergics
- CNS depressants
- oral contraceptives
- cardiac glycosides
- other ergot drugs (such as methysergide)
- TCAs. (See *Adverse reactions to ergotamine alkaloids*.)

Benzodiazepines

Benzodiazepines are used primarily to ease anxiety. Although they aren't effective in treating acute pain, they have some value in easing muscle spasms.

Benzodiazepines include:

- alprazolam
- diazepam
- lorazepam
- midazolam
- oxazepam.

Pharmacokinetics

Benzodiazepines are well-absorbed from the GI tract and distributed widely in the body. Some agents may be given parenterally.

All benzodiazepines are metabolized in the liver and excreted primarily in the urine.

Pharmacodynamics

Benzodiazepines increase availability of the neurotransmitter GABA to brain neurons. At low doses, they ease anxiety by acting on the limbic system and related brain areas that help regulate emotional activity. At higher doses, they show sleep-inducing properties.

Pharmacotherapeutics

In pain management, benzodiazepines are used mainly for short-term relief of acute musculoskeletal pain characterized by muscle spasms. (When used for longer periods, these drugs have sedating affects that impede the patient's functional status.)

A variety show

Other uses for benzodiazepines include preoperative sedation and treatment of anxiety disorders.

Adverse reactions to ergotamine alkaloids

Dihydroergotamine mesylate and ergotamine tartrate and may cause:
- nausea and vomiting
- abnormally fast or slow heartbeat
- numbness and tingling in the fingers and toes
- weakness in the legs
- muscle pain
- itching
- localized swelling.

Downright dangerous
Women who are pregnant or who plan to become pregnant should avoid these drugs because they can stimulate the uterus or retard intrauterine growth. (Intrauterine death has occurred in animals.)

Other patients who should avoid ergotamine alkaloids are those with:
- renal or hepatic impairment
- coronary artery disease
- hypertension.

Don't get too dependent
Drug dependency can occur with extended use of ergotamine alkaloids. When discontinuing the drug, a dependent patient will experience withdrawal symptoms.

Drug interactions

Benzodiazepines interact with few drugs, except for other CNS depressants. When they're used concomitantly with CNS depressants, sedative and other depressant effects are enhanced. Possible consequences may include motor skill impairment, respiratory depression and, with high doses, death. (See *Adverse reactions to benzodiazepines*.)

Psychostimulants

Psychostimulants are used mainly to treat such disorders as Parkinson's disease and attention deficit hyperactivity disorder. In pain management, they may be used adjunctively to manage acute or chronic pain disorders.

Psychostimulants include:
- caffeine
- dextroamphetamine
- methylphenidate.

Pharmacokinetics

Absorption time and half-life vary with the specific drug.

Pharmacodynamics

Psychostimulants appear to act on the cerebral cortex, stimulating the nervous system by promoting nerve impulse transmission.

Pharmacotherapeutics

Dextroamphetamine has an analgesic affect in patients with postoperative pain. Methylphenidate helps ease pain associated with Parkinson's disease and cancer. It also reduces opioid-induced sedation and cognitive impairments associated with opioid use.

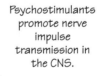

Psychostimulants promote nerve impulse transmission in the CNS.

Drug interactions

Excessive CNS stimulation may occur if caffeine is used with beta-adrenergic agonists, cimetidine, fluoroquinolones, oral contraceptives, theophylline, phenylpropanolamine, or caffeine-containing beverages.

Crisis mode

Dextroamphetamine can interact with many drugs. For instance, when taken within 14 days of an MAOI, hypertensive crisis may

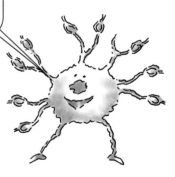

Adverse reactions to psychostimulants

Like other stimulants, caffeine, dextroamphetamine, and methylphenidate may cause:
- rapid heartbeat
- hypertension
- excessive urination
- nausea and vomiting
- restlessness and anxiety
- tremors
- difficulty sleeping.

Dextro dangers
Dextroamphetamine may cause:
- fast or irregular breathing
- a false feeling of well-being
- hallucinations
- skin rash
- dizziness
- poor coordination
- headache
- changes in sex drive or sexual function
- diarrhea or constipation
- appetite and weight loss.

More with methyl
Besides classic stimulant effects, methylphenidate may cause:
- seizures
- arrhythmias
- thrombocytopenia
- leukopenia
- serious skin reactions such as erythema multiforme.

occur. Caffeine-containing beverages may increase the drug's psychostimulant effects.

Methylphenidate also can cause hypertensive crisis when used with an MAOI. Also, this drug may interact with centrally acting antihypertensives to cause decreased antihypertensive effects. Caffeine-containing beverages may increase its psychostimulant effects. (See *Adverse reactions to psychostimulants*.)

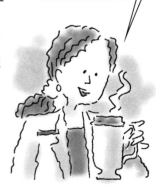

Go slow on the cup of Joe. Too much coffee can make you especially hyper if you're taking psychostimulants.

Cholinergic blockers

Cholinergic blockers are used to treat spastic or hyperactive conditions of the GI tract. They relax muscles and decrease GI secretions.

Major cholinergic blockers are the belladonna alkaloids, which include belladonna and scopolamine hydrobromide.

Pharmacokinetics

Belladonna alkaloids are absorbed from the eyes, GI tract, mucous membranes, and skin. They have low to moderate binding with serum proteins. Metabolized in the liver, they're excreted by the kidneys as unchanged drug and metabolites.

Pharmacodynamics

Cholinergic blockers interrupt parasympathetic nerve impulses in the central and autonomic nervous systems. They stop acetylcholine from stimulating cholinergic receptors.

Pharmacotherapeutics

Cholinergic blockers are given by injection to relax GI muscles before such procedures as endoscopy or sigmoidoscopy. They're also used to:
- treat muscular rigidity
- prevent nausea and vomiting from motion sickness
- help treat peptic ulcer disease and other GI disorders
- decrease secretions before surgery.

Putting the brakes on peristalsis

Cholinergic blockers may be useful adjunctive agents in malignant bowel obstruction because they reduce peristalsis and secretions. The transdermal scopolamine patch is the drug of choice for this purpose.

Octreotide, a cholinergic blocker used to treat malignant bowel obstruction, reduces gastric and pancreatic secretions by reducing GI motility. Anecdotal reports suggest it also has an analgesic effect.

Drug interactions

By decreasing gastric motility and delaying gastric emptying, cholinergic blockers may increase absorption of other drugs. Also, delayed gastric emptying keeps the drugs in prolonged contact with the GI mucosa, which can increase their adverse effects.

Reduction in absorption

Cholinergic blockers may be affected adversely by antacids and antidiarrheal agents, which may reduce drug absorption. (See *Adverse reactions to cholinergic blockers.*)

Corticosteroids

Corticosteroids are used to treat pain and inflammation. Based on their activity, they fall into two groups: mineralocorticoids and glucocorticoids.

The mineral variety

Mineralocorticoids regulate electrolyte and fluid homeostasis. They include:
* cortisone
* fludrocortisone acetate
* hydrocortisone.

The glucose connection

Glucocorticoids regulate the body's reaction to inflammation, stimulate conversion of fat and protein into glucose by the liver, and regulate the immune response to diverse stimuli. These agents include:
* betamethasone
* dexamethasone
* methylprednisolone
* prednisone
* triamcinolone.

Pharmacokinetics

Corticosteroids may be given orally, epidurally, or intra-articularly. Oral corticosteroids are absorbed rapidly. The duration of action ranges from 12 to 36 hours. The half-life varies with the specific drug and the administration route.

Distribution is systemic. Corticosteroids are metabolized by the liver and excreted in urine and stool.

Pharmacodynamics

Corticosteroids decrease inflammation by limiting influx of neutrophils and macrophages to the inflammation site. Apparently, they do this at an earlier stage than NSAIDs.

Go figure

Glucocorticoids suppress hypersensitivity and the immune response by a process that isn't well understood. They also suppress redness, edema, heat, and tenderness associated with inflammation and the pain.

Mineralocorticoids bind to mineralocorticoid receptors in the hippocampus, kidney, colon, salivary glands, and sweat glands. Aldosterone is converted to cortisone, which affects electrolyte and water balance.

Lesson in suppression

Glucocorticoids suppress the inflammatory response by stabilizing the lysosomal membrane (a cell structure that contains digestive enzymes). As a result, the cell doesn't release its store of hydrolytic enzymes into the cells.

These agents also prevent plasma exudation, suppress the migration of polymorphonuclear leukocytes, inhibit phagocytosis, and decrease antibody formation in injured or infected tissues.

Drug interactions

Corticosteroids diminish the effects of insulin and oral hypoglycemic agents. They also may decrease the effects of oral anticoagulants.

Barbiturates, phenytoin, rifampin, cholestyramine, colestipol, and antacids may reduce corticosteroid potency. Estrogen prolongs corticosteroid half-life. (See *Adverse reactions to corticosteroids.*)

Drug administration routes

Drugs can be delivered through many routes. Each route has advantages and drawbacks.

No switching allowed

Keep in mind that administration routes aren't therapeutically interchangeable. The administration route influences a drug's absorption and distribution — in turn, affecting drug action and patient response.

For instance, when given orally, the anxiolytic diazepam is readily absorbed. When given I.M., it's absorbed slowly and erratically.

Oral administration

For most patients, oral administration is the most convenient and easiest way to take analgesics. Oral pain medications generally are available in tablet, capsule, and liquid forms.

Adverse reactions to corticosteroids

Systemic corticosteroids affect almost all body systems. Adverse reactions include:
- insomnia
- sodium and water retention
- increased potassium excretion
- suppressed immune and inflammatory responses
- osteoporosis
- intestinal perforation
- peptic ulcers
- impaired wound healing.

Earmark the endocrine system

Endocrine system reactions can be especially serious. These may include:
- diabetes mellitus
- hyperlipidemia
- adrenal atrophy
- hypothalamic-pituitary axis suppression
- cushingoid signs and symptoms.

Put a gradual end to it

Oral doses must be tapered gradually in patients who have taken corticosteroids for more than 10 days. Abrupt withdrawal may cause fatal adrenal insufficiency.

Upping the absorption

After ingestion, tablets and capsules are absorbed by the GI system. How extensively and quickly absorption occurs depends on such factors as whether the drug is formulated for immediate or controlled release. Also, liquid preparations are absorbed faster.

Liquid pain medications are absorbed faster than tablets and capsules.

Sublingual administration

Sublingual medications are placed under the tongue, providing rapid and convenient analgesia. Most sublingual medications are rapidly disintegrating tablets and soft gelatin capsules filled with a liquid drug. High drug concentration is achieved in the sublingual region before being absorbed by the mucosa.

Transdermal administration

Transdermal administration refers to the use of drugs that come as ointments or transdermal patches. Lipid-soluble, they're absorbed through the skin, bypassing the GI tract.

Many specially compounded creams, gels, and ointments can be applied to the skin for pain relief. Fentanyl, lidocaine, and clonidine are available in transdermal systems, typically called patches.

A potent patch

The transdermal fentanyl patch (Duragesic), for instance, is 75 times more potent than morphine. Transdermal fentanyl has a slow onset of action—approximately 16 hours. It's rarely used in patients who haven't built up a tolerance to opioids.

Lidocaine patches are particularly useful for herpetic pain syndromes. Typically, the doctor prescribes a dosing schedule of 12 hours with the patch on, followed by 12 hours with it off.

Don't get this complex

Clonidine patches are used to relieve hyperalgesia in patients with complex regional pain syndrome. This syndrome involves pain caused by injury to an arm or a leg; rarely, it follows surgery, myocardial infarction, or some other medical problem.

Buccal administration

Buccal medications are inserted between the cheek and mouth. The patient closes his mouth and holds the tablet against his cheek until it's absorbed. Because the buccal mucosa is less permeable than the sublingual area, absorption is slower and drug availability is somewhat decreased.

Break through the pain

The buccally administered drug Actiq (oral transmucosal fentanyl citrate) is a flavored lozenge on a stick. Originally used to treat cancer breakthrough pain in opioid-tolerant patients, it has also been found to be useful in treating acute pain.

Onset of action occurs from use over a 15-minute period. Pain relief may take up to 45 minutes after finishing the dose; duration is 1 to 2 hours. However, because of patient variations in sucking, drug delivery may be inconsistent.

> That's right. Insert the buccal medication between the cheek and mouth.

S.C. administration

Subcutaneous drugs are injected into the fatty tissue beneath the skin. Drug absorption and action depend on the specific drug and its properties. S.C. administration usually provides rapid pain relief.

Pumping away the pain

Subcutaneous medications can be given through single injections or through a patient-controlled analgesia (PCA) pump. With PCA, a catheter is implanted under the skin and attached to an external electronic pump. The patient self-administers basal (continuous) and bolus (additional) doses as needed. Disadvantages of PCA include possible discomfort and irritation at the injection or infusion site.

I.M. administration

I.M. injections deliver medication deep into muscle tissue. Typically, the I.M. route is used when S.C., oral, or I.V. access isn't available or possible. Absorption and action of I.M. drugs depend on the specific drug and various patient factors.

Pretty fast against pain

Drugs given I.M. have a faster onset than oral drugs, but a slower onset than I.V. drugs. Pain and irritation at the injection site are common.

I.V. administration

Delivering a drug directly into a vein allows rapid onset because the drug enters the bloodstream quickly. The I.V. route is a good choice if the patient can't swallow, has persistent nausea and vomiting, or needs rapid onset.

On the down side, I.V. administration may cause drug infiltration and infection at the catheter site.

They're fast but they don't last

I.V. drugs are absorbed rapidly but have a short duration of action. Almost all opioids can be given I.V. PCA is also available for I.V. drugs.

Intranasal administration

Intranasal administration (typically using a nasal spray) may be indicated for patients who can't tolerate the oral route. The vascular nasal mucosa absorbs medication rapidly.

Intranasally administered pain medications include butorphanol, lidocaine, and sumatriptan succinate.

Epidural administration

A drug may be administered into the epidural space to provide local relief to irritated nerves in patients with chronic or acute pain. Epidurally administered pain medications include local anesthetics, narcotics, and steroids.

An epidural injection achieves pain relief within 2 to 10 days, on average. Duration of action ranges from days to months, depending on the patient's diagnosis and response.

Let's talk pumps again

Continuous and intermittent epidural medication delivery can be achieved by placing a catheter in the epidural space and attaching it to a pump. Catheters usually are placed temporarily for increased joint mobilization or intense physical therapy or to assess the patient's response to drug therapy. Pain relief occurs within minutes, although finding the dose that brings optimal relief may take a few days.

Drawbacks of epidural delivery include potential infection, local bleeding, and site tenderness.

Intrathecal administration

Intrathecal administration refers to delivery of a drug into the subarachnoid space of the spinal canal. This method is used to administer drugs that don't readily cross the blood-brain barrier. Drugs that may be given intrathecally include morphine, baclofen, clonidine, and ziconotide.

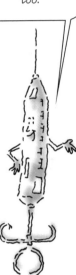

Unfortunately, just the sight of me has instilled fear in countless children — and some adults, too.

You're going to inject what into where?!

Some anesthetics may be given intrathecally to achieve regional anesthesia, as in spinal anesthesia or epidural block or to treat patients with chronic pain (by injecting a neurolytic agent into the cerebrospinal fluid [CSF]).

Even more about pumps

Sometimes, intrathecal drugs are delivered through an implanted pump to allow precise delivery of continuous doses. The pump is embedded below the skin and a catheter is tunneled to the precise location of pain in the spine. The drug enters the CSF and then the spinal cord, where it acts on the targeted site.

Five years isn't bad for a battery

Intrathecal administration typically allows smaller doses of pain medication and causes fewer adverse reactions. When a pump is used, it must be refilled with medication every 1 to 3 months, depending on the delivery rate. Typically, the pump must be replaced every 5 years because of limited battery life.

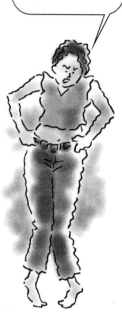

Intrathecal pumps have to be replaced every 5 years or so...Like a certain pair of jeans I know.

Rectal administration

Medications given rectally (as a gelatin or waxy suppository capsule) have a slow onset and variable absorption. Because absorption varies, the degree of pain relief with this administration route also varies. Although cost-effective, rectal administration isn't widely accepted.

Opioids, such as morphine, oxymorphone, and hydromorphone, are sometimes given rectally when other routes can't be tolerated.

Intra-articular administration

Intra-articular administration delivers drugs directly to the synovial joint cavity to relieve pain, reduce inflammation, and produce localized numbness. Drugs given by this route include corticosteroids, local anesthetics, and hyaluronic acid derivatives (used to treat osteoarthritis of the knee).

Shock absorbers

Intra-articular drugs absorb shock and lubricate the joint. Duration depends on the specific agent. For instance, hylan G-F 20 is given weekly for 3 weeks; sodium hyaluronate is given weekly for 5 weeks.

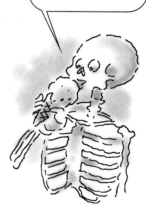

I'm celebrating! I just got an intra-articular administration and my joint pain is gone!

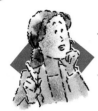

Quick quiz

1. Which statement about acetaminophen is *true*?
   A. The maximum recommended daily dose is 4,000 mg.
   B. Having six alcoholic drinks daily cuts the maximum recommended dose almost in half.
   C. Analgesic action occurs through drug effects on the hypothalamus.
   D. The drug has no effect on anticoagulants.

Answer: A. The maximum recommended daily dose of acetaminophen is 4,000 mg. Higher doses can cause severe hepatotoxicity.

2. Drugs that may be used as adjuvant analgesics include all of the following *except:*
   A. anticonvulsants.
   B. opioids.
   C. antidepressants.
   D. antihistamines.

Answer: B. Opioid analgesics are used as primary, not adjuvant, analgesics.

3. Which of the following statements about intrathecal drug delivery is *true*?
   A. It allows lower doses than other administration routes.
   B. It causes more adverse effects than other administration routes.
   C. It's usually noninvasive.
   D. It may involve use of a pump with a battery life of 10 years.

Answer: A. Because intrathecal administration delivers the drug directly into the CSF, a lower dose of the drug is needed to bring pain relief.

Scoring

✩✩✩ If you answered all three questions correctly, marvelous! You obviously received a bolus injection of knowledge from this chapter.

✩✩ If you answered two questions correctly, good for you! Pain medications haven't given you any complications.

✩ If you answered only one question correctly, chill out. Take two aspirin and give the chapter another whirl.

Nonpharmacologic pain management

Just the facts

In this chapter, you'll learn:

♦ physical therapies used in pain management

♦ roles of alternative and complementary therapies in relieving pain

♦ cognitive and behavioral approaches to pain management

♦ optimal use of nonpharmacologic techniques.

A look at nonpharmacologic approaches

Managing pain doesn't necessarily involve capsules, syringes, I.V. lines, or medication pumps. Many nonpharmacologic therapies are available, too — and they're gaining popularity among the general public and health care professionals alike.

What accounts for this trend? For one thing, many people are concerned about the overuse of drugs for conventional pain management. For another, some people simply prefer to self-manage their health problems.

Something for everyone

Collectively speaking, nonpharmacologic approaches offer something for nearly everyone. They range from the relatively conventional (whirlpools, hot packs) to the electrifying (vibration, electrical nerve stimulation), the sensual (aromatherapy, massage), the serene (meditation, yoga), and the high-tech (biofeedback).

These therapies fall into three main categories:
• physical therapies
• alternative and complementary therapies

> They won't be needing me in this chapter. Looks like I can catch a few Zzzzzz...

- cognitive and behavioral therapies.

Many of them can be used either alone or combined with drug therapy. A combination approach may improve pain relief by enhancing drug effects and allow lower dosages.

Plenty of perks

Nonpharmacologic approaches have other benefits besides pain management. They help reduce stress, improve mood, promote sleep, and give the patient a sense of control over pain.

Opt for more options

By understanding how these techniques work and how best to use them, you can provide additional options for patients who experience pain.

Although the techniques discussed in this chapter can be effective for a wide range of patients, they're best administered, prescribed, or taught by licensed practitioners or experienced, credentialed lay people. A few require a doctor's order.

> Many of the therapies you'll read about in this chapter can be used alone — or combined with analgesic drugs.

Physical therapies

Physical therapies use physical agents and methods to aid rehabilitation and restore normal functioning after an illness or injury. These therapies are relatively cheap and easy to use. With appropriate teaching, patients and their families can use them on their own, which helps them participate in pain management.

Physical therapies include:
- hydrotherapy
- thermotherapy
- cryotherapy
- vibration
- transcutaneous electrical nerve stimulation (TENS)
- exercise
- immobilization.

Therapeutic goals

The goals of physical therapies are to:
- promote health
- prevent physical disability
- rehabilitate patients disabled by pain, disease, or injury.

Besides easing pain, physical therapies reduce inflammation, ease muscle spasms, and promote relaxation.

Hydrotherapy

Hydrotherapy uses water to treat pain and disease. Sometimes called the ultimate natural pain reliever, water comforts and soothes while providing support and buoyancy.

Depending on the patient's problem, the water can be hot or cold, and liquid, solid (ice), or steam. It can be applied externally or internally.

Most commonly prescribed for burns, hydrotherapy relaxes muscles, raises or lowers tissue temperature (depending on water temperature), and eases joint stiffness (as in rheumatoid arthritis or osteoarthritis). In pain management, hydrotherapy is most often used to treat acute pain — for instance, from muscle sprains or strains.

Now this is what I call hydrotherapy!

Jet set

Whirlpool baths — bathtubs with jets that force water to circulate — aid in rehabilitating injured muscles and joints. Depending on the desired effect, the water can be either hot or cold. The water jets act to massage soothing muscles. (See *Pools that ease pain,* page 90.)

Whirlpools and certain other hydrotherapy treatments can be done at home. But the more intensive forms are best done in a supervised clinical setting, where both the treatment and the patient response can be monitored.

Other types of hydrotherapy

In a *neutral bath,* the patient is immersed fully (up to the neck) in water that's near body temperature. This soothing bath calms the nervous system.

In a *sitz bath,* the pelvic area is immersed in a tub of water to relieve perianal pain, swelling, or discomfort; boost circulation; and reduce inflammation.

How hydrotherapy works

Hydrotherapy's pain-relieving properties are related to the physics and mechanics of water and its effect on the human body. When a body is immersed in water, the resulting weightlessness reduces stress on joints, muscles, and other connective tissues. This buoyancy may relieve some types of pain instantly.

Hot-water hydrotherapy eases pain through a sequence of events triggered by increased skin temperature. As skin temperature rises, blood vessels widen and skin circulation increases. As resistance to blood flow through veins and capillaries drops, blood pressure decreases. The heart rate then rises to maintain blood pressure. The result: a significant drop in pain and greater comfort.

Peak technique

Pools that ease pain

Hydrotherapy often takes the form of a whirlpool bath, which uses water jets to help ease pain.

Pool tips
- When administering whirlpool therapy, keep water temperature between 52° and 109° F (11° and 43° C), depending on the body surface area being treated and the patient's physical condition.
- Use a hydraulic chair to help the patient get into and out of the whirlpool tub.
  This illustration shows a patient whose leg injury is being treated in a whirlpool.

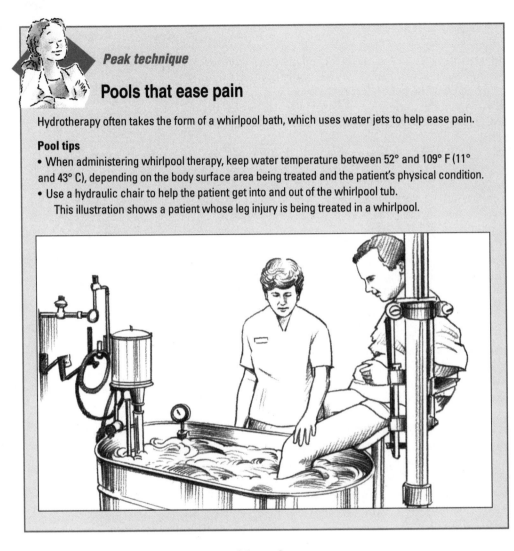

Special considerations
- Be aware that hydrotherapy may cause burns, falls, or light-headedness.
- Stop the treatment session if the patient feels light-headed, dizzy, or faint.
- Don't keep the patient in a heated whirlpool for more than 20 minutes.
- Instruct the patient to wipe his face frequently with a cool washcloth so he won't get overheated.
- Know that hydrotherapy isn't recommended for pregnant women, children,

A hot bath eases pain as it lowers blood pressure and speeds the heart rate.

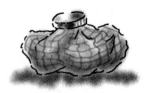

elderly patients, or patients with diabetes, hypertension, hypotension, or multiple sclerosis.

Thermotherapy

Thermotherapy refers to application of dry or moist heat to decrease pain, relieve stiff joints, ease muscle aches and spasms, improve circulation, and increase the pain threshold.

Dry heat can be applied with a hot water bottle, a K-pad, or an electric heating pad. Moist heat can be applied with a hot pack, a warm compress, or a special heating pad. (See *Heaping on the hot packs.*)

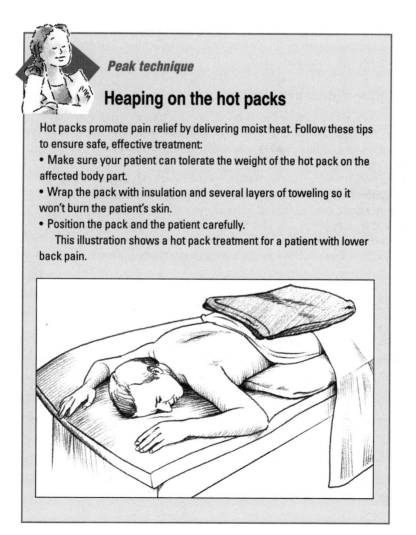

Peak technique

Heaping on the hot packs

Hot packs promote pain relief by delivering moist heat. Follow these tips to ensure safe, effective treatment:
• Make sure your patient can tolerate the weight of the hot pack on the affected body part.
• Wrap the pack with insulation and several layers of toweling so it won't burn the patient's skin.
• Position the pack and the patient carefully.

This illustration shows a hot pack treatment for a patient with lower back pain.

Both dry and moist heat involve conductive heating—heat transfer that occurs when the skin directly contacts a warm object.

What's the use?

Thermotherapy is used to treat pain caused by:
• headache
• muscle aches and spasms
• earache
• menstrual cramps
• temporomandibular joint (TMJ) disease
• fibromyalgia (a syndrome of chronic pain in the muscles and soft tissues surrounding joints).

Thermotherapy on trial

Trial and error may be needed to find the best thermotherapy method for your patient. If he's hospitalized, he'll need a doctor's order to receive thermotherapy.

How thermotherapy works

Thermotherapy enhances blood flow, increases tissue metabolism, and decreases vasomotor tone. It produces analgesia by suppressing free nerve endings. It also may reduce the perception of pain in the cerebral cortex.

Regional heating—heat therapy of selected body areas—can bring immediate temporary pain relief. This method may have a systemic effect, too, resulting from autonomic reflex responses to localized heat application. The reflex-mediated responses may raise body temperature, enhance blood flow, and cause other physiologic changes in areas distant from the heat application site.

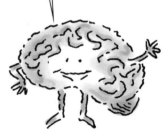

My cortex isn't perceiving much pain right now. I just love those hot packs!

Special considerations

• Before administering thermotherapy, determine the patient's awareness level and ability to communicate his response to the treatment.
• If the patient has a cognitive impairment, measure the temperature of the heating agent before applying it. It should be 104° to 113° F (40° to 45° C) when it contacts the skin.
• Be aware that some patients may prefer a slightly lower (or higher) temperature. Keep the heating agent at a temperature that's comfortable for the patient.

Wrap it up

• Wrap the heating agent so it doesn't directly contact the patient's skin.

• Regularly assess skin at the heat application site for irritation and redness.
• Frequently evaluate the patient's response to treatment and his pain level.

Halt the heat

• Stop the treatment if the patient's pain increases.
• Don't apply heat to an area that's infected, bleeding, or receiving radiation therapy or where oil or menthol has been applied.
• Know that thermotherapy is contraindicated in patients with vascular insufficiency, neuropathy, skin desensitization, or neoplasms.

Cryotherapy

Cryotherapy involves applying cold to a specific body area. Besides reducing fever, this technique can provide immediate pain relief and help reduce or prevent edema and swelling.

Packs, bags, massage

Cryotherapy methods include cold packs, ice bags, and ice massage. Ice massage has a temporary anesthetic effect and is used during brief painful procedures. (See *Reducing pain with ice massage*, page 94.)

Quite a contrast

In another cryotherapy technique, *contrast therapy*, cold and heat application are applied alternately during the same session. Contrast therapy may benefit patients with rheumatoid arthritis and certain other conditions.

Typically, the session begins by immersing the patient's feet and hands in warm water for 10 minutes. Next come four cycles of cold soaks (each lasting 1 to 4 minutes) alternating with warm soaks (each lasting 4 to 6 minutes).

Freezing out pain

Cryotherapy often is used for acute pain — especially when caused by a sports injury (such as a muscle sprain). It may also be indicated for pain resulting from:
• acute trauma
• joint disorders such as rheumatoid arthritis
• headache such as migraine
• muscle aches and spasms
• incisions
• surgery.

Think it's cold now? Wait 'til you get an ice massage!

Peak technique

Reducing pain with ice massage

Normally, ice shouldn't be applied directly to the skin because it may damage the skin surface and underlying tissues. But when carefully performed, this technique, called ice massage, may help patients tolerate brief, painful procedures, such as bone marrow aspiration, lumbar puncture, and chest tube or suture removal.

Get ready...
Prepare for ice massage by gathering the ice, a porous covering to hold it (if desired), and a cloth for wiping water off the patient's skin as the ice melts.

Get set...
Just before the procedure begins, rub the ice over the appropriate area to numb it. Assess the site frequently; stop rubbing immediately if you detect signs of tissue intolerance.

Go!
To start the procedure, rub the ice over a point near — but not at — the affected site. This distracts the patient and gives him another stimulus on which to concentrate.

If the painful procedure lasts longer than 10 minutes or if you think tissue damage may occur, move the ice to a different site and continue the massage. If you know in advance that the procedure will last longer than 10 minutes, massage the site intermittently — 2 minutes of massage alternating with a rest period until the skin regains normal color.

Alternatively, you can divide the area into several sites and apply ice to each one for several minutes at a time.

How cryotherapy works

Cryotherapy constricts blood vessels at the injury site, reducing blood flow to the site. This, in turn, thickens the blood, resulting in decreased bleeding and increased blood clotting.

Cold application also slows edema development, prevents further tissue damage, and minimizes bruising.

Cooler endings

Cryotherapy also decreases sensitivity to pain by cooling nerve endings. It eases muscle spasms by cooling muscle spindles — the part of the muscle tissue responsible for the stretch reflex. (See *Applying cold to a muscle sprain.*)

Contrast therapy is thought to stimulate endocrine function, reduce inflammation, decrease congestion, and improve organ function.

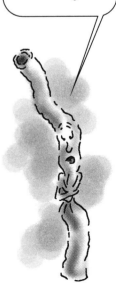

Brrr... Cryotherapy is so cold it constricts me at the injury site and reduces bleeding.

Peak technique

Applying cold to a muscle sprain

Cryotherapy helps reduce pain and edema when used during the first 24 to 72 hours after an injury. For best results, follow the guidelines below.

Method and materials
• Apply cold to the painful area four times daily for 20 to 30 minutes each time.
• Use enough crushed ice to cover the area.
• Place the ice in a plastic bag, and place the bag inside a pillowcase or a large piece of cloth, as shown below. Then apply the bag over the painful area for the specified treatment time.

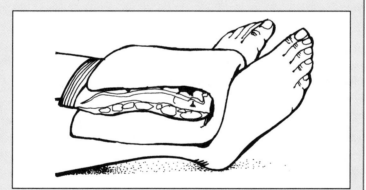

The old switcheroo
• After 24 to 72 hours, when swelling has subsided or when cold can no longer help, switch to thermotherapy.

Wise words
• Inform the patient that ice eases pain in a joint that has begun to stiffen—but caution him not to let the analgesic effect lull him into overusing the joint.

Special considerations
• As appropriate, encourage your patient to try cold application. Many patients aren't aware that cold relieves pain.
• Before applying cold, assess the pain or injury site and the patient's pain level. Evaluate him for impaired circulation (such as

from Raynaud's disease), inability to sense temperature (as from neuropathy), extreme skin sensitivity, and inability to report the response to treatment (for instance, a young child or a confused elderly patient).

Temper the temperature

• If the patient has a cognitive impairment, measure the temperature of the cooling agent. It should be no colder than 59° F (15° C).
• When administering moist cold, keep in mind that moisture intensifies cold.
• Wrap cold packs so they don't directly contact the patient's skin. Keep them at a comfortable temperature.

Numbness is a bummer

• Stop the treatment if the patient's skin becomes numb.
• Use caution when applying ice to the elbow, wrist, or outer part of the knee. These sites are more susceptible to cold-induced nerve injury.

Colder than ice

• Be aware that refreezable gel packs and chemical packs may be colder than ice. Also, they may leak.
• Regularly assess the patient for adverse effects, such as skin irritation, joint stiffness, numbness, frostbite, and nerve injury.
• Don't apply cold to areas that have poor circulation or have received radiation.

Stop cryotherapy if the patient's skin goes numb.

Vibration

Vibration therapy eases pain by inducing numbness in the treated area. This technique, which works like an electric massage, may be effective in such disorders as:
• muscle aches
• headache
• chronic nonmalignant pain
• cancer pain
• fractures
• neuropathic pain.

Hospitalized patients need a doctor's order to use a vibrating device. Outpatients may choose from various devices available without a prescription.

I'm pickin' up good vibrations

A vibrating device can be stationary or handheld. Stationary devices range from vibrating cushions to full beds and recliners. The patient lies or sits on the device and receives the treatment passively.

With a handheld vibrator, the patient or a caregiver moves the device over the painful area. Some handheld vibrators are battery-operated; others plug into a wall outlet.

Handheld vibrators come in many shapes and sizes. Some are relatively heavy and may be hard for frail or arthritic patients to use.

How vibration therapy works

Vibration therapy reduces pain by numbing the stimulated area. It also has a soothing effect.

Special considerations

• Before using vibration therapy, teach your patient about this method, including how it works and when it should and shouldn't be used.
• Tell the patient he may feel a warm sensation initially.
• Apply the vibrator to an area above or below the pain site.

Step on the gas

• For more effective pain relief, use the highest vibration speed the patient can tolerate.
• Apply the vibrating device for 1 to 15 minutes at a time, two to four times daily, or as ordered.
• Determine the length of treatment needed to achieve adequate pain relief. Continue to assess the patient's response to treatment.
• Stop the treatment if the patient experiences discomfort, pain, or excessive skin redness or irritation.
• Don't use vibration therapy if the patient has thrombophlebitis or bruises easily.
• Don't apply the vibrator over burns, cuts, or incision sites.

A lesson in assessin'

• If the patient will self-administer this therapy, provide appropriate teaching. Advise him to assess his pain level before the session, immediately afterward, and at a later time to assess how long pain relief lasts. This helps determine the optimal length of treatment. (Usually, the longer the session, the longer the duration of pain relief.)

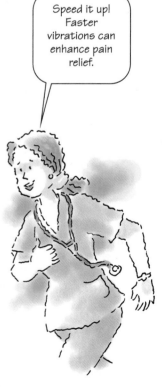

Speed it up! Faster vibrations can enhance pain relief.

TENS

In transcutaneous electrical nerve stimulation (TENS) therapy, a portable, battery-powered device transmits painless alternating electrical current to peripheral nerves or directly to a painful area. Used postoperatively and for patients with chronic pain, TENS reduces the need for analgesic drugs and helps the patient resume normal activities. TENS therapy must be prescribed by a doctor.

Belt it on

The patient usually wears the TENS unit on a belt. Units have several channels and lead placements. The settings allow adjustment of wave frequency, duration, and intensity. (See *Positioning TENS electrodes*.)

Typically, a course of TENS therapy lasts 3 to 5 days. Some conditions (such as phantom limb pain) may require continuous simulation. Others, such as a painful arthritic joint, call for shorter treatment periods—perhaps 3 to 4 hours.

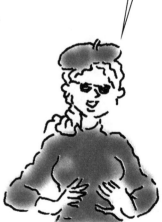

This TENS thing is cool! It really delivers the juice.

Top TENS list

TENS can provide both temporary relief of acute pain (such as postoperative pain) and ongoing relief of chronic pain (such as in sciatica).

Specific pain problems that have responded to TENS include:
- chronic nonmalignant pain
- cancer pain
- bone fracture pain
- low back pain
- sports injuries
- myofascial pain
- neurogenic pain (as in neuralgias and neuropathies)
- phantom limb pain
- arthritis
- menstrual pain.

How TENS works

Although TENS has existed for about 30 years, experts still aren't sure exactly how it relieves pain. Some believe that it works according to the gate control theory, which proposes that painful impulses pass through a "gate" in the brain. According to this theory, TENS alters the patient's perception of pain by closing the gate to painful stimuli.

Special considerations

• To ensure that your patient is a willing and active participant in TENS therapy, provide complete instructions on using and caring for the TENS unit.

Peak technique

Positioning TENS electrodes

In transcutaneous electrical nerve stimulation (TENS), electrodes placed around peripheral nerves or an incision site transmit mild electrical impulses, which presumably block pain messages.

Perfect placement

Electrode placement usually varies, even for patients with similar complaints. Electrodes can be placed in several ways:

• to cover or surround the painful area, as for muscle tenderness or spasm or painful joints
• to capture the painful area between electrodes, as for incisional pain.

The illustrations below show combinations of electrode placement (dark squares) and areas of nerve stimulation (shaded strips) for low back and leg pain.

Placement tips

• If the patient has peripheral nerve injury, place electrodes proximal to the injury (between the brain and the injury site) to avoid increasing his pain.
• If a site lacks sensation, place electrodes on adjacent dermatomes (areas of skin innervated by sensory fibers from a single spinal nerve).
• Don't place electrodes in a hypersensitive area. Doing so can increase pain.

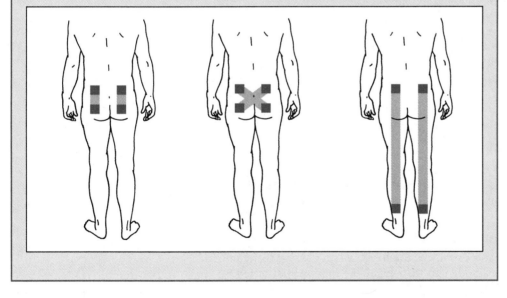

• Before TENS therapy begins, assess the patient's pain level and evaluate for skin irritation at the sites where electrodes will be placed.
• Be aware that the safety of TENS during pregnancy hasn't been established.

Three taboos

• Don't use TENS if the patient has undiagnosed pain, uses a pacemaker, or has a history of heart arrhythmias.
• Don't apply a TENS unit over the carotid sinus, an open wound, or anesthetized skin.
• Don't place the unit on the head or neck of a patient who has a vascular disorder or seizure disorder.

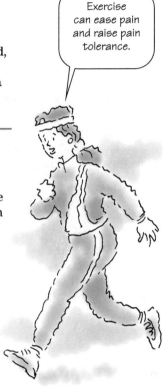

Exercise can ease pain and raise pain tolerance.

Exercise

Exercise can be a valuable therapy for patients with either acute or chronic pain. In most successful pain management programs, mobilization through exercise is an important component. Active exercise—muscle contraction entirely through the patient's own efforts—is the best way to achieve early mobilization and normal function.

A bevy of benefits

Appropriate exercise provides these benefits:
• builds muscle strength
• improves endurance
• enhances joint flexibility
• improves posture
• increases range of motion (ROM)
• improves coordination and balance
• raises pain tolerance
• promotes a sense of control over one's pain and physical functioning.

Exercise often is the treatment of choice in fibromyalgia and other chronic pain conditions.

Exercise good judgment

Be sure to choose an exercise program that's appropriate for your patient. The program may range from simple stretching exercises to low-impact aerobic exercises such as walking.

ROM exercises are even better than a lube job for keeping me limber.

Range-of-motion exercises

ROM exercises are a simple yet encompassing technique for moving a body part through all the motions permitted by the involved joint. Each joint has a normal ROM. To maintain a normal ROM, the joint must be moved regularly.

Limited ROM can lead to increased pain by impeding functional status (such as the ability to ambulate) and causing physical complications (such as skin breakdown).

Besides maintaining normal joint movement, ROM exercises decrease pain caused by stiffness and muscle spasms. Plus, they help the patient maintain or increase flexibility and preserve muscle strength (especially important if he can't exercise actively on his own).

Go through the motions

ROM exercises take muscles and joints through all natural movements — extension, flexion, rotation, pronation, supination, abduction, adduction, eversion, and inversion. (See *Joints in motion*, page 102.)

ROM exercises can be done passively, actively, or in an active-assistive manner.

Passive ROM

Passive ROM refers to movement of a joint through its entire range without active muscle contraction. Another person moves the patient's limb (or other body part) for him.

However, many patients can be trained to self-apply this technique. Also, passive ROM can be done with an electrically powered continuous passive motion device.

Active ROM

In active ROM, the patient contracts his muscles through his own efforts. Compared to passive ROM, active ROM exercises more effectively return the body to normal functioning.

Active-assistive ROM

In early healing stages, a patient may be unable to move the body part actively through the complete ROM and may benefit from an active-assistive routine. This type of ROM incorporates an additional passive force, applied by either a caregiver or the patient, along with the patient's own active efforts.

How exercise works

Exercise may reduce pain by boosting the release of endorphins (the body's natural painkillers), which promotes a sense of comfort and alters the perception of pain. Moving about also increases the patient's self-esteem and gives him a sense of control.

ROM exercises stretch the muscles, ligaments, and tendons surrounding a joint. They promote increased joint flexibility and movement and may reduce joint pain and stiffness from arthritis and other painful disorders.

OK — so I'm not doing ROM exercises. But you can't say I'm not passive!

Joints in motion

ROM exercises take the muscles and joints through all natural movements. Range of motion refers to movement of a joint through its entire range. The illustrations below show joint movements.

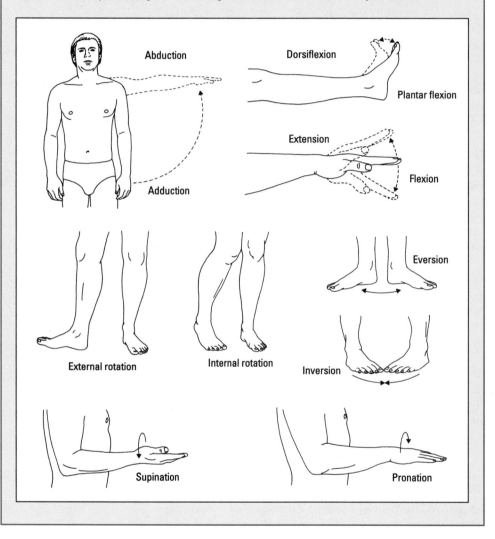

Special considerations

• Teach the patient about the benefits of exercise in pain management.

• Consult an occupational or physical therapist, as appropriate, to develop an exercise program tailored to the patient's abilities and interests.

- Let the patient pace his activities according to his pain level.
- Before an exercise session, assess the patient's pain level and mobility limitations.
- If your patient has chronic pain, explain that increased pain during exercise doesn't necessarily mean harm is being done. Point out that pain may result simply from using muscles that have become weakened from disuse.

Goal for the day

- Encourage a patient with chronic pain to set a daily exercise or activity goal and to record progress toward that goal. Advise him to rest only after completing the specified activity, instead of when pain occurs.
- Reassess the patient if exercise worsens his pain.
- During an episode of acute pain, limit the patient's exercise to self-administered ROM.
- Instruct a patient at risk for fractures to avoid weight-bearing exercises.

For ROM exercises

- Determine the joints that need ROM exercises, and consult the doctor or physical therapist about limitations or precautions for specific exercises.
- Be aware that some patients benefit from heat or cold application before ROM exercises.

Three ROMS daily

- Be aware that patients should do ROM exercises three times daily.
- Hold the arm or leg directly above and below the joint to be exercised. Keep a firm — but not tight — grip.
- Perform passive ROM exercises slowly, gently, and to the end of the normal ROM or to the point of pain — but no further.
- If a muscle spasm occurs, move the joint to the point of tightness and hold.
- Stop passive ROM exercises if the patient's pain increases.

> Before an exercise session, evaluate your patient's pain level and mobility limitations.

Immobilization

Immobilization is used to restrict movement of one or more body parts. It's most often ordered during the acute stage of an injury. Methods include traction, casting, and bracing (orthotics).

Immobilization may be indicated for:
- relief of acute pain
- fracture stabilization
- support of painful, weakened joints during activity.

Traction

Traction applies a distracting force to the spine or limbs. It usually involves weights and a pulley system.

Traction may be indicated to stabilize limb fractures or treat vertebral fractures and dislocations with associated spinal cord injury.

A gentler pull

Management of pain—especially cervical or lumbar spine pain—may call for reduced-intensity traction. This type of traction, which applies a gentle pulling force, causes soft-tissue stretching and relieves muscle spasms.

> Traction sure looks funny, but it applies a distracting force that stabilizes injuries.

Can you stand the suspense?

Spinal traction may be applied through weights and a pulley system—or by suspending the body itself to produce its own traction effect. Suspension or inversion of a patient in a traction frame uses the body's weight as a distraction force on the spine.

Traction also can be applied by an electrically driven distracting force.

Casting

Casting refers to fracture immobilization using casting material. Various materials are available for casting, some more lightweight and comfortable than others.

Bracing

Braces and orthotic devices are used to selectively immobilize and align body parts for treatment of fractures and soft-tissue and joint injuries. Bracing an injured or weakened joint, for instance, protects the joint and allows the patient to be up and about.

> This suit of armor isn't exactly a brace. But believe me, it's quite immobilizing.

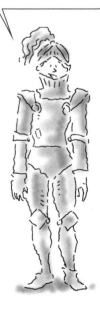

A brace against pain

By immobilizing the affected body part, bracing devices reduce pain and improve function. They can be used on a temporary or long-term basis.

Braces may be indicated for pain associated with various cervical and lumbar spine conditions. Spinal braces relieve back and neck pain and decrease the risk of further injury.

Braces are available for all body areas and come in many sizes and forms. A patient who needs a brace must be properly fitted and instructed in how to use and care for it. (See *Common cervical, thoracic, and lumbosacral braces.*)

How immobilization works

The various immobilization methods help reduce pain in different ways.

• Traction maintains optimal body alignment for healing. The distraction force separates normally contingent bony surfaces or enlarges the space within a joint without rupturing or displacing the associated ligaments.

• Bracing or casting a painful or injured body part, such as a knee, provides support during activities and helps prevent further pain and injury.

Common cervical, thoracic, and lumbosacral braces

Braces (also called orthoses) reduce pain by immobilizing a body part. These illustrations show three common types of braces, including cervical, thoracic, and lumbosacral.

Hard (Philadelphia) collar
The illustration below shows a patient wearing a typical hard cervical orthosis, also known as a Philadelphia collar. Made of rigid plastic, this collar holds the patient's neck firmly, keeping it straight, while the chin remains slightly elevated and tucked in.

Cervical brace (SOMI design)
The illustration below shows a patient wearing a typical cervical-thoracic brace. This design is the sternal occipital mandibular immobilizer (SOMI).

Thoracic lumbosacral brace
The illustrations below show rear and side views of a patient wearing a thoracic lumbosacral brace. This design controls flexion, extension, rotation, and lateral motion of the thoracic, lumbar, and sacral spine.

Hard (Philadelphia) collar

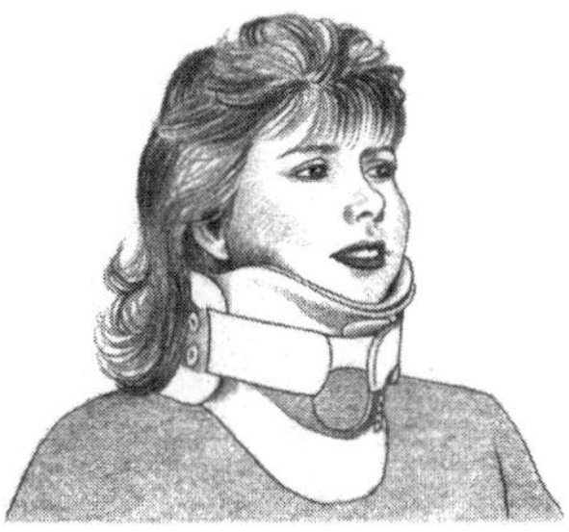

Cervical brace (SOMI design)

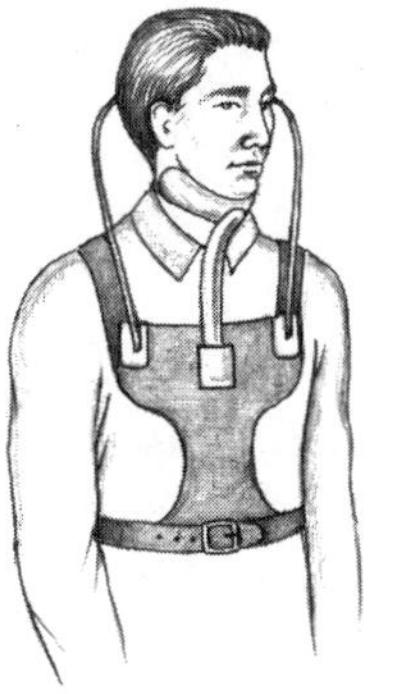

Thoracic lumbosacral brace

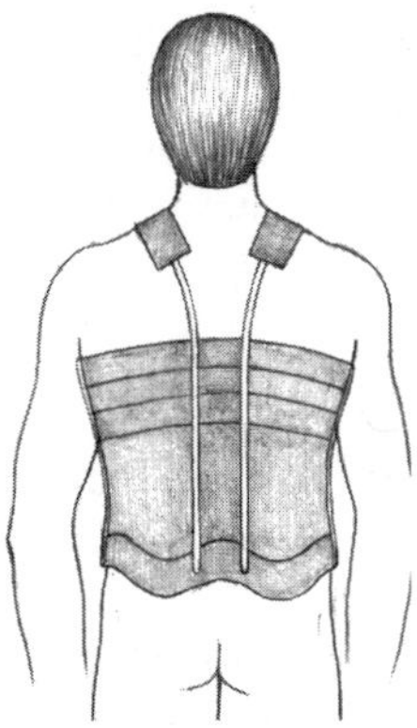

Rear view 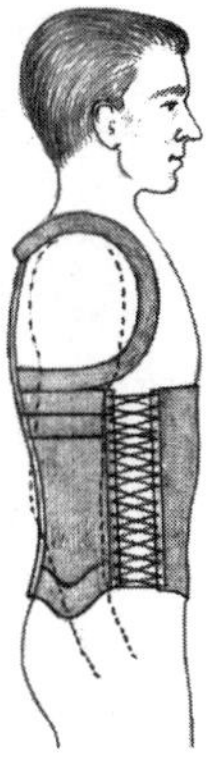   Side view

Special considerations

- Whether your patient is using traction, a cast, or a brace, be sure to assess the affected area for signs and symptoms of circulatory impairment. Regularly assess his pain level, and report worsening of pain, decreased circulation, skin irritation, or increased swelling.

Take it to the max — not!

- Know that joints should be braced in their position of optimal — not maximal — function.
- Caution the patient not to adjust a brace that has been prescribed for him.

No sharing allowed

- Advise the patient not to lend his brace to another person for self-treatment of painful injuries.
- Never apply traction to an artificial joint.
- Keep in mind that prolonged immobilization may lead to joint contractures and muscle tissue damage.
- Be aware that traction may be unsafe for patients with certain underlying skeletal abnormalities, such as metastatic cancer or multiple myeloma.

> Traction shouldn't be applied to an artificial joint. It also may be dangerous for patients with skeletal abnormalities.

CAUTION!

Alternative and complementary therapies

Alternative and complementary therapies greatly expand the range of therapeutic choices for patients suffering pain. Today, patients are increasingly seeking these therapies — not just to treat pain but also to address many other common health conditions.

Various theories have been offered to explain the increased interest in alternative and complementary therapies. (See *Understanding the alternative trend.*)

Wholly holistic

Regardless of the problem for which they're used, alternative and complementary therapies address the whole person — body, mind, and spirit — rather than just signs and symptoms.

Defining the terms

Although alternative and complementary therapies are usually discussed together, they aren't exactly the same.

• *Alternative* therapies are those used *instead of* conventional or mainstream therapies—for example, the use of acupuncture rather than analgesics to relieve pain.
• *Complementary* therapies are those used *in conjunction with* conventional therapies—such as meditation used as an adjunct to analgesic drugs.

East meets West

Some of the alternative and complementary therapies practiced today have been used since ancient times and come from the traditional healing practices of many cultures—particularly in the Eastern part of the world.

I'll be using alternative and complementary therapies? Groovy!

Now I get it!

Understanding the alternative trend

Why are more and more people turning to alternative and complementary therapies to treat health problems? For one reason, most of these therapies are noninvasive and cause few adverse effects.

People with certain chronic conditions may be drawn to these therapies because conventional medicine has few, if any, effective treatments for them. Also, many people are encouraged by research that documents the effectiveness of specific therapies, such as acupuncture, meditation, and yoga.

Hoopla about holism
Another reason for increased interest may be the holistic approach of alternative medicine. Whereas conventional medicine tends to treat only signs and symptoms, alternative and complementary therapies focus on the whole person.

Time—and more time
Many people also value the extra time alternative practitioners spend with the patient and the attention they pay to the patient's temperament, behavioral patterns, and perceived needs. In an increasingly stressful world, people are searching for someone who will take the time to listen to them and treat them as people, not just bodies displaying signs and symptoms.

Spiritual hunger
Some people view modern society as spiritually malnourished and hungry for meaning. Alternative practitioners seem to be more responsive to this need.

Cultural connections
Finally, in a culturally diverse country such as the United States, a wide variety of traditional healing practices and beliefs exist. Some are based on the same principles that underlie alternative and complementary therapies.

Documented research reveals that yoga is effective in treating various health problems.

Many mainstream Western doctors have become more open-minded about these therapies. In fact, some medical doctors even administer them. But others still object to them on the grounds that they aren't based solely on empirical science.

Pain relief prospects

Nonetheless, alternative and complementary therapies can frequently relieve some types of pain that don't respond to Western techniques. They may prove especially valuable when a precise cause evades Western medicine, as often occurs with chronic low back pain.

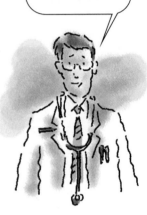

Some mainstream doctors now administer alternative and complementary therapies themselves.

Aromatherapy

Used since ancient times to heal the body, mind, and spirit, aromatherapy refers to the inhalation or application of essential oils distilled from various plants. Health care providers say the technique reduces stress, prevents disease, and even treats certain illnesses.

Aromatherapy has been used for:
- headaches
- muscle disorders
- arthritis
- shingles
- premenstrual syndrome.

From the ground up

Aromatherapy oils come from many parts of the plant, including the leaf, stem, flower, seed, bark, and root. This transference of the life force is a crucial component of aromatherapy.

Specific oils are thought to have either relaxing or stimulating effects. Oils that supposedly reduce pain include basil, eucalyptus, chamomile, geranium, lavender, rosemary, and tea tree.

How do you prefer your oil?

Aromatherapy may be self-administered or administered by a trained health care provider. The oil can be applied on the skin through gentle massage, added to bath water, or inhaled through an aerosol device.

A carrier oil, such as grapeseed or almond oil, may be used with the essential oil for better application. Using the essential oil with massage may stimulate the circulation, which in turn may relieve pain.

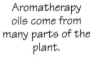

Aromatherapy oils come from many parts of the plant.

How aromatherapy works

When absorbed by body tissues, essential oils are thought to interact with hormones and enzymes to produce changes in blood pressure, pulse rate, and other physiologic functions.

Aromatherapists also believe smells can affect physiologic function through their effects on the limbic system—the part of the brain associated with emotion and memory.

I smell a memory

Odors stimulate receptors in the nose. These receptors convert the odors to nerve impulses that travel to the limbic system, where they may trigger memories associated with the odors.

According to aromatherapy researchers, the emotions evoked—joy, sadness, anger, anxiety—can affect heart rate, blood pressure, breathing, brain wave activity, and release of hormones that regulate insulin production, body temperature, stress, metabolism, and hunger.

Odors also may stimulate release of neurotransmitters and endorphins in the brain, affecting emotional well-being and the perception of pain.

Special considerations

• Be aware that essential oils must be diluted carefully according to the distributor's instructions.
• Caution your patient never to massage essential oils into open or excoriated skin or to ingest the oils.
• Instruct the patient to wash essential oil off the skin before venturing into the sun; some oils are highly photosensitive.

Oils aren't for eyes

• Warn the patient to keep essential oils away from the eyes and mucous membranes. If contact occurs, he should flush the eyes or mucous membranes copiously with water. If this doesn't relieve pain, he should get prompt medical attention.
• Many essential oils are toxic to children under age 5. Rose and eucalyptus oils have an especially high potential for toxicity.
• Know that aromatherapy is contraindicated in pregnancy because many essential oils pose a toxic risk to the mother and fetus. A few spontaneous abortions have occurred.

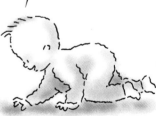

Mom says I should stay away from essential oils. They can be toxic to cute little kids like me.

Music therapy

A form of sound therapy, music therapy takes advantage of the universal appeal of rhythmic sound to communicate, relax, encourage healing, and create a feeling of well-being.

Music therapy can take the form of:
- listening to music
- creating music
- singing
- moving to music
- music and imagery exercises.

Music therapy is offered in various settings — general and psychiatric hospitals, rehabilitation facilities, mental health centers, senior centers and nursing homes, hospices, halfway houses, and substance abuse clinics. More than 5,000 registered music therapists practice in the United States today.

Musical uses

Music therapy can be effective in reducing chronic pain and as an adjunctive therapy for patients with burns, cancer, cerebral palsy, stroke and other brain injuries, Parkinson's disease, and substance abuse problems.

Studies show that music decreases pain associated with dental and medical procedures.

Wanted: health care musicians

As a treatment for pain, music can be as formal or as informal as the patient's situation requires. Health care providers can provide the music themselves, which benefits both the giver and the receiver of care.

Titrate the tempo

A comfortable environment and enjoyable music are the two necessary ingredients for music therapy. The music should be appropriate for the patient and the session goal. As you might expect, fast music stimulates and slow music calms.

Music selection can also be based on the patient's ethnic, cultural, or religious background. Whatever the choice, the music should be meaningful to the patient.

How music therapy works

Various theories attempt to explain how music affects the body. One proposes that the resonance emitted by sound waves restores the body's natural rhythm and encourages healing.

Another theory proposes that the brain reacts to sound waves by sending out instructions to control the heart rate, respiratory rate, and other body functions. These effects may lower blood pressure and decrease muscle tension.

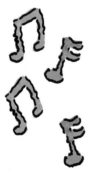

I'll be signing autographs after I finish my gig on the unit today.

Also, sound impulses may trigger release of endorphins, which help relieve pain and lift the mood. This combination of factors may create a state of total relaxation, possibly allowing the body to heal itself.

Don't worry, be happy

In some cases, music therapy may work simply by conjuring up happy memories in the listener. The memories produce positive emotions, which may reduce stress and enhance feelings of well-being.

Reharmonize the chakras

In the Ayurvedic system of medicine, sound waves are thought to balance energy centers within the body known as *chakras*. According to this philosophy, the body has seven chakras, which vibrate at different frequencies (similar to the notes on a scale).

When stress or disease disrupts the chakras, the frequencies are thrown off. Music can reharmonize the chakras, allowing the body to heal itself.

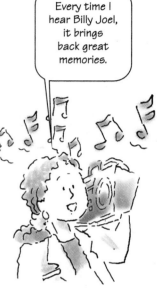

Every time I hear Billy Joel, it brings back great memories.

Special considerations

• After a music therapy session, encourage the patient to discuss the feelings he had while listening to the music.
• If a musical selection brings back an unpleasant memory or experience, comfort the patient and help him change his focus to more pleasant thoughts.

Therapeutic Touch

Developed in the 1970s, Therapeutic Touch is a widely used complementary therapy, developed by and for health care providers in an attempt to bring a more humane and holistic approach to their practice. It's best known for its use in relieving pain and anxiety.

It's universal

Central to Therapeutic Touch is the concept of a universal life force, which is thought to permeate space and sustain all living organisms. Practitioners believe that in healthy people, this vital energy flows freely in and through the body in a balanced way that nourishes all body organs — and that when a person gets sick, it's because the energy field is out of equilibrium.

No touching required

Despite its name, Therapeutic Touch doesn't require actual physical contact during a treatment. In most cases, the health care provider's hands remain several inches above the patient's body.

A typical session lasts 10 to 30 minutes. The patient lies fully clothed on a massage table or hospital bed. The session starts with the health care provider "centering" himself and ends after he completes "interventions" aimed at balancing the energy field and removing obstructions. (See *Basic steps of Therapeutic Touch*.)

> Even though it's called Therapeutic Touch, I won't be touching you during the session.

How Therapeutic Touch works

Therapeutic touch is founded on the premise that the body, mind, emotions, and intuition form a complex, dynamic human energy field. During periods of health, the energy field is governed by pattern and order. During periods of stress and dis-

---

Now I get it!

Basic steps of Therapeutic Touch

A Therapeutic Touch practitioner applies her hands to the energy field around a patient's body. This method involves several steps.

Centering
In the first step, called centering, the practitioner achieves a calm, meditative state that helps her sense the patient's signs and symptoms and perceive subtle changes in the patient's energy field.

Assessment
Next, the practitioner begins her assessment. She slowly moves her hands over the patient's body, 2" to 6" (5 to 15 cm) away from the skin surface, to detect alterations in the energy field, such as cold, heat, vibration, or blockages.

Unruffling
Depending on assessment findings, the practitioner then performs interventions aimed at balancing the energy field and removing any obstructions. Typically, these interventions involve "unruffling," which attempts to restore order to the patient's energy field.

To perform unruffling, the practitioner uses hand movements from the midline while continuing to move her hands in a rhythmic, symmetrical, head-to-toe fashion. Where an energy deficit occurs, energy is thought to transfer from the practitioner's hands to the patient.

Other interventions include eliminating "congestion" or acting as a conduit to direct the "life energy" from the environment into the patient.

Closure
The last step, closure, ends the treatment. Using intuitive judgment, the practitioner determines when to end the session. Cues come largely from continuous reassessment of the patient's energy field during the treatment to determine balance and obtain feedback.

ease, it's unbalanced and disordered. (See *The human energy field.*)

Manipulative power

By using their hands to manipulate the energy field above the patient's skin, practitioners say they can restore equilibrium, which reactivates the mind-body-spirit connection and empowers the patient to fully participate in his own healing.

The human energy field

Practitioners of Therapeutic Touch and other energy-based therapies believe the human body emits several energy fields, as shown in the illustration below.

However, the layers aren't as separate as the illustration suggests. Rather, each successive layer encompasses some of the preceding one.

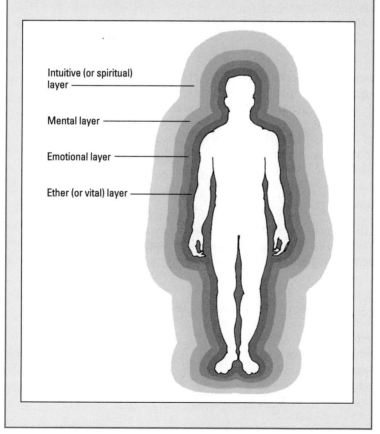

Intuitive (or spiritual) layer

Mental layer

Emotional layer

Ether (or vital) layer

I bet a piece of chocolate candy would enhance my energy field.

Although the existence of a human energy field remains unproven, practitioners claim they can feel something best described as energy when performing the technique.

Balancing away pain

Pain is thought to create a disorder in the person's energy field. Therapeutic Touch is said to reduce pain by restoring balance to the energy field. Many patients who receive Therapeutic Touch report that the treatment helps them feel deeply relaxed and reduces their pain.

> Therapeutic Touch is said to ease pain by restoring balance to the patient's energy field.

Special considerations

• Therapeutic Touch rarely causes complications. However, practitioners must take care to moderate the length and strength of the treatment for elderly patients and young children because of their more fragile physiology.
• Be aware that restlessness during or after a session is a common sign of overtreatment.

Yoga

One of the oldest known health practices, yoga integrates physical, mental, and spiritual energies to promote health and wellness. Its basic components are proper breathing, movement, meditation, and posture.

Yoga is based on the Hindu principle of mind-body unity, which holds that pain or chronic restlessness results in poor health and decreased mental clarity.

So versatile

Numerous studies show that yoga helps reduce pain, relieve stress and anxiety, lower blood pressure, slow the respiratory rate, improve respiratory function, enhance motor skills, and produce brain waves indicating deep relaxation.

Uses for yoga

Yoga is used to relieve pain and anxiety in such disorders as:
• heart disease
• diabetes
• migraine headaches
• hypertension
• cancer
• arthritis
• back and neck pain.

The Hatha path

Various yoga styles exist. Hatha yoga, the type most often taught in the West, encompasses a unique combination of physical postures and exercise (known as asanas), breathing techniques (pranayamas), relaxation, diet, and proper thinking.

Hatha yoga focuses on removing toxins from the body, cleansing the mind, energizing and realigning the body, releasing muscle tension, and increasing strength and flexibility.

How yoga works

While practicing specific postures, the person closely observes his breathing, exhaling at certain times and inhaling at others. Yoga breathing techniques are believed to help maintain the postures as well as to promote relaxation and enhance the flow of vital energy, known as prana. (See *Understanding yoga.*)

Now I get it!

Understanding yoga

Yoga practitioners believe that *prana,* or the life force, circulates throughout the body in a system of 72,000 subtle nerves. Improper diet, stress, or toxins can interrupt the flow of *prana,* affecting a person's physical or mental health. Chronic blockages can lead to illness.

By promoting an even flow of *prana* and removing blockages, yoga breathing exercises are thought to maintain and restore health.

A boost to body systems

Other yoga practices are believed to stimulate the endocrine and nervous systems.
• Assuming certain body positions and contracting specific muscles during particular postures supposedly boosts circulation to the glands.
• Breathing exercises manipulate the respiratory system and presumably benefit the nervous system.

Relaxation response

Many scientific studies show that practicing yoga regularly can produce the same physiologic changes as meditation. Called the *relaxation response,* these changes include:
• decreased heart and respiratory rates
• improved heart and respiratory function
• lower blood pressure
• reduced oxygen consumption
• brain wave changes found only during deep meditation.

I'm practicing my asanas and pranayamas.

Special considerations

• Advise your patient to consult the doctor before starting a yoga program. Some yoga postures can be stressful to people with certain pain disorders.
• Be aware that yoga may cause muscle injury if done improperly or if the patient tries to force his body into a certain position. Advise him to try the various postures cautiously.

It isn't a cinch

• Inform the patient that yoga requires regular practice to be effective and that few people can perform all the movements in the beginning.
• Tell the patient that the effects of yoga are cumulative.
• Remind the patient that yoga is a complementary therapy — not a cure for pain or disease. Instruct him to continue conventional treatments.

Massage

Massage involves rubbing and kneading of soft tissues for therapeutic purposes. As a therapy for pain relief and relaxation, massage has existed throughout history in almost all cultures. Different systems of therapeutic massage have been developed and are increasingly available today.

Therapeutic massage is used mainly for stress reduction and relaxation. It also serves as a complementary therapy for a broad range of conditions. Pain-related disorders that may benefit from massage include:
• mild, moderate, or severe pain
• muscle spasms
• fibromyalgia
• headache
• arthritic joints
• back and shoulder pain.

Oh, this feels soooooo good!

Distraction tactic

Relaxation and stimulation from massage distract the patient from pain. In some cases, massage is used to stretch fibrous scar tissue that's causing pain.

Inga will see you now

Most massage therapists in the United States practice some variation of Swedish massage, applying several basic strokes to the body's soft tissue. Beyond this, many individual therapists have their own style and technique.

How massage therapy works

The main physiologic effect of massage is improved blood circulation. Kneading and stretching of muscles increases blood return to the heart. It also aids removal of lactic acid and other toxins from the muscle tissues for excretion from the body.

Improved circulation enhances tissue perfusion and oxygenation. When more blood circulates through the brain, thinking becomes clearer and the person feels more alive. Improved perfusion and oxygenation of other organ systems leads to better digestion and elimination and speeds wound healing.

> We were doing fine here in the muscle tissues, but this massage will surely get rid of us toxins. We're outta here!

Uncorking the endorphins

Massage may relieve pain by stimulating specific parts of the body or by shutting the "gate" to transmission of pain messages to the brain. Some researchers suspect massage also triggers endorphin release.

Special considerations

• To avoid causing pain or discomfort, closely observe the patient's body language and note his verbal responses.
• Don't perform massage within 6″ (15 cm) of a bruise, cyst, skin break, or broken bone.
• Know that massage is contraindicated in patients with diabetes, varicose veins, phlebitis or other vascular problems, pitting edema, or swollen limbs.
• Avoid massaging the abdomen of a patient with hypertension or gastric or duodenal ulcers.

May I see your license?

• Advise patients seeking a massage therapist to get recommendations from others who have been satisfied with their treatment. Tell them to make sure the therapist is properly trained and licensed.

Chiropractic treatment

Chiropractic is a therapeutic system based on the belief that most medical problems result from vertebral misalignments and can be corrected by spinal manipulation (called adjustments).

Health care providers believe chiropractic has two main benefits:

- It relieves musculoskeletal pain and disability.
- It reestablishes internal organ function.

Typically, chiropractors assess the source of pain and determine whether chiropractic treatment is an appropriate therapeutic choice. If the patient's problem requires medical care, the chiropractor makes referrals.

Age is no object

Chiropractic treatment may be useful in managing pain in patients of all ages—especially those with:

- neck and shoulder pain
- headaches
- sports injuries
- work-related injuries such as carpal tunnel syndrome.

Chiropractical magic?

Chiropractic medicine approaches health from a preventive point of view. One of its main tenets is that the human body seeks to maintain a state of homeostasis and has an innate ability to heal itself. This "innate intelligence" regulates all body functions through the nervous system.

Surrender your subluxation

Because the nerves originate in the spine, displaced vertebrae are thought to disrupt nerve transmission—a condition called a *subluxation*. The chiropractor aims to eliminate subluxations so the body can carry out its job of maintaining equilibrium unimpeded.

Detect and correct

Conventional medical doctors repudiated chiropractic for many years because it viewed nearly every disease as caused (ultimately) by subluxations and treatable through spinal manipulation. Although few chiropractors today adhere to this theory, the core of the chiropractic profession remains detecting and correcting vertebral misalignment.

> I'm no chiropractor, but I'd say your spinal vertebrae look a tad misaligned.

> It says here that the chiropractor will try to fix my subluxations.

Now I get it!

Understanding spinal manipulation

Early theories of how chiropractic spinal adjustment worked relied on the anatomic understanding of the time. Misaligned vertebrae were thought to put pressure on spinal nerves, blocking the flow of nerve impulses. Spinal manipulation (adjustment) restored the free flow of neural impulses, relieving symptoms.

Because patients commonly reported significant relief of their complaints and increased function after an adjustment, this explanation was deemed satisfactory for many years. But better understanding of anatomy and physiology over the years has made this explanation less acceptable.

No X-ray evidence

Another problem with the original explanation is that positive changes in health status aren't always reflected in vertebral alignment. That is, an adjustment may cause immediate and dramatic pain relief—but X-rays may show no detectable change in spinal alignment.

Also, no clearly demonstrated physiologic link exists between spinal manipulation and the organ responses they sup-

posedly cause. Because of these problems with the original explanation, alternative theories of how chiropractic achieves results have been proposed.

Fixating on a new theory

Currently, the most widely accepted theory is that of intervertebral motion and segmental dysfunction. This theory centers on loss of correct spinal joint mobility, not vertebral misalignment. Neighboring pairs of vertebrae and their surrounding tissues consist of a motion segment. Loss of mobility within a segment is called a *fixation*. These fixations are most amenable to spinal manipulative therapy.

Recent neurophysiologic advances may explain how spinal manipulation can lead to visceral organ responses. Studies show that spinal adjustment initiates nerve signals that travel to internal organs through autonomic nervous system pathways. These signals provide a physiologic link between spinal manipulation and visceral organs.

How chiropractic works

Today, the most widely accepted theory of how chiropractic works centers on intervertebral motion and segmental dysfunction. (See *Understanding spinal manipulation*.)

Special considerations

• If your patient is seeking chiropractic care, explain the nature of chiropractic medicine and advise him on how to find a licensed practitioner.
• Tell your patient that chiropractic hasn't been proven effective in treating serious illnesses such as cancer.
• Be aware that chiropractic physicians are formally educated through accredited schools of chiropractic medicine and are licensed by the state in which they practice. All 50

I don't detect a change in your spinal alignment.

states have licensure, granted after successful completion of a state board exam. The scope of chiropractic practice, however, differs from state to state.

• Know that chiropractic manipulation is contraindicated in patients with a condition that might worsen with spinal adjustment, such as osteoporosis.

Acupuncture

Acupuncture involves inserting thin metal needles just under the skin at specific points. Typically, the needles stay in place for 20 to 30 minutes. To enhance their intended benefits, they may be set in motion or connected to low-voltage electric generators.

Needling away pain

The World Health Organization lists 100 conditions that may benefit from acupuncture. Pain-related conditions on the list include:
• arthritis
• back pain
• carpal tunnel syndrome
• dental pain
• fibromyalgia
• headache
• menstrual cramps
• postoperative pain
• peripheral neuropathy
• trigeminal neuralgia.

May the qi be with you

A key component of traditional Chinese medicine, acupuncture dates back nearly 5,000 years. It's based on the existence of a vital life force, called *qi*, which circulates in the body through channels known as meridians.

Used to diagnose and treat, the meridians act as a road map that helps the practitioner find specific acupuncture points. The 12 major meridians are thought to be connected to specific organ systems.

Meridians act as a road map, helping the practitioner find specific acupuncture points.

Early warning system

According to the Chinese theory, an organ experiencing an energy imbalance or disease may manifest signs or symptoms at its corresponding meridian. Such symptoms may include pain or aching, sensitivity to touch, or changes in skin temperature, texture, or color.

Now I get it!

Insight into acupuncture

Various theories provide a possible explanation for how acupuncture works.

Endorphin stimulation

According to the endorphin stimulation theory, acupuncture needles stimulate peripheral nerves, triggering release of endorphins and enkephalins (the body's natural painkilling chemicals). Researchers have found that during acupuncture analgesia, endorphin levels rise in the blood and cerebrospinal fluid and fall in specific brain regions.

Neurotransmitter effect

The neurotransmitter theory proposes that acupuncture affects levels of serotonin and norepinephrine, neurotransmitters that help relay nerve impulses across brain synapses.

Gate control

The popular gate control theory proposes that pain perception is controlled by a "gate"—a part of the nervous system that regulates pain impulses. When bombarded by too many impulses, as during acupuncture, the gate becomes overwhelmed and closes.

Inserting acupuncture needles is thought to "close the gate" on the nerve fibers that carry pain impulses to the brain.

Electrical conductance

The electrical conductance theory hinges on findings that acupuncture points (acupoints) have a higher level of electrical conductance than other sites. Some scientists theorize that acupoints amplify minute electrical signals as they travel through the body and that acupuncture needles interrupt that flow. This effect then blocks transmission of pain impulses.

Enhanced immunity

Some researchers suspect acupuncture may raise the white blood cell count and increase prostaglandin, gamma globulin, and overall antibody levels.

Circulation control

The circulation control theory proposes that acupuncture works by narrowing or widening blood vessels, possibly through control of vasodilators.

These symptoms help the practitioner determine which organ systems are affected and, thus, which "acupoints" to use in treatment. Needle stimulation of acupoints is thought to balance, release, or enhance the flow of qi, relieving pain or restoring health.

Needles aren't always needed

Some acupuncturists don't use needles at all. Instead, they use electrostimulation, ultrasonic waves, or laser beams.

In acupressure, a related therapy, the practitioner applies deep finger pressure to the acupoints.

Suction-cup method

Some acupuncturists use a supplementary technique called cupping. They place glass or bamboo cups on the patient's skin to create a vacuum suction, which is thought to draw out pathogenic substances.

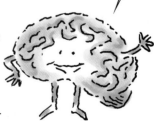

Acupuncture "closes the gate" on nerve fibers that carry pain impulses to me.

How acupuncture works

Although acupuncture is one of the most thoroughly researched alternative therapies, Western scientists aren't sure how it works. Various theories have been proposed. (See *Insight into acupuncture*, page 121.)

Special considerations

• If your patient's considering acupuncture, advise him to get a practitioner referral from the National Commission for the Certification of Acupuncturists.

• Be aware that acupuncture has a lower incidence of adverse effects than many accepted medical procedures used for the same conditions. Nonetheless, some types of acupuncture carry a slight risk of life-threatening reactions, such as pneumothorax.

• Know that some third-party payers cover acupuncture treatments by a qualified practitioner. However, inability to pay continues to be a problem for many patients seeking acupuncture and other alternative treatments.

Cognitive and behavioral approaches

Cognitive approaches to pain management focus on influencing the patient's interpretation of the pain experience. *Behavioral* approaches help the patient develop skills for managing pain and changing his reaction to it.

Cognitive and behavioral approaches to managing pain include meditation, biofeedback, and hypnosis. These techniques improve the patient's sense of control over pain and allow him to participate actively in pain management.

Meditation

Meditation—focusing one's attention on a single sound or image or the rhythm of one's own breathing—has been found to have positive effects on health. By directing attention away from pain and other negative stimuli, it reduces stress, which often accompanies or worsens pain.

Desperately seeking stresslessness

Stress reduction has a wide range of physiologic and mental health benefits, ranging from decreased oxygen consumption and slower heart and respiratory rates to improved mood, spiritual calm, and heightened awareness.

The health benefits of meditation have been long recognized in the East. But in the West, meditation has become widely accepted only in the past 25 years. Besides helping patients cope better with pain and anxiety, meditation may enhance immune function in patients with cancer, AIDS, and autoimmune disorders.

Strictly a side dish

Meditation may be especially helpful in chronic pain. But it should be considered strictly an adjunct to pain management—not a substitute for medical treatment—because it doesn't always decrease pain intensity.

Meditation modes

Most meditation techniques fall into one of two categories: concentrative or mindful.
• In *concentrative* meditation, the person focuses on an image, a sound, or his own breathing. The goal is to achieve a state of calm and heightened awareness.
• In *mindful* meditation, the person remains aware of all sensations, feelings, images, thoughts, sounds, and smells that pass through his mind—but doesn't actually think about them. The goal is a calmer, clearer, nonreactive mental state.

A simple type of meditation combines breathing with sounds or images. (See *The mindful breath.*)

> I feel positively celestial when I meditate.

Peak technique

The mindful breath

When teaching your patient the proper technique for relaxation and breathing to promote pain relief, cover these points:
• Sit in a comfortable position with eyes closed.
• Focus on a sound or an image (such as an image of a peaceful scene or of white light entering the body).
• Breathe in through the nose to a count of 4.
• Hold your breath for a count of 2.
• Breathe out through your mouth for a count of 6.
• Repeat this cycle for 30 seconds to 5 minutes.

How meditation works

Meditation is thought to relieve stress and reduce pain through an effect called the *relaxation response*—a natural protective mechanism against overstress. Learning to activate the relaxation response through meditation may offset some of the negative physiologic effects of stress.

> Meditation has a restful effect on the heart and other organs.

Transcend the pain

Transcendental meditation, for instance, has been shown to reduce oxygen consumption, slow the heart and respiratory rates, lower blood lactose levels, increase alpha waves (brain waves indicating a deeply relaxed state), and ease hypertension.

Special considerations

• Know that teaching meditation and other relaxation exercises to patients, family members, and other caregivers is considered an independent health care activity. (See *Progressive relaxation*.)

Peak technique

Progressive relaxation

Progressive relaxation is a simple and widely used technique for relaxing the body and calming the mind. It involves tensing and relaxing the muscles in a progressive manner. To teach your patient this technique, follow these guidelines.

Get tense, then loose
Instruct the patient to tense a specific muscle group for several seconds—and then to stop tensing. Tell him to notice how it feels when the muscles relax as the tension flows away.

Instruct him to repeat this tensing-and-relaxing process with each muscle group. When using the common toe-to-head pattern, for instance, tell him to first relax and tense the muscles in his feet and then progress upward, sequentially relaxing and tensing the muscles in his calves, thighs, abdomen, chest, back, arms, neck, and head.

Willful relaxation
Through repetitive practice, he can quickly learn to recognize how muscle tension and relaxation feel. Once he learns this technique, he can induce muscle relaxation at the first sign of the tension that accompanies anxiety or pain.

No substitutions
If your patient wants to use progressive relaxation, advise him that this technique doesn't replace medical treatment. If he's taking prescribed drugs, tell him to continue to take them.

> By teaching your patient about progressive relaxation, you're relaxing his body and calming his mind.

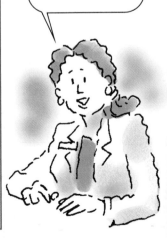

- Before providing teaching, assess what the patient knows and how he feels about meditation.
- Inform the patient that learning to meditate takes some practice.
- Be aware that patients with respiratory problems may have difficulty with meditation techniques that focus on breathing.

Biofeedback

Biofeedback uses electronic monitors to teach patients how to exert conscious control over various autonomic functions. By watching the fluctuations of various body functions (such as breathing, heart rate, or blood pressure) on a monitor, patients eventually learn how to change a particular body function by adjusting thoughts, breathing pattern, posture, or muscle tension.

As they learn to modify vital functions at will, patients may develop the ability to control pain and certain other conditions without using drugs or other conventional medical treatments.

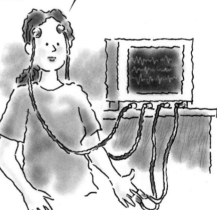

Can this biofeedback machine read my mind, too?

Great for control freaks

Biofeedback is used to treat various chronic pain states, such as headache, back pain, TMJ, stress-related disorders, and GI disorders. Approved by both conventional and alternative practitioners, it's popular with patients because it gives them a sense of control over their health problem.

Common types of biofeedback used to treat pain disorders include:
- electromyography (EMG), which measures muscle tension
- thermal biofeedback, which measures skin temperature.

EMG biofeedback

In EMG biofeedback, the patient is connected to a device with electrodes that pick up signals from muscles. The device changes the signals into a form the patient can understand, such as flashing lights or beeping, when the muscles tense up. A biofeedback practitioner interprets the signals and guides the patient in mental and physical exercises that help him achieve the desired result.

Eventually, the patient trains himself to control physiologic functions by adjusting muscle tension. Decreasing muscle tension can reduce pain.

No strings attached

With experience, patients become increasingly more self-aware and can learn how to relax muscle groups even without the device attached.

Thermal biofeedback

Used most often to treat migraine, thermal biofeedback measures skin temperature (usually of a finger) as an indication of changes in peripheral blood flow. (See *Biofeedback: Behind the curtain.*)

How biofeedback works

Scientists aren't sure how biofeedback produces its positive effects. Early investigators believed it directly reduced maladaptive physiologic processes associated with pain.

But several studies have shown that biofeedback can be beneficial when no physical changes occur, or even when the patient learns to increase muscle tension.

How do you explain it?

One possible explanation is that for some people, biofeedback reduces maladaptive physiologic activity, whereas for others it in-

Now I get it!

Biofeedback: Behind the curtain

In biofeedback, the patient learns to change a specific body function, such as heart rate or skin temperature, by changing his thoughts, breathing pattern, posture, or muscle tension.

Halting a migraine
To treat a patient with a migraine, for example, a special probe monitors skin temperature, which reflects the amount of blood flowing beneath the skin. Temperature changes, reflecting vasoconstriction and vasodilation, indicate the stress response.

As skin temperature fluctuates, lights on the monitor indicate the patient's response: black if he's tense, blue if he's relaxed. (Environmental conditions must be constant when monitoring skin temperature.)

Open to interpretation
The therapist helps the patient interpret the signals and teaches him relaxation and imagery techniques designed to maintain a blue light. The patient repeats this process until he achieves the desired response—migraine relief.

stills the belief that they can exert some control over their bodies and symptoms. This belief might lead to other coping behaviors that reduce emotional distress and help relieve pain.

Special considerations

- If your patient is seeking biofeedback therapy, help him find a qualified practitioner. Practitioners should be licensed, board-certified, or both. They may come from a variety of disciplines and have varying levels of education.
- Instruct the patient to keep taking prescribed medications while receiving biofeedback training.
- Minimize distractions during the biofeedback session because they can prevent the patient from focusing and gaining optimal results.
- Know that biofeedback is contraindicated in patients with hypotension, psychiatric disorders, impaired memory, or dementia.

Hypnosis

Hypnosis harnesses the power of suggestion and altered levels of consciousness to produce positive behavior changes and treat various health conditions. Under hypnosis, a patient typically relaxes and experiences changes in respiration, which may lead to a positive shift in behavior and a greater sense of well-being.

You're getting sleepy...

Defined as a state of attentive and focused concentration, hypnosis leaves a person relatively unaware of surroundings and highly susceptible to suggestion.

However, he must be willing to follow the suggestions offered. He can't be hypnotized to follow suggestions that go against his wishes.

... and your pain is vanishing

Hypnosis aids pain management by helping the patient gain control over the fear and anxiety that may accompany pain. It has been used to treat:
- chronic pain
- headaches
- rheumatoid arthritis
- menstrual pain.

> **Now I get it!**
>
> ## Fathoming hypnosis
>
> Hypnosis and hypnotic techniques have become recognized as powerful methods for effective relief of many acute and chronic pain conditions.
>
> **Pretty dramatic**
> Although hypnosis isn't magic, the results can be dramatic. For example, hypnotized patients have experienced analgesia with little or no pain medication while undergoing surgery, burn debridement, and childbirth.
>
> One study found that hypnosis relieves pain not only through an effect on the higher brain centers responsible for perception and interpretation of stimuli but also by reducing afferent nerve impulse transmission at the spinal cord level.

How hypnosis works

The hypnotic state may increase the patient's control over autonomic nervous system functions ordinarily considered beyond conscious control.

Physiologic changes that occur during hypnosis include:
- decreased sympathetic nervous system activity
- reduced oxygen consumption
- lower blood pressure
- slower heart rate
- increases in certain types of brain wave activity.

These physiologic effects are similar to those seen in other states of deep relaxation.

Do you hear what I hear?

Exactly how this state of relaxation makes a person more receptive to suggestion isn't known. But research shows that the brain's left side (the center for verbalization) is less active under hypnosis and that the brain's right side then "hears" messages that can be used to transform the body. (See *Fathoming hypnosis*.)

Special considerations

- Because hypnosis deals with the subconscious mind, it may elicit disturbing emotions or memories. If the patient becomes upset or aggressive or exhibits strong negative feelings, the hypnotherapist should redirect him to a safe memory and end the session.

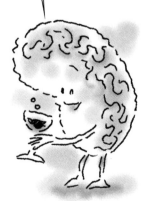

My left side conks out while my right side hears messages? Sounds like what happens when I drink too much.

• Be aware that some patients experience light-headedness or psychological reactions to hypnosis.
• Know that patients with organic psychiatric conditions, psychosis, or antisocial personality disorders shouldn't be treated with hypnosis.

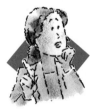

Quick quiz

1. Thermotherapy causes which of the following effects?
  A. Vasoconstriction
  B. Paresthesia
  C. Vasodilation
  D. Vasocompression

Answer: C. Thermotherapy causes vasodilation, which enhances blood flow to the affected area.

2. Which statement best describes Therapeutic Touch?
  A. It's thought to relieve pain by rebalancing the patient's energy force.
  B. It entails hands-on massage to remove pain from the patient's energy field.
  C. It involves use of the hands to eliminate painful forces from the patient's energy field.
  D. It involves placing warm, scented water on the patient.

Answer: A. Therapeutic Touch is thought to relieve pain by rebalancing the patient's energy force.

3. Massage promotes increased circulation and softening of connective tissues. It also has which of the following effects?
  A. Narrows blood vessels
  B. Causes hyperventilation
  C. Eases muscle spasms
  D. Widens blood vessels

Answer: C. Massage decreases muscle tension, thereby easing muscle spasms.

4. Which of the following is *not* a usual effect of exercise?
  A. Joint inflexibility
  B. Muscle strengthening
  C. Greater ROM
  D. Endorphin release

Answer: A. Exercise makes the joints more flexible.

5. After an injury, cyrotherapy helps reduce pain and edema when used for:

  A.   1 week.
  B.   the first 24 to 72 hours.
  C.   the first 12 hours only.
  D.   3 to 4 days

Answer: B. Cryotherapy helps reduce pain and edema when used during the first 24 to 72 hours after an injury. After 72 hours, switch to thermotherapy.

Scoring

☆☆☆   If you answered all five questions correctly, excellent! You're acing the many nonpharmacologic approaches to treating pain!

☆☆   If you answered three or four questions correctly, fantastic! You're beginning to understand that relieving pain can be painless!

☆   If you answered fewer than three questions correctly, don't suffer in pain! Go get a massage and review this chapter again!

Acute pain

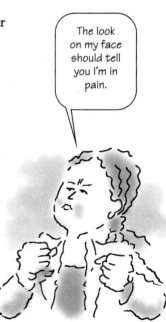

The look on my face should tell you I'm in pain.

Just the facts

In this chapter, you'll learn:

♦ the causes of acute pain

♦ approaches to assess acute pain

♦ pharmacologic and nonpharmacologic ways to manage acute pain

♦ analgesic administration routes and schedules

♦ management of selected acute pain disorders.

A look at acute pain

Acute pain—pain of recent onset and short duration—is a predictable physiologic response to harmful thermal, mechanical, or chemical stimuli. Acute pain has a protective effect and often evokes a withdrawal reflex.

Causes of acute pain include:

• trauma
• burns
• inflammation
• infection
• exacerbations of chronic medical disorders
• surgical and diagnostic procedures.

Short — but not sweet

Acute pain may last from moments to weeks. (Most pain experts classify pain lasting beyond 6 weeks as chronic.)

Acute pain typically triggers physiologic responses, such as elevated blood pressure, increased pulse, and diaphoresis. It also causes behavioral responses, including guarding, grimacing, and verbalizations of pain.

Blame it on management

Although acute pain usually can be controlled and sometimes even prevented, all too often it goes undertreated.

Some health care professionals, for instance, think the proper way to manage postoperative and postprocedural pain is to give I.M. analgesics on an as-needed basis. But according to most pain experts, this regimen is inadequate for many patients because of individual differences in the way people experience and tolerate pain. Also, I.M. injections themselves can be painful.

Gimme some relief!

Unrelieved acute pain can lead to pneumonia, myocardial infarction (MI), blood clots, and delayed return of gastric and bowel function. It can even predispose the patient to a debilitating chronic pain syndrome, such as phantom limb pain, postmastectomy pain, or postthoracotomy pain.

Unrelieved acute pain may have other consequences, too—including social withdrawal, increased photosensitivity, and a delayed recovery.

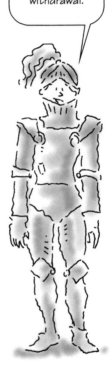

Stay away from me! Unrelieved pain may lead to social withdrawal.

Assessing acute pain

If your patient experiences an acute pain episode, perform a baseline pain assessment and ask him whether he's currently taking analgesics. This information will help you and other health care team members develop an appropriate pain management plan.

Stoic, shmoic

Ask the patient to rate his pain intensity using an objective tool such as a pain rating scale. Doing so helps the patient avoid both stoicism and exaggeration. (For pain assessment tools, see chapter 2, Assessing pain.)

Anxiety on the side

If he seems anxious, have him rate his emotional distress separately from his pain, but on a similar scale—for instance, a scale of 0 to 10, with 0 representing no anxiety and 10 representing the worst anxiety possible.

Mismatch

If the patient's self-rated pain intensity doesn't match his behaviors—say, if he rates his pain a 0 but grimaces frequently—try to identify the reason. Keep in mind that some patients come from cultures that discourage verbalizing pain.

Myth busters

Misconceptions about addiction

Outdated ideas about drug addiction may cause needless suffering in patients experiencing pain. Read on to get the facts on two of the most common myths.

Myth: Patients who receive opioids for pain relief often become addicted.

Fact: The risk of addiction among these patients is less than 1%.

Myth: Drug addiction is the same thing as physical drug dependence or drug tolerance.

Fact: Drug addiction is a neurobehavioral disease characterized by compulsive drug use, psychological dependence, and continuing drug use despite harm. It isn't the same as physical drug dependence or drug tolerance.

> Sometimes things don't add up. Be suspicious if the patient's self-rating of pain doesn't match his behavior.

It's also common for patients to fear that if they report pain, they'll be prescribed — and grow addicted to — pain pills. (See *Misconceptions about addiction*.)

Before...during...after

Throughout the acute pain episode, reassess the patient continuously. If he's scheduled for surgery or another procedure, assess his pain before, during (if appropriate), and after the procedure.

Check the rule book

If you work in a facility accredited by the Joint Commission on Accreditation of Healthcare Organizations (JCAHO), be sure to comply with JCAHO standards for pain assessment, management, and documentation. (For details, see chapter 2, Assessing pain.) For instance, to meet JCAHO standards, you must record pain assessment data in a way that promotes reassessment.

In any case, you should assess the patient's pain at least as often as you assess his vital signs.

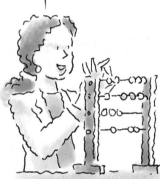

Developing a pain management plan

Whenever possible, the patient's pain management plan should focus on preventing pain. Ideally, the plan should be developed *be-*

fore the patient undergoes surgery or another procedure likely to cause pain.

An important goal of the plan is for the patient to identify a target pain level—a level of pain that's tolerable enough for him to comfortably perform such self-care activities as getting out of bed or using an incentive spirometer.

> Have the patient identify a target level of pain that will allow her to get out of bed without much discomfort.

Cover all the bases

When developing the plan, consider additional patient problems, such as concurrent cancer pain or opioid tolerance. Discuss with the patient and family such issues as treatment alternatives, potential risks of analgesic drugs, dosage adjustments, and adjunctive therapies.

Teaching time

Before the patient has surgery or another procedure, provide appropriate teaching. Be sure to cover both pharmacologic and nonpharmacologic options for managing pain, such as meditation or other relaxation methods.

Whenever possible, teach these methods before pain arises. (See chapter 4, Nonpharmacologic pain management.)

Pharmacologic management

Pharmacologic management of acute pain may involve:
- nonopioid analgesics
- opioid analgesics
- adjuvant analgesics
- local or topical anesthetics
- epidural analgesia.

Nonopioid analgesics

For patients with acute pain of mild to moderate intensity, drug treatment typically starts with a nonopioid analgesic. The three major types of nonopioids are:
- nonsteroidal anti-inflammatory drugs (NSAIDs) such as ibuprofen
- acetaminophen
- salicylates.

Now I get it!

Preemptive strikes against pain

Preemptive analgesia aims to stop pain before it even starts. This clinical concept evolved from research showing that peripheral pain receptors are more sensitive after exposure to pain-causing stimulation than before such exposure. (That explains why pain is harder to suppress than prevent.) Preemptive analgesia prevents this receptor sensitization.

Beating pain to the punch

With preemptive analgesia, dosing begins before the predicted onset of noxious stimuli. Surgery is the perfect setting because the presence and timing of postoperative pain are predictable. But preemptive analgesia also should be considered for patients scheduled for other painful procedures or whenever pain management is expected to be difficult.

Typically, analgesics are given before, during, and after surgery via I.V. opioids, local anesthetic infiltration, nerve blocks, subarachnoid block, or epidural blocks. The most effective regimens are those that limit neurologic sensitization throughout the entire perioperative period.

Less pain, much gain

Researchers found that surgical patients who received preemptive analgesia requested pain medication later—and were discharged earlier—than those who received only general anesthesia.

Make the first move

NSAIDs commonly are used in surgical patients for preemptive (preventive) analgesia. Ketorolac, for instance, frequently is used preemptively. (See *Preemptive strikes against pain.*) For many patients, NSAIDs also provide effective pain relief after noninvasive surgical procedures.

Balanced analgesia

Although most patients with moderate to severe postoperative pain need opioids, nonopioids given in combination with opioids may allow for lower opioid dosages. This, in turn, reduces the likelihood of adverse opioid effects.

In fact, combining opioids with nonopioids often provides more effective analgesia than does giving either drug class alone. This approach, called *balanced analgesia*, uses multiple pain management methods—for instance, multiple types of drugs or multiple administration routes.

Combating pain even before it occurs can prevent pain from making inroads later.

An early edge

Patients receiving balanced analgesia usually ambulate, tolerate full diets, participate in recovery activities, and get discharged earlier than patients who receive just one class of analgesic.

Opioid analgesics

Opioid analgesics are the cornerstones of postoperative pain management—especially for patients who have undergone extensive surgery that causes moderate to severe pain. Even when not given preemptively, opioids usually control postoperative pain effectively.

Opioid doses should be based on the patient's analgesic response and any adverse effects that occur. Remember that patients vary greatly in their dose requirements and responses to these drugs. Although equianalgesic charts (which show analgesic equivalents) are useful in choosing appropriate starting doses, ongoing patient monitoring is crucial to tailor the drug regimen to your patient's individual needs.

Ordinary opioids

Commonly used opioid analgesics include:
- codeine
- fentanyl citrate
- hydrocodone
- hydromorphone
- meperidine
- methadone
- morphine
- oxycodone
- proproxyphene.

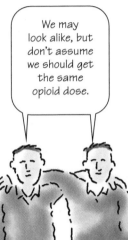

We may look alike, but don't assume we should get the same opioid dose.

Adjuvant analgesics

Adjuvant analgesics are drugs with other primary indications that are used to relieve pain in some circumstances. They may be used alone or in combination with opioids or nonopioids.

Mixin' it up

A wide variety of drugs can be used as adjuvant analgesics, including:
- anticonvulsants
- benzodiazepines
- cholinergic blockers
- corticosteroids

- ergotamine alkaloids
- muscle relaxants
- serotonin 5-HT$_1$ agonists
- selective serotonin reuptake inhibitors
- psychostimulants
- tricyclic antidepressants.
    For more information on adjuvant analgesics, see chapter 3, Pharmacologic pain management.

Anesthetics

Anesthetics stop pain transmission by blocking nerve conduction. These drugs may be given locally, topically, or epidurally.

Local anesthetics work by impeding sodium-potassium exchange across the nerve cell membrane.

Local anesthetics

Local anesthetics are used to manage pain associated with many different types of procedures—from minor ones (laceration repair) to major ones (bone marrow aspiration). They're inexpensive, easy to use, and generally safe.
    Local anesthetic agents include:
- bupivacaine
- lidocaine
- ropivacaine.

No exchanges

Local anesthetics block depolarization by interfering with sodium-potassium exchange across the nerve cell membrane. This prevents generation and conduction of nerve impulses.

How nervy

Local anesthetics are injected intradermally or subcutaneously at nerve ending sites to anesthetize the localized area of concern. They're absorbed quickly into the circulation. If they're required for a long procedure, drug concentration must be adjusted.

Don't inject digits

Don't use local anesthetics on end-arteriole tissues, such as the fingers and toes. Also, be aware that these drugs can cause dizziness, blurred vision, and decreased hearing.

Topical anesthetics

Applied directly to the skin or mucous membranes, topical anesthetics are used to relieve pain from such procedures as venipuncture and laceration repair.

Commonly used topical anesthetics include:
• benzocaine
• dibucaine
• lidocaine
• nupercainal
• tetracaine.

Ion injection

Topical anesthetics sometimes are delivered by iontophoresis — a process that uses a mild electrical current to "inject" electrically charged ions into the skin. Anesthesia occurs within 10 minutes and lasts for 15 minutes.

Although often effective, iontophoresis is underused — perhaps because it's expensive and can't be applied to large body surface areas.

Combination preparations

Combinations of local anesthetics can be used topically. These preparations include:
• lidocaine, epinephrine, and tetracaine (LET)
• eutectic mixture of local anesthetics (EMLA), which consists of lidocaine and prilocaine.

LET's prevent pain

LET is cost-effective and comes as a gel or solution. It's safe for children under age 2.

LET can be used only on nonmucosal skin lacerations. It contains epinephrine, so it shouldn't be applied on fingers, toes, or other end-arteriolar parts.

EMLA's a gem

Available as a cream, EMLA delivers a higher anesthetic concentration. It's applied to intact, nonmucosal skin and covered with a clear dressing to promote penetration into the skin. Effects last for 1 to 2 hours after application and continue for 30 to 60 minutes after removal.

Because of its variable penetration, EMLA shouldn't be applied to the palms or soles. Although it's effective on extremity lacerations, repair must be delayed for 90 minutes after cream application.

Adverse reactions include blanching or redness at the application site. Infants less than 3 months old may experience methemo-

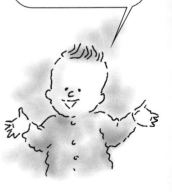

In infants less than 3 months old, EMLA may cause a dangerous condition called methemoglobinemia.

globinemia—a potentially fatal disorder that can cause such symptoms as cyanosis, headache, fatigue, ataxia, tachycardia, drowsiness, and coma.

Epidural analgesia

Opioids or local anesthetics commonly are given epidurally to manage postoperative pain or various forms of acute or chronic pain. In this method, an analgesic or anesthetic drug is injected into the epidural space. Located between a tough ligament and the dura mater (the spinal cord's outermost covering), the epidural space contains a venous network, fat, and nerve extensions.

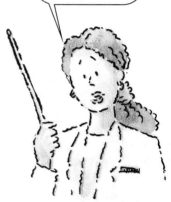

An epidural block delivers drugs directly to the spinal nerves that transmit pain signals.

Block around the clock

Opioids and local anesthetics injected into the epidural space produce an *epidural block.* An indwelling catheter may be placed preoperatively to deliver analgesics into the epidural space. This technique produces profound analgesia by delivering drugs directly to the spinal nerves involved in transmitting pain signals.

Breathing a little easier

Postoperative epidural analgesia has dramatically changed the care of intrathoracic and intra-abdominal surgical patients. It speeds postoperative recovery and respiratory function. Unburdened by pain, patients who receive epidural analgesia can take deep breaths and cooperate with respiratory care staff during postoperative recovery.

Soothing synergy

An opioid and a local anesthetic may be delivered simultaneously to the epidural space to produce a synergistic effect. This combination provides more efficient analgesia with fewer adverse effects, such as respiratory depression and motor blockade, compared to equianalgesic doses of either agent alone. (See *Using a permanent epidural catheter*, page 140.)

Nerve blocks

Injections of a local anesthetic on or near a nerve, nerve blocks are used to block nerve fibers that carry pain sensations—while leaving sensory and motor function relatively intact. Bupivacaine (Marcaine) is the anesthetic most commonly used in nerve blocks.

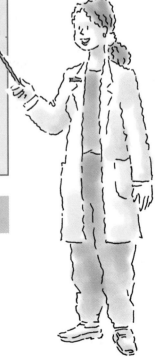

Rein in the pain

Using a permanent epidural catheter

If your patient will receive an epidural catheter for analgesic administration, explain that the catheter will be implanted beneath the skin and inserted near the spinal cord at the selected interspace. The insertion site selected depends on where the pain is located. The first lumbar (L1) interspace is shown in the illustration below.

For analgesic therapy that will last less than 1 week, the catheter may exit directly over the spine and be taped up the patient's back to the shoulder. For prolonged therapy, it may be tunneled subcutaneously to an exit site on the patient's side or abdomen or over his shoulder.

Dial down the dose

The most common complications of epidural infusion are numbness and leg weakness. These may occur after the first 24 hours and are drug- and concentration-dependent. As ordered, titrate the dosage until the drug provides adequate pain control without causing excessive numbness and weakness.

Other possible complications include respiratory depression during the first 24 hours, pruritus, nausea, and vomiting.

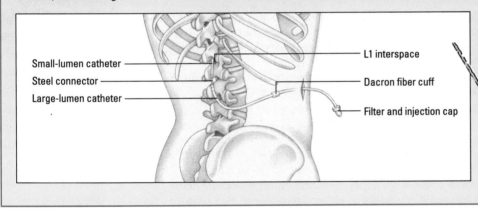

Small-lumen catheter

Steel connector

Large-lumen catheter

L1 interspace

Dacron fiber cuff

Filter and injection cap

Administration routes

Pain medications are most often given by the oral, I.M., subcutaneous (S.C.), and I.V. routes. They also can be delivered sublingually, dermally, or rectally.

Hurray for PCA

Patient-controlled analgesia (PCA), which lets the patient self-administer doses, has become a popular way to control acute postoperative pain and certain other types of pain.

Oral administration

The oral route is the most convenient and least expensive route — and the one most often prescribed in ambulatory surgery centers. Oral analgesic therapy should begin as soon as the patient can tolerate oral intake.

> I.V. analgesics are preferred for patients who can't take oral medications.

I.M. and S.C. routes

The I.M. route commonly is used to deliver pain medication to postoperative and postprocedural patients.

Both I.M. and S.C. administration carry an increased risk of infection from repeated injections and muscle tissue fibrosis. Also, they can be painful. What's more, opioids given by I.M. or S.C. injection have erratic absorption, resulting in poor pain management.

I.V. administration

I.V. administration is preferred when the patient can't take oral medications. I.V. delivery allows more accurate dosing because the entire dose enters the bloodstream immediately, producing an immediate drug effect.

Sublingual, dermal, and rectal administration

When oral or I.V. access isn't an option, drugs may be delivered by the sublingual route, dermal route (as with a fentanyl patch), or rectal route.

As with all other administration routes except I.V., these routes involve a lag time between administration and onset of drug action.

> PCA lets the patient rein in his own pain.

Patient-controlled analgesia

An interactive pain management method, PCA lets patients tailor pain relief to their individual needs and pain tolerance through self-administration of analgesic doses.

Self-controlling pain

Based on the concept that only the patient knows how much pain he's in and when he needs an analgesic dose, PCA gives the patient a sense of control over pain. Instead of having to rely on a caregiver's assessment of his pain level, the patient determines his own medication needs.

Pump away the pain

A PCA device, which can be either battery-operated or mechanically operated, holds a syringe or I.V. bag of medication, which attaches directly to the patient's I.V. line. A small pump delivers a prescribed amount of drug when the patient presses a button.

Demand and supply

Small boluses of opioid administered on demand let the patient titrate the medication to his own needs. The PCA prevents overdoses through a timing feature that imposes a lock-out time (usually 6 to 10 minutes) between doses.

No lagging

PCAs reduce or eliminate the time lag between the desire for pain relief and medication delivery. Also, by allowing small but frequent doses, PCAs help reduce adverse effects caused by high systemic opioid levels.

Less than perfect

Despite their high patient satisfaction rate, PCAs aren't perfect. For example, when patients with PCAs go to sleep, they may awaken in severe pain if they haven't been receiving the analgesic continuously.

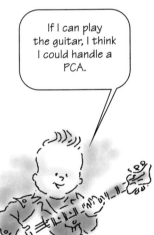

If I can play the guitar, I think I could handle a PCA.

Candidates for PCA

To be considered for PCA, the patient must be mentally alert and able to understand and comply with instructions and procedures.

Patients shouldn't be denied access solely on the basis of age. Children as young as age 5 have used PCAs effectively and safely.

When patients won't or can't self-administer analgesics, family-controlled analgesia or nurse-activated dosing may be used. (See *Watching for PCA problems.*)

Dosing methods

Most PCAs can deliver both constant maintenance (basal) infusions and on-demand boluses. A typical I.V. PCA uses a series of loading doses repeated every 5 minutes until initial postoperative pain diminishes. A low-dose basal infusion also may be given.

> ### Rein in the pain
> ## Watching for PCA problems
>
> If your patient can't self-administer his patient-controlled analgesia (PCA) pump, family and friends can activate it for him after discharge.
>
> **Teach and watch**
> Be sure to provide adequate teaching to all caregivers. Teach them how to use the PCA device, and watch them practice with a sample device.
>
> Tell them what adverse effects to watch for. Respiratory depression is the main adverse effect of opioid analgesics. Sedation also can occur. Explain that the patient should receive enough analgesic to relieve acute pain but not enough to cause drowsiness.

The starting prescription is an estimate of what the patient will need. When morphine is prescribed, on-demand doses typically add 1 mg of morphine every 6 minutes, up to a preset maximum. When the patient can take oral medication, the basal infusion is discontinued.

Patient assessment

If your patient has a PCA device, assess his pain level regularly. Based on assessment findings, titrate the dosage as necessary to maintain adequate analgesia with minimal adverse effects.

Unlocking memories

If the patient reports inadequate pain relief while using PCA, evaluate him at once. Adjust doses if the patient reports a pain level consistently above the designated goal or experiences intolerable adverse effects. Besides the patient's report, check the information in the PCA history, which is retained in the pump's memory.

Health care provider's role

Remember — even though your patient is using PCA, you're still his primary pain manager. Simply telling him to press the PCA button doesn't constitute acceptable pain management.

Dosing schedules

Unless your patient is using PCA, he'll receive pain medication according to one of two schedules:
- around-the-clock dosing
- p.r.n. (as needed) dosing.

Around-the-clock dosing

Around-the-clock dosing is indicated when pain is expected to occur for more than 12 out of 24 hours. Giving the primary analgesic around the clock helps the patient maintain stable blood drug levels and thus helps prevent pain. (See *The pitfalls of dose skipping.*)

Ban the breakthrough

Additional analgesics should be available to treat breakthrough pain—a transient flare-up of moderate to severe pain in a patient whose pain is otherwise controlled. The pain breaks through the patient's regular pain medication.

Additional doses used to treat breakthrough pain are sometimes called rescue doses.

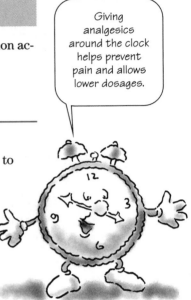

p.r.n. dosing

A p.r.n. dosing schedule may be appropriate for patients with intermittent pain or those in later stages of postoperative recovery. Such dosing provides pain relief while decreasing the risk of adverse effects.

Now for the bad news

Unfortunately, p.r.n. dosing forces the patient to ask for each dose—and some patients are reluctant to ask for painkillers.

What's more, p.r.n. dosing usually involves a delay in pain control while the health care provider unlocks the narcotic drawer and prepares the drug for administration. Another delay occurs after the patient receives the dose; before the drug takes effect, it must travel to its site of action and combine with cellular drug receptors.

If your patient must receive p.r.n. analgesics, be sure to teach him to ask for analgesics *before* pain becomes severe.

Rein in the pain

The pitfalls of dose skipping

If your patient is scheduled to receive around-the-clock analgesic doses, don't let him skip doses during the sleep hours. Otherwise, he may wake up in intense pain because his blood analgesic levels have declined.

Right of refusal

In some cases, the doctor may use a variation of p.r.n. dosing by writing drug orders that let the patient refuse a dose when appropriate.

For example, morphine may be given every 4 hours around the clock for the first 36 hours after surgery to help manage severe postoperative pain. But the patient can refuse the dose if he isn't in pain or doesn't wish to be awakened.

Nonpharmacologic interventions

Nonpharmacologic interventions used to control acute pain include transcutaneous electrical nerve stimulation and relaxation techniques such as meditation. For more information on these techniques, see chapter 4, Nonpharmacologic pain management.

Managing acute pain disorders

Besides postoperative and postprocedural pain, the most common types of acute pain include:
- acute abdominal pain
- acute chest pain
- burn pain
- acute orthopedic pain
- pain from blunt and penetrating injuries.

Acute abdominal pain

Acute abdominal pain may arise from the abdominal viscera or peritoneum, or it may be referred from another site.

It's not unusual

Abdominal pain is the primary complaint in roughly 25% of patients admitted for general surgery. It's also a common reason for visits to emergency departments (EDs), accounting for roughly 5% to 10% of annual ED visits in the United States (about 5 million patients).

Scores of sources

Causes of acute abdominal pain include:
- appendicitis
- dissecting abdominal aortic aneurysm
- duodenal and gastric ulcers
- ectopic pregnancy

- endometriosis
- gallstones
- gastroenteritis
- intestinal obstruction
- renal calculi
- liver disease
- pancreatitis
- myocardial infarction
- splenic rupture.

What to look for

Acute abdominal pain often is accompanied by reflex guarding, tenderness and, in many cases, nausea and vomiting. Other characteristics depend on the pain's origin:
- Pain from visceral organs is predominately dull and poorly localized (because of smooth muscle spasms in the hollow organs).
- Somatic or peritoneal pain is sharp and may be localized or referred.

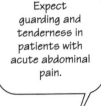

Expect guarding and tenderness in patients with acute abdominal pain.

Assessing acute abdominal pain

When assessing a patient with acute abdominal pain, obtain a thorough history and perform a physical examination. Evaluate the onset, location, severity, duration, and quality of pain. Find out whether anything makes it worse or better. Pay close attention to the patient's pain description. (See *Abdominal pain: Types and locations.*)

Been there, done that

Determine whether the patient has had previous episodes of abdominal pain. Also ask whether he has any preexisting medical conditions.

Although the main goal is to determine whether the patient needs surgery, this goal shouldn't interfere with appropriate pain management.

Don't withhold

Many health care professionals have been taught to withhold analgesics in patients with acute abdominal pain for fear the medication could mask important signs or symptoms.

But recent studies suggest that giving opioids to patients with acute abdominal pain doesn't alter diagnostic accuracy or delay surgery. Patients who received morphine reported greater pain relief than those who received a placebo. Also, morphine didn't mask physical findings such as peritoneal signs. (See *Myths about managing abdominal pain*, page 148.)

Abdominal pain: Types and locations

Abdominal pain can occur in many different types and locations. This chart describes the affected organ and the type of pain.

Affected organ	Visceral pain	Parietal pain	Referred pain
Appendix	Periumbilical area	Right lower quadrant	Right lower quadrant
Distal colon	Hypogastrium and left flank for descending colon	Over affected area	Left lower quadrant and back (rare)
Gallbladder	Middle epigastrium	Right upper quadrant	Right subscapular area
Ovaries, fallopian tubes, and uterus	Hypogastrium and groin	Over affected area	Inner thighs
Pancreas	Middle epigastrium and left upper quadrant	Middle epigastrium and left upper quadrant	Back and left shoulder
Proximal colon	Periumbilical area and right flank for ascending colon	Over affected site	Right lower quadrant and back (rare)
Small intestine	Periumbilical area	Over affected site	Midback (rare)
Stomach	Middle epigastrium	Middle epigastrium and left upper quadrant	Shoulders
Ureters	Costovertebral angle	Over affected site	Groin: scrotum in men, labia in women (rare)

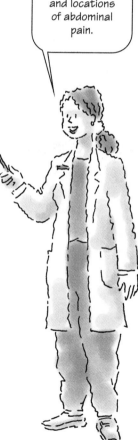

Here you'll find the different types and locations of abdominal pain.

Managing acute abdominal pain

Interventions for acute abdominal pain depend on the underlying cause, as revealed by laboratory tests, abdominal ultrasound, abdominal computed tomography (CT) scans, abdominal and chest X-rays, excretory urography, and other studies.

As ordered, administer drugs, such as NSAIDs, opioids, or antiemetics. Monitor the patient for changes in bowel sounds, abdominal tenderness, and distention. Determine whether his symptoms are worsening or improving.

Myth busters

Myths about managing abdominal pain

Myths about abdominal pain can pose a serious hindrance to pain management. To separate myth from fact, read what follows.

Myth: Giving opioids to a patient with abdominal pain could mask important signs and symptoms such as localized tenderness.

Fact: No study shows that effective pain management hampers diagnosis of abdominal pain. In fact, opioids relax the patient and may make examination easier.

Myth: Giving opioids preoperatively to a patient with abdominal pain inactivates his informed consent.

Fact: Recent judicial opinions state that withholding pain medication until the patient gives consent to treatment is tantamount to coercion.

Myth: Meperidine is superior to morphine for patients with suspected biliary colic.

Fact: Meperidine and morphine cause roughly the same rise in intrabiliary pressure. What's more, the increased pressure has no clinical significance.

Memory jogger

What should you do when you encounter a patient with ischemic chest pain? Think of the acronym MONA:

Morphine

Oxygen

Nitroglycerin

Aspirin

Acute chest pain

Because chest pain often signals myocardial ischemia or MI, any patient with acute chest pain must be evaluated immediately. In fact, chest, jaw, or arm pain may indicate myocardial ischemia even if the patient rates his pain intensity as low.

Besides myocardial ischemia or MI, acute chest pain may stem from:
- cardiomyopathy
- cholecystitis
- dissecting aortic aneurysm
- esophagitis
- hiatal hernia
- mediastinitis
- pancreatitis
- pericarditis
- pneumonia
- pneumothorax
- pulmonary embolism.

What to look for

Chest pain may arise suddenly or gradually. It may radiate to the arms, neck, jaw, or back. It may be steady or intermittent, mild or acute.

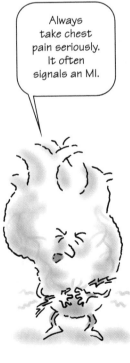

Always take chest pain seriously. It often signals an MI.

Character test

Acute chest pain can range in character from a sharp, shooting sensation to a feeling of dullness, heaviness, fullness, or even indigestion. Stress, anxiety, exertion, deep breathing, or eating certain foods may provoke chest pain.

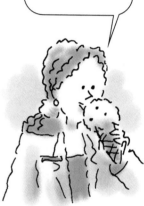

Eating certain foods may trigger chest pain. In my opinion, though, ice cream is worth it.

Assessing acute chest pain

Initially, the cause of chest pain may be hard to determine. The patient's description of the pain is crucial to accurate diagnosis. Ask about pain onset, duration, severity, nature, location, radiation (especially to the arms), aggravating or alleviating factors, and prior episodes.

Be sure to have the patient rate his pain intensity using a pain rating scale. (See chapter 2, Assessing pain.)

Managing acute chest pain

If the doctor suspects MI as the cause of chest pain, interventions should begin immediately — even before the initial history and physical examination are completed. Expect to give oxygen along with aspirin and nitroglycerin (in sublingual or spray form).

If nitroglycerin proves ineffective, the patient typically receives morphine I.V. A patient who doesn't respond to conventional treatment may require thoracic epidural analgesia.

Burn pain

Initial pain from a burn results from the body's response to tissue damage. Pain fibers (nociceptors) and chemicals involved in the inflammatory response signal that an injury has occurred. These chemicals also promote healing.

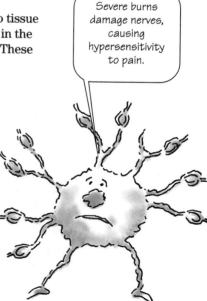

Severe burns damage nerves, causing hypersensitivity to pain.

Lingering pain

During the healing process, pain persists because newly formed tissues and nerves are hypersensitive. Severe burns damage nerves and may cause large areas of hypersensitivity in and around the burn wound. Such stimulation leads to greater pain sensitivity and a high risk of persistent, neuropathic pain even after the burn has healed.

What to look for

Burns cause excruciating pain. The deeper the burn, the more extensive the damage to nerve tissue — and the more intense the pain.

Patients typically describe burn pain as aching or burning. Some patients also have neuropathic pain (such as paresthesia), sensations of numbness or burning, or shooting pains.

Painful cures

Unfortunately, the procedures the burn patient must undergo to promote healing and rehabilitation—dressing changes, debridement, physical therapy, skin grafting, and reconstructive surgery—can also cause severe pain.

Assessing burn pain

Make every effort to perform a comprehensive pain assessment. Have the patient rate his pain intensity on a pain rating scale.

Keep in mind that burn severity is determined by the depth and extent of the burn and the presence of other factors, such as age, complications, and coexisting illnesses.

It gets complicated

Assessing burn patients can pose a challenge because these patients have complex physical and emotional needs. For instance, some patients may be too upset to cooperate because of traumatic memories of the incident, being in a strange environment, or fear of painful treatments and procedures. Also, young children and infants may be unable to verbalize pain severity.

Managing burn pain

Poor pain management can hamper recovery from a burn. The injury causes a stress response that triggers catecholamine release, in turn worsening the hypermetabolism (increased energy expenditure) that follows a serious burn.

Hypermetabolism decreases blood flow to the skin and soft tissues, impairing wound healing. At the same time, excessive pain triggers release of endogenous endorphins, possibly leading to hemodynamic instability and immunosuppression.

High anxiety

Pain relief is a priority and should begin immediately. Untreated pain is hard to control and may cause a conditioned anxiety response. Effective pain relief also reduces the risk of posttraumatic stress disorder.

Analgesic analysis

The analgesic type, dose, and administration route depend on pain severity and frequency (constant or intermittent). Morphine and hydromorphone are the

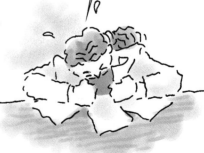

Untreated pain may cause a conditioned anxiety response.

drugs of choice (usually given using a PCA infusion pump) for patients who can't tolerate oral intake.

In a patient who can tolerate oral intake, controlled-released morphine or oxycodone may be given orally to relieve constant moderate to severe pain.

Try to give analgesics as painlessly as possible. Avoid injections because they may cause pain and unpredictable drug absorption.

Adjuvant action

Quick, short-acting I.V. fentanyl or remifentanil may be used to control intense pain of short duration, such as procedural pain. Adjuvant drugs, such as clonidine and anticonvulsants, may be useful for neuropathic pain associated with burns.

Benzodiazepines help reduce anxiety. Neuroleptics may be prescribed to treat intensive care psychosis, a psychological condition associated with serious burns.

Dress for less pain

Dressings and creams promote healing and pain relief. Biocclusive dressings have an analgesic effect, protecting the area from inadvertent touch and breezes and decreasing the need for debridement.

Sulfadiazine (Silvadene) cream is an antimicrobial agent used to treat severe burns. Researchers have infused this cream with morphine in an attempt to reduce burn pain. Another option is to apply local anesthetics to burn sites.

Inhalation anesthetics may be used during dressing changes, debridement, skin grafting, and reconstructive surgery. Nitrous oxide is sometimes used for minor procedures.

A spell on pain

Nonpharmacologic pain management techniques, such as hypnosis and relaxation techniques, may be helpful for some burn patients.

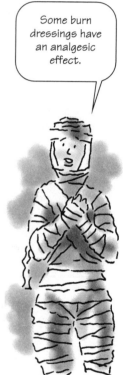

Some burn dressings have an analgesic effect.

Acute orthopedic pain

Acute orthopedic pain usually results from trauma or excessive exercise. Acute musculoskeletal injuries involve muscles, ligaments, tendons, joints, and bones. Acute low back pain is one of the most common types of orthopedic pain. (See *The lowdown on low back pain*, page 152.)

Orthopedic pain results from pain fibers responding to the pressure or distortion of the injured structure — along with re-

The lowdown on low back pain

Few of us get through life without experiencing low back pain (pain below the costal margin and above the inferior gluteal folds). This pain may be accompanied by muscle spasms, tension, stiffness, and sciatica—pain along the course of the sciatic nerve, typically radiating into the buttock or leg.

Typecasting
Low back pain falls into three main categories:
• acute pain, which lasts a few days to a few months
• primary pain, caused by a derangement of muscular, ligamentous, fascial, or joint structures
• secondary pain, stemming from a primary disorder such as kidney stones, cancer, aortic aneurysm, infection, or bone fracture.

Most patients with primary or mechanical back pain are ages 20 to 50. In persons younger than age 20 or older than 50, suspect that acute back pain is secondary to another condition.

Assess it
Obtain a thorough history and perform a physical examination, including a neurologic exam. Be sure to examine the entire trunk. Ask the patient to rate her pain using a pain intensity scale (such as a 0-to-10 scale).

If she has signs or symptoms of progressive neurologic deficits—for instance, fever, bowel or bladder incontinence, or progressive sensorimotor deficits—suspect a serious emergent problem. If she has constitutional symptoms, such as weight loss or nocturnal back pain, thoroughly evaluate her for an underlying cause.

Manage it
Usually, acute nonspecific back pain (with or without leg radiation) is self-limiting and resolves spontaneously. Exercise, drug therapy, and nonpharmacologic pain management approaches are often effective.

Typically, the doctor orders short periods of bed rest, analgesics, and local physical measures. In most cases, muscle relaxants should be used for only a brief period. Behavioral therapy and multidisciplinary treatment programs also may have some benefit.

Get the patient out of bed
Research shows that using nonsteroidal anti-inflammatory drugs and staying active speed recovery and reduce chronic problems. Bed rest—once a mainstay of treatment—is no longer advised.

lease of chemical mediators, such as prostaglandins, at the injury site. Pain severity varies with injury location and extent.

Footwear factor

Causes of or contributors to orthopedic pain include:
• poor conditioning
• poor body mechanics
• acute physical disorders
• unstable footwear.

Teen tendencies

Adolescents experience the highest rates of orthopedic injuries. For males, high-risk sports include:
• basketball
• football
• lacrosse
• soccer

Low back pain is inevitable. Read on to find out how to assess, manage, and treat it.

- track
- wrestling.
    For females, high-risk activities include:
- basketball
- cheerleading
- gymnastics
- soccer
- softball
- track
- volleyball.

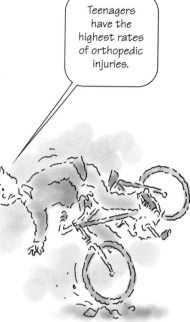

Teenagers have the highest rates of orthopedic injuries.

What to look for

Bone pain is deep, aching, and continuous. Except with fractures, movement rarely exacerbates bone pain.

Muscle pain, on the other hand, tends to get worse with movement. Patients commonly describe muscle pain as stiffness, soreness, aching, spasms, or cramps. The area may be swollen, with loss of function.

Close neighbors

Because muscles, tendons, and ligaments are in close proximity to one another, the precise injury site may be hard to determine. What's more, pain localization may be poor, and pain may be referred. For instance, pain from an arthritic hip may be referred to the thigh or knee.

Joint pain is more easily localized. It's commonly accompanied by stiffness and limited movement.

Assessing acute orthopedic pain

Obtain the patient's history, and ask him to rate his pain intensity on a pain rating scale. If his pain is severe, give analgesics, as ordered, before performing a detailed examination.

Unlike muscle or tendon pain, joint pain usually is easy to localize.

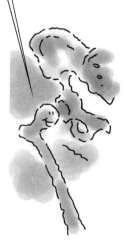

Seek the source

To help determine the source of the pain, the doctor may order various radiologic studies, such as X-rays, fluoroscopy, CT scans, magnetic resonance imaging, or bone scans.

Laboratory studies help determine whether infection or inflammation is present. Diagnostic joint fluid aspiration also may be done.

Managing acute orthopedic pain

Despite beliefs to the contrary, giving analgesics to a patient with an acute orthopedic injury doesn't interfere with diagnosis or treatment. In fact, early treatment of orthopedic pain can help reduce complications.

Soft-tissue orthopedic injuries usually are treated with rest, ice, compression, and elevation. If the patient has a ligament or tendon injury, he may need prolonged analgesic therapy because these structures have poor vascularization and heal slowly.

Get moving

Within 5 days to 3 weeks of the injury, the patient should begin to move the injured area — gently, of course — to promote collagen regeneration.

Pharmaceuticals for fractures

Pain from a fracture may warrant NSAIDs, opioids, cold application, and splinting. Surgical immobilization, fusion, resection, or reconstruction can provide further pain relief.

Blunt and penetrating injuries

Most blunt and penetrating injuries result from work-related accidents, motor vehicle accidents, or violent crimes involving weapons. Although little has been written about managing pain in patients with traumatic injuries, pain control is paramount. Severe pain can potentiate shock or cause other problems that jeopardize the patient.

What to look for

Blunt and penetrating injuries cause acute onset of severe pain, requiring immediate medical attention. Typically, penetrating injuries result in localized pain, whereas blunt injuries cause pain over a wider area.

Assessing pain from blunt and penetrating injuries

If the patient is conscious and cooperative, use standard pain assessment tools. Be sure to have him rate his pain intensity on a pain-rating scale.

If he's incapable of reporting pain, you'll need to gauge his pain level through observation, especially noting any behavioral signs. Ask family members or friends for assistance.

To detect underlying injuries, the doctor may order such diagnostic tests as X-rays, ultrasound, and CT scans.

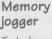

Memory jogger

To help you remember what to do if your patient has a soft-tissue injury, think of the acronym RICE-M:

Rest. Have the patient rest the injured part for 24 to 48 hours.

Ice. Apply ice to the injury site every 1 to 4 hours for 20 minutes at a time. Ice eases pain, edema, and inflammation.

Compression. Compress (squeeze) the injured area to limit swelling and internal bleeding. An elastic wrap is unbeatable for this purpose.

Elevation. Elevate the injured area for the first 24 hours. This action limits circulation, decreases swelling, and reduces internal bleeding.

Motion. Have the patient perform range-of-motion exercises after the initial rest period to reduce edema and prevent muscle spasms and contractures.

Delay for diagnosis?

Some doctors delay pain management for these patients, believing analgesics mask certain abdominal signs and symptoms. In essence, they use untreated pain as a diagnostic tool.

Although serial physical exams may be needed to diagnose certain conditions, studies show that analgesics don't mask physical findings (such as peritoneal signs), alter diagnostic accuracy, or delay surgery.

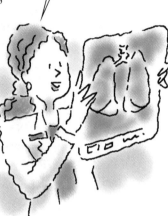

X-rays can be crucial in evaluating damage from a blunt or penetrating injury.

Managing pain from blunt and penetrating injuries

During the urgent phase of care, goals of pain management include:
- helping the patient tolerate diagnostic tests
- reducing the risk of complications
- decreasing anxiety
- increasing patient cooperation
- improving patient satisfaction.

If the patient is hemodynamically unstable, the doctor may order midazolam along with fentanyl or ketamine (both thought to be superior to other opioids). Avoid giving NSAIDs in this situation because of the risk of hemorrhage.

Regardless of which opioid is used, titrate the dosage carefully and monitor the patient closely to achieve pain control without compromising patient safety.

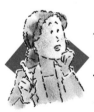

Quick quiz

1. What does preemptive analgesia refer to?
   A. Starting pain management before painful stimuli occur
   B. Using more than one class of analgesics for pain control
   C. Avoiding opioids in patients with substance abuse disorders
   D. Using NSAIDs alone to control pain

Answer: A. Preemptive analgesia is used to prevent pain — especially before painful procedures. It's based on the concept that pain is easier to prevent than to control.

2.   What's the preferred administration route for pain medications?

A.   I.M.
B.   Oral
C.   I.V.
D.   Intradermal

Answer: B. Oral administration is the most convenient and least expensive route. If the oral route isn't an option, I.V. administration is preferred. I.M. administration can be painful, and I.M. drugs may be absorbed erratically.

3.   Which statement about epidural analgesia is *true*?

A.   It's noninvasive.
B.   It allows lower opioid doses.
C.   It always provides complete pain relief.
D.   It carries no infection risk.

Answer: B. Epidural analgesia allows lower opioid doses for pain control, thereby reducing the risk of adverse effects.

4.   When pain is expected to occur for more than 12 out of 24 hours, which type of dose schedule is indicated?

A.   p.r.n.
B.   Once a day
C.   Twice a day
D.   Round the clock

Answer: D. Giving the primary analgesic around the clock helps the patient maintain stable blood drug levels and helps prevent pain.

Scoring

☆☆☆   If you answered all four questions correctly, awesome! You're managing acute pain topics with ease!

☆☆   If you answered three questions correctly, congrats! This chapter is obviously not causing you pain!

☆   If you answered fewer than three questions correctly, keep your chin up and take a look at this chapter one more time!

Chronic nonmalignant pain

A look at chronic nonmalignant pain

Chronic nonmalignant pain (CNP) is the most common type of pain. Individuals who experience this pain suffer for months and even years. CNP is defined as pain that has lasted for more than 6 months and isn't caused by a life-threatening condition. When CNP has progressed to the point that it has become the focus of a patient's life and interferes with social relationships and work, it's sometimes called CNP syndrome. Some common causes of CNP include fibromyalgia, herpes zoster, osteoarthritis, peripheral neuropathy, and rheumatoid arthritis.

Chronic — not so, ah, cute

CNP differs from acute pain because it's an ongoing process — sometimes evolving over years — that can interfere with an individual's quality of life. Acute pain is pain that comes on suddenly after trauma, surgery, or an acute disease and lasts from a few days to a few weeks. Acute pain may be constant, intermittent, or both. Acute pain resolves when

> Osteoarthritis can produce chronic nonmalignant pain that lasts for years — even with regular lube jobs.

Comparing acute and chronic pain

While acute pain and chronic pain may have some similarities, it's important to know their differences when treating patients with chronic nonmalignant pain. Here's a summary of how acute pain and chronic pain differ.

Acute pain	Chronic pain
• Followed by a specific precipitating event	• Possibly no identifiable pathophysiologic reason or precipitating event
• Easily identified pattern of onset (for example, procedural pain and orthopedic pain)	• Irregular pattern of onset with recurrence that continues for at least 6 months
• Usually accompanied by identifiable tissue damage, which indicates an underlying disorder or causative procedure	• Commonly no correspondence with identifiable tissue damage
• Behavioral signs that consist of guarding at the pain site, facial grimacing, the patient's inability to think of anything else, and vital signs changes such as increase in blood pressure, pulse, and respirations	• Possibly no behavioral signs of pain experience (due to learned methods of coping with chronic pain)
• Satisfactory pain relief with pharmacologic intervention (such as nonopioids, opioids, adjuvant medications, and anesthetics) or nonpharmacologic intervention (such as transcutaneous electrical nerve stimulation and relaxation)	• Commonly unalleviated by one pharmacologic intervention in normal dosage range or nonpharmacologic intervention without concomitant pharmacologic treatment

the cause is diagnosed and treated or analgesics are administered. (See *Comparing acute and chronic pain.*)

Survey says...

A 1999 survey by the American Pain Society states that more than 4 of every 10 people with moderate to severe chronic pain have yet to find adequate relief. The survey also revealed that CNP sufferers commonly don't receive the care experts consider necessary, even though nearly half of those in the study had switched physicians at least once and more than 50% had pain rated as 5 or higher on a scale of 10 for more than 5 years. Only 22% of the individuals in the survey had been referred to a specialized pain program.

> Most CNP sufferers don't receive adequate care for their pain, despite seeking health care providers.

Vicious cycle of CNP

Most patients with chronic nonmalignant pain (CNP) experience a vicious cycle of sleep disturbance, pain, and depression that has far-reaching implications for their lifestyle, social relationships, and self-image. The diagram below helps illustrate this cycle and explain the frustration and despair experienced by many patients with CNP.

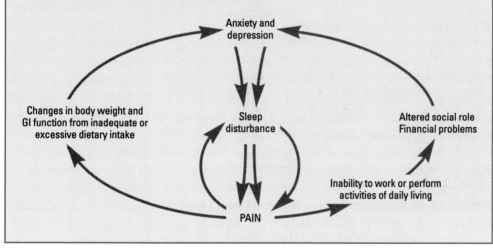

To relieve, know what they perceive

The perception of pain is the result of a complicated process. It begins in the peripheral nervous system when a nociceptor sends a signal along its axon to the spinal cord or cells leading to the cranial nerves. However, CNP seems to be the result of nociceptive pain as well as neuropathic pain. It can begin at the nociceptor, which is activated by an external stimulus such as a laceration (nociceptive pain). However, it can also come from chronically activated tissues in the spine and brain, due to a dysfunction in the tissue itself, such as from a damaged blood vessel (neuropathic pain).

The health care provider must simultaneously address the physiologic and psychological manifestations of CNP. All pain has an emotional component. With CNP, the emotional toll is significant. The energy required to withstand pain is tremendous and, when pain lasts for months, energy reserves dwindle. People with CNP are physically and emotionally fatigued by the time they seek help; many have begun to lose hope as they're increasingly unable to work and their social relationships are affected. (See *Vicious cycle of CNP*.)

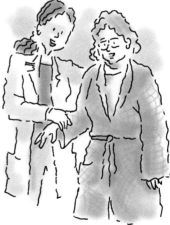

By the time they seek help, many CNP sufferers have begun to lose hope that they'll find relief.

Assessing CNP

Many patients with CNP have misguided assumptions about their pain and its causes. Some fear unconfirmed disease or malignancies to be the cause of their pain. Others also worry excessively about reinjury. In addition, some patients suspect that they haven't been informed of their true condition. Finally, sufferers worry that the pain will never end or may worsen.

Start with the whole person

In a challenging situation like this, a holistic analysis of CNP is essential. Begin with a thorough health history and physical examination, and stay alert for undiagnosed underlying organic disease. This information is vital to forming a pain management plan tailored to the patient's specific needs.

Obtaining a health history

A thorough health history provides a baseline from which to measure the effect of treatment. First, it's important to ask for all available records of previous treatment of the patient's pain. Because these records can provide valuable information, review them carefully before formulating a pain management plan.

Getting back to nature

To complete the history, question the patient about the nature of his pain. Asking specific questions about the pain can help diagnose a specific pain disorder or formulate the first step in a pain management plan. Ask the patient about the location, onset, intensity, and duration of his pain as well as what aggravates it or relieves it (for example, with medications or alternative therapies). Key criteria to look for include history of smoking, lack of exercise, and caffeine intake. The data collected will determine if further diagnostic testing or a referral to a specialist is needed.

In addition, be sure to gather information about coexisting medical conditions. Such diseases as diabetes, stroke, osteoporosis, and heart disease may be clues to possible tissue dysfunction or neurologic impairments that impact your pain assessment.

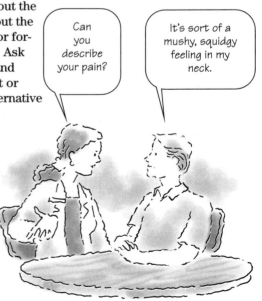

Can you describe your pain?

It's sort of a mushy, squidgy feeling in my neck.

Examining the patient with CNP

A comprehensive physical examination provides additional information about the patient and his pain. Diagnostic tests rule out organic disease and may help to diagnose the pain syndrome (although many syndromes don't have specific pathologies to test). Because CNP has long-term effects on a patient's physical and emotional well-being, it's important to assess the patient's psychological status and the risk of suicide.

Psychological evaluation

Because of the emotionally debilitating effects of CNP, psychological evaluation can help identify depression and coping mechanisms. It can also help target situations and stressors in the patient's life that may interfere with his ability to carry out the pain management plan. The Minnesota Multiphasic Personality Inventory is used to predict the patient's response to pain interventions.

Risk of suicide

CNP may cause hopelessness and depression and, therefore, carries with it a suicide risk. The practitioner should always ask the patient if he has thought of suicide. If he responds affirmatively, the practitioner should ask if the patient has thought about or devised a plan. A well thought out plan indicates that the patient is at a higher risk for suicide. Access to the means to carry out the plan also increases the risk. If the risk seems imminent, appropriate personnel should be notified and hospitalization might be necessary.

Role of a lifetime

It can be very uncomfortable for a nurse when a patient responds that he has considered suicide. It's a good idea to have practiced how to respond in this case, after consulting expert sources on the health care team, such as a psychologist, psychiatrist or mental health practitioner, or social services. Role playing exercises and other forms of practice will help the nurse respond in a way that's honest and reassuring.

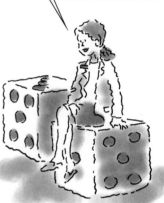

Don't gamble with your patient's emotional health. Assessing the psychological effects of his pain is an important step in preventing suicide.

Role playing can help you respond to your patients with honesty and reassurance. I'm ready for my close-up, Mr. DeMille.

Developing a pain management plan

Developing a pain management plan for the patient with CNP involves engaging in a professional, collaborative relationship with the patient and the pain management team. Along with the patient, the team must establish goals. Some of the most common goals in this type of plan include:
- reducing pain whenever possible
- improving or restoring function
- developing coping skills
- decreasing depression, anxiety, and other emotional problems
- improving relationships with family members and caregivers.

> Establishing a professional, collaborative relationship with the health care team is important for the success of every pain management plan.

Specify, measure, and achieve!

The pain management plan should outline goals in specific, measurable, and achievable ways. Patient compliance is the key to a successful plan. To ensure compliance, the practitioner must enable the patient to achieve the goals outlined in the plan. To do so, the health care provider must:

- understand the degree to which the patient has accepted his condition
- discern the patient's level of motivation to achieve goals
- identify the patient's ability to follow the plan independently
- be aware of the patient's financial and social resources and incorporate participation of the caregiver or significant others into the plan, if warranted (due to physical disability, for example)
- ensure that the patient participates fully in setting goals and is confident in his ability to achieve them
- be attentive and open-minded about the patient's account of his pain experience. (See *Tips for developing a CNP management plan.*)

Noncompliance: A hard pill to swallow

Sometimes a patient isn't willing or able to follow through on the plan's recommendations. In such a case, the health care provider may prescribe pain medications that are appropriate for CNP management, such as oxycodone (OxyContin) and valproic acid (Depakene). The provider should also give the patient information on CNP resources, such as the American Academy of Pain Medi-

---

Tips for developing a CNP management plan

The health care provider, along with the pain management team, should formulate an individualized pain management plan to ensure success when treating the patient with chronic nonmalignant pain (CNP). This list describes the holistic process involved in formulating this plan:

• Establish a trusting and therapeutic relationship with the patient.
• Involve the patient as an integral member of the pain management team and encourage him to help establish goals, evaluate responses, and make care decisions.
• Assess associated emotional problems, including anxiety, and implement necessary intervention along with pain assessment. Psychologists and other trained therapists are essential team members who can help the patient gain control of his life. In addition, because financial considerations are usually the biggest source of anxiety for the patient with CNP, these team members can also identify community resources to help pay for treatment.
• Always respect a person's report of his pain experience. Discounting the patient's pain experience is counterproductive. Although it may seem that the patient is reporting his pain incorrectly (whether intentionally or not), the pri-

ority in this situation is building a trusting relationship with the patient, including supporting his account of pain.
• Ensure that the medications offered to alleviate pain are given in sufficient doses to relieve pain but avoid harmful adverse effects.
• Understand the role of opioid therapy, which has been shown to be effective in treating CNP. Concerns over the development of dependence are legitimate; however, if carefully administered, opioids can allow the patient to regulate his dose to control pain and achieve a higher level of function.
• All recommendations to the patient as well as the rehabilitation plan should be specific, detailed, and offered in writing.
• Include patient education on self-help and self-management skills, including relaxation and cognitive and behavioral therapies, to reduce anxiety and depression and, consequently, lower the risk of suicide.

---

cine (*www.painmed.org*) and the American Board of Anesthesiology (*www.abanes.org*).

Patient education

Patients with CNP have usually seen a number of health care providers for their pain. Unfortunately, many patients' pain is undertreated or treated inappropriately by well-intentioned general practitioners who aren't trained in pain management. Commonly, CNP sufferers are prescribed opioids regardless of their complaint or, conversely, are prescribed acetaminophen for severe pain.

Barriers to CNP management

It's important for the health care provider to be aware of the negative impact pain has on the patient experiencing chronic nonmalignant pain (CNP). There are several barriers to successful management of CNP, including an uncommunicative patient, practitioner prejudice, clinical knowledge gaps about effective treatments, and factors contributing to altered social relationships for the patient with CNP.

Patient reticence

Patients might not be willing to share their pain experience as fully as is necessary for adequate assessment. Some patients might be inhibited by cultural norms that prohibit "complaining." Other patients might fear more pain from possible treatments. Older patients especially might be vague about the extent of their pain for fear of losing their independent lifestyle. In general, patients with CNP experience great frustration due to inappropriate treatments or ineffective pain management plans and may feel hopeless about finding relief.

Misinterpretation of pain by practitioners

Practitioners generally are trained to treat acute pain rather than chronic pain. Thus, many treat the CNP patient with inappropriate procedures or insufficient pain relief medication. What's more, practitioners tend to question the patient's pain experience when no obvious pathology can be detected.

Addiction knowledge gap

Unlike acute pain, CNP is ongoing, so no time limit can be set on medication administration. Health providers' fears of patient addiction from opioid use make them less willing to prescribe a dose that's adequate for CNP relief. Fortunately, these fears are unfounded. Because opioids improve the patient's ability to function, he's better able to control his use of opioids, unlike the substance abuser who's trying to achieve an alteration in mood and can't control his use.

Altered social relationships

Because CNP isn't well understood by society in general, many patients with CNP feel cut off from social interaction. Because chronic pain is, by its nature, ongoing, society views it as less severe than other forms of pain such as from trauma. Underestimating the patient's pain experience isolates him from society by labeling him as a "hypochondriac" or "depressed."

No more wait and see

Because chronic pain is so misunderstood, patients also receive a lot of misinformation about their pain and chronic pain in general. Many become frustrated with the "trial and error" approach they experience with many untrained practitioners. Therefore, it's important to take the time to clear up misconceptions and offer honest, detailed explanations of pain management plans. (See *Barriers to CNP management.*)

It isn't just a physical thing

Commonly, a patient focuses on the physical aspects of pain and doesn't want to discuss emotional aspects. Encourage the patient to confide in you about the emotional and social effects of his pain. It may help if you cite current research showing that successful CNP management is associated with plans that ad-

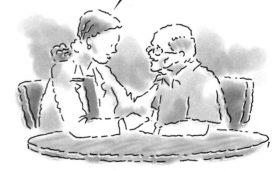

To help you achieve your pain management goals, we need to explore the emotions you're experiencing as well as your physical pain.

dress the patient's psychological and social challenges as well as the physical effects of his pain.

Pharmacologic management

Medications are the mainstay of treatment in most CNP disorders. These therapies consist of local anesthetics and nonopioid, opioid, epidural, and adjuvant analgesia.

Local anesthetics

Local anesthetics are used to provide temporary pain relief. Examples of local anesthetics are sympathetic blocks, nerve blocks, and neurolysis.

I may look like a blockhead, but I can be very sympathetic, really I can.

Sympathetic blocks

Sympathetic blocks are injections of local anesthetic into the paraspinal sympathetic ganglion (a cluster of nerve cell bodies just adjacent to the spinal column), where pain perception is thought to occur. A sympathetic block also stops autonomic function, such as smooth muscle contraction and vasoconstriction. Skeletal muscle control and sensation remain intact.

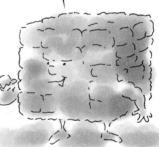

Nerve blocks

Nerve blocks are injections of local anesthetic that infiltrate the area within or around the nerve trunk and temporarily deaden the nerve. If the pain is relieved, it's clear that the source of the pain is peripheral.

If it works...

If the nerve block is effective, a follow-up injection may be given using a long-acting steroid to decrease inflammation and break up fibrosis.

What can go wrong

Nerve blocks can provide rapid and complete relief. However, because they block out all nerve function, the patient may experience motor or sensory innervation in the area beyond the block. In addition, in long-standing pain, the central nervous system becomes involved in pain perception. In these cases, a nerve block won't relieve the pain.

Neurolysis

Neurolysis is an injection of alcohol or phenol into the trigeminal ganglion (5th cranial nerve), the celiac plexus (first lumbar vertebra), or the lumbar sympathetic chain (in the spinal cord). The goal of neurolysis is to destroy nerve function for weeks, months or, possibly, longer. If neurolysis is effective, it's an indication that nervectomy for long-term relief may be effective.

Nonopioid analgesics

Nonopioid analgesics are the most widely used drugs for pain. Their effectiveness is generally limited to mild pain of short duration. Occasionally, they may be used in mild cases of some CNP disorders, such as osteoarthritis and back pain.

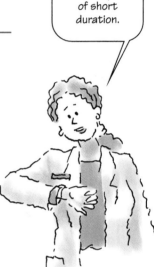

Nonopioids are effective for mild pain of short duration.

NSAIDs

Pain and swelling are caused by prostaglandins released at the site of tissue injury. Nonsteroidal anti-inflammatory drugs (NSAIDs) are useful for producing analgesia and reducing inflammation because they're prostaglandin inhibitors. They're effective analgesics for mild to moderate pain in skin, muscle, and connective tissues. They're also used in conjunction with opioid analgesics to potentiate pain relief.

Acetaminophen

Acetaminophen is useful to relieve mild pain, such as muscle aches, and general pain. Unlike NSAIDs, however, acetaminophen doesn't have an anti-inflammatory effect.

Opioid analgesics

Opioid therapy for CNP has become an accepted avenue of treatment when other types of therapy (pharmacologic and nonpharmacologic) have failed. The American Academy of Pain Medicine and the American Pain Society have endorsed the use of opioids in selected patients with CNP. It's important for the clinician working with these patients to understand and comply with applicable laws regarding opioid medication for CNP.

Know the risks

Before beginning opioid therapy for CNP, patients should be informed of the risks of therapy: adverse effects, physical dependence, and the potential for withdrawal symptoms if the medicine is discontinued abruptly. The health care provider and the patient should agree on how the medications will be administered (orally, transdermally, epidurally, or intrathecally).

Rescue from breakthrough

The practitioner must also reach an agreement with the patient on treatment for breakthrough pain. Breakthrough pain is pain experienced despite adherence to the established analgesic dosing schedule. "Rescue" doses may be prescribed to address this breakthrough pain, which may occur during initial medication periods, when dosages are speculative and may not be set at a therapeutic level, or when a particular therapy interferes with the effects of the analgesia (as in radiation therapy). The health care provider and the patient should discuss and agree on the number of rescue doses or adjustments than can be made for breakthrough pain. If frequent rescue dosing is required, the health care provider should reexamine the scheduled analgesic dosage and adjust accordingly.

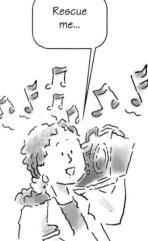

Rescue me...

One practitioner, one pharmacy

A single provider should be in charge of coordinating and prescribing opioids, and a specific pharmacy should be used consistently to fill those prescriptions. Provider and pharmacy should follow their state's regulations regarding opioid therapy for CNP.

Monitor the patient for responsible use of the medication. Requests for doses beyond those outlined in the pain management plan must be reviewed carefully. It may be necessary to discontinue opioid therapy if the patient's functional level deteriorates.

My longer half-life can help a patient get a good night's sleep.

More morphine, please!

Long-acting, or controlled release, forms of opioids are most effective in treating CNP. When taken as directed, they don't usually produce euphoric effects. Their longer half-life allows patients to obtain better sleep at night and reduces the frequency of dosing. Morphine preparations, such as MS Contin or Oramorph SR, are used frequently. Sedation may occur at first, but if it persists beyond a few days, be on the lookout for other causes.

Many other preparations are used, such as oxycodone (OxyContin) and hydrocodone (Hycodan). All have the same basic mode of action and differ mainly in duration of action, the strength of the analgesic effect, and adverse effects.

Epidural analgesia

An implanted epidural analgesia device (a form of intraspinal anesthesia) may be used to provide continuous pain control. To control breakthrough pain, intermittent bolus doses may be administered.

Adjuvant analgesics

Adjuvant analgesics are medications that have other primary indications but can also be used as analgesics to treat some conditions, including CNP. These analgesics may be given in combination with opioids or alone. Adjuvant therapies can help maximize pain control and lower the required dose of opioids.

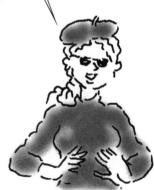

Antidepressants may put your patient in a groovy mood but, more importantly, they help relieve certain types of chronic pain.

Tricyclic antidepressants

Tricyclic antidepressants (TCAs), such as amitriptyline (Elavil) and nortriptyline (Pamelor), are especially useful in treating pain from nerve damage. The reason for their effectiveness isn't known; however, it's probably related to their ability to block the reuptake of certain neurotransmissions at nerve endings and in the spinal cord. Regardless, it's clear that they have intrinsic analgesic effects, in addition to any positive effect on the patient's mood.

Antidepressants are also more effective than benzodiazepines or other tranquilizers in long-term help for sleep disturbances due to CNP. Antidepressants aren't dependence-forming like benzodiazepines; however, sudden withdrawal after prolonged use can occasionally result in convulsions.

It isn't how you feel; it's what you feel

Many people are under the mistaken impression that antidepressants are given to pain sufferers only to relieve depression. Health care providers should counsel patients that the antidepressant isn't treating their mood, but their pain.

And now, the bad news

Drawbacks of TCAs are their unpleasant adverse effects — especially dry mouth, which doesn't go away even with prolonged use. Another major adverse effect is sedation, which interferes with the patient's ability to perform daily activities. Other less common but no less unpleasant adverse effects are visual disturbances, constipation, and weight gain. Any of these adverse effects can ultimately cause the patient to stop taking the medication.

Hypotension, arrhythmias, glaucoma — oh, my!

In addition, the anticholinergic effects of TCAs can exacerbate other illnesses. These drugs can cause acute urine retention in men with prostatic enlargement, cardiac arrhythmias, and postural hypotension. In addition, TCAs have been known to precipitate narrow-angle glaucoma.

Anticonvulsants

Anticonvulsants are effective in treating neuropathic pain, especially pain classified as stabbing or lancinating. The medicine has a membrane-stabilizing effect, diminishing the output from the pain receptors (nociceptors). Be sure to warn the patient to avoid abruptly discontinuing anticonvulsant medication because acute withdrawal can result in seizures. The most common anticonvulsants used to treat CNP are carbamazepine (Tegretol), sodium valproate (Depakene), gabapentin (Neurontin), phenytoin (Dilantin), and clonazepam (Klonopin).

Carbamazepine

Carbamazepine is the most commonly used anticonvulsant, although not everyone can tolerate its adverse effects. To try to prevent these effects, the drug is usually started at low doses (such as 100 mg/day) and increased very gradually, allowing 2 weeks to elapse before increasing the dose. Some patients will need as much as 400 mg three times per day to achieve analgesia. In addition, the pain has been known to return after a period of effectiveness.

You are getting sleepy (and nauseous and dizzy and ...)

The adverse effects of carbamazepine are sedation, GI upset, and ataxia (problems with balance). Monitoring blood counts is necessary because of rare instances of bone marrow depression and thrombocytopenia.

Sodium valproate

An alternative to carbamazepine, sodium valproate is better tolerated, although GI upset occasionally occurs, and alopecia has been known to occur as well. Fortunately, these adverse effects reverse when the drug is stopped. Rarely, hepatic function is affected, so liver enzyme levels must be monitored.

Gabapentin

An increasingly popular anticonvulsant drug is gabapentin, which was originally developed as an ad-

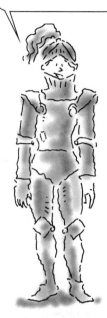

Did someone say lancinating? Sounds like the perfect job for an anticonvulsant.

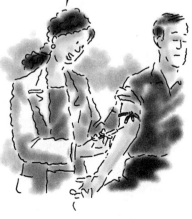

Be sure to monitor blood count in your patient taking carbamazepine to detect possible bone marrow depression or thrombocytopenia.

junct for anticonvulsant therapies. It's especially effective in alleviating pain from peripheral neuropathy and reflex sympathetic dystrophy. It has a low incidence of adverse effects, which are generally similar to those of other anticonvulsant medications.

Phenytoin

Phenytoin is effective in stopping the shooting pain of nerve damage. It has a long half-life and a narrow therapeutic range, and its rate of metabolism is affected by other medicines. It causes a number of unpleasant adverse effects, including skin reactions, nystagmus, and GI upset. Although fairly common in the past, it's now rarely used for pain management; its primary use is for seizure disorders.

> The most popular drugs never cause any trouble. I mean, who wants Chloe Nazepam when you can take Gabby Pentin?

Clonazepam

Clonazepam, a benzodiazepine, has also been used with some success. However, it causes significant sedation, so much so that most patients can't tolerate it in therapeutic doses. Also, because it's a benzodiazepine, dependence is highly likely and withdrawal can produce a host of problems.

Surgical interventions

The decision to pursue surgery to treat CNP must take into account the patient's present condition and the long-term benefits weighed against the possible risks. The patient's quality of life is the most important variable. There are two common surgical interventions used to treat CNP: cordotomy and neurectomy.

> Always weigh the long-term benefits against the risks of surgery to treat CNP.

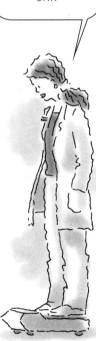

Cordotomy

Cordotomy unilaterally or bilaterally severs the nerve fibers in the spinal cord. Doing so prevents nerve impulse transmission to the brain, thus blocking the pain pathway. Because pain and the sensation of temperature travel the same pathway, patients who undergo this procedure will experience temperature sensation impairment as well.

Neurectomy

Neurectomy resects one or more peripheral branches of the cranial or spinal nerves. It's a safe, quick procedure requiring only local or regional anesthesia. Even so, peripheral nerves control motor and sensory output, so motor loss occurs concomitantly with the loss of pain sensation. In addition, pain relief is commonly temporary. For these reasons, neurectomy isn't common practice, although peripheral neurectomy is performed as a last resort to treat trigeminal neuralgia.

> Fasten your seat belt. We're entering the dorsal root entry zone!

Dorsal root entry zone

Dorsal root entry zone (DREZ) is a surgical procedure that involves making a series of lesions in the DREZ of the spinal cord. This procedure is indicated for such CNP disorders as postherpetic neuralgia, phantom limb pain, and severe facial pain. It requires laminectomies and general anesthesia. The postoperative period requires 2 to 4 days of bed rest followed by intensive physical therapy. Common complications are wound infection, ataxia, and cerebrospinal fluid (CSF) leakage. Patients who have pain in an extremity with intact motor function may suffer from a transient incoordination postoperatively because the spinal cerebellar tract is crossed by the electrode. This resolves in a few weeks to a few months. However, if the procedure isn't successful at first, repeated procedures may make this condition a permanent problem.

Rhizotomy

Rhizotomy is the selective destruction of the dorsal root of a spinal nerve to relieve pain. Indications for rhizotomy include a limited pain area and a normal life expectancy. Selective nerve blocks are administered first to determine if rhizotomy will be effective. If the patient obtains relief from selective nerve block, a rhizotomy should relieve pain. Rhizotomy results in complete sensory loss; no pain, temperature, or pressure sensations are present.

> Relax. They said "rhizotomy," not "rhinotomy"!

You win some, you lose some

Because this procedure interrupts sensory input, loss of motor function can be a direct result. Therefore, rhizotomy is indicated for thoracic and high cervical pain relief and isn't recommended for pain in extremities or low lumbar areas. Rhizotomy has been successful in

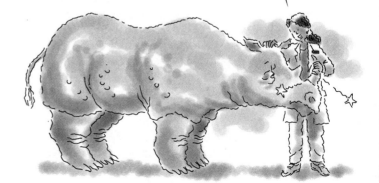

relieving sacral pain resulting from malignancies as well as postra-
diation pain.

Thalamotomy

Thalamotomy involves making lesions stereotactically
in the thalamus, resulting in the interruption of the
spinothalamic tract and absence of pain and temperature sensation in the area opposite and below the level of the lesions. The most common indication for
thalamotomy is cancer pain. Pain relief is obtained
early in the postoperative period but diminishes with
time. Complications of this procedure include intracranial hemorrhage and infection. Ataxia and mild
apathy may also occur postoperatively.

> Rhizotomy may
> help relieve
> postradiation pain.

Nonpharmacologic interventions

Nonpharmacologic interventions to treat CNP include several
forms of physical therapy:
- thermotherapy (most common)—increases collagen extensibility and blood flow and decreases inflammation and joint stiffness
- cryotherapy—causes vasoconstriction of the superficial blood
vessels and decreases the blood flow to the affected area
- transcutaneous electrical nerve stimulation (TENS)—helps relieve low back pain, reflex sympathetic dystrophy, and phantom
limb pain by closing the gate to painful stimuli and, thus, altering
the patient's perception of pain
- strengthening and exercise—restores tone, strength, and length
of muscles.

> Darn that TENS!
> How can I cause pain
> when this stupid gate
> is closed?!

It's complementary, my dear Watson

Alternative and complementary therapies also play a role in
CNP management. These therapies include:
- acupuncture—traditional Chinese treatment based on a
belief in the existence of vital life forces (qi) circulating in
the body that applies needles to an individual's "acupoints"
to influence the circulation of qi and aid in pain management
- relaxation therapy—meditative practice in which the patient focuses on an image, a sound (mantra), or his own
breathing to achieve a state of calm and heightened awareness that, when combined with a comprehensive pain management plan, can help reduce stress and, thus, pain severity

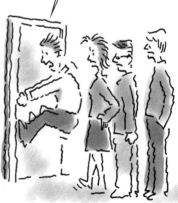

• biofeedback—process in which a person learns to control his physiologic response to pain, such as using relaxation techniques to control heart and respiratory rates and to reduce the overall fatigue and pain resulting from such reactions as tensing muscles.

Psychosocial concerns

The psychological impact of CNP is significant. The health care provider should be aware of three main problems that affect the patient's overall quality of life:

- depression

- anxiety

- sleep disturbance.

Blues clues

Depression can arise from the loss of social role functioning and the depletion of energy reserves. It commonly causes or is caused by sleep disturbances. Depression can be treated through antidepressants and psychotherapy as well as methods tailored to the individual's needs but generally geared to improving his mentation, energy level, and ability to work.

Taking the edge off

Cognitive therapeutic techniques, such as relaxation therapy, distraction, and desensitization, focus on influencing the patient's interpretation of the pain experience. These therapies are common, effective ways to help the patient cope with anxiety. Behavioral therapies, such as biofeedback, help the patient develop skills to manage and change his reaction to pain. These therapies are adjuncts to medication and can help the patient reduce anxiety by feeling more in control of his pain experience.

To sleep, perchance to rest

Sleep is necessary for many psychological functions, including concentration, stress management, and performance of activities of daily living (ADLs) despite pain. In the past, benzodiazepines were prescribed to induce sleep; however, these quickly produce dependence and cause significant sedation. Now, greater focus is placed on optimizing analgesic and antidepressant dosing to allow the patient to sleep more restfully.

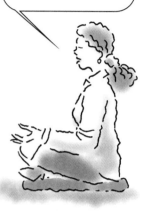

Relaxation therapy can help reduce pain severity through a heightened state of awareness and calm. Ooomm...

Help patients develop skills to manage their reaction to pain. They'll feel more in control when they know how to rein in the pain. Yee Haw!

CNP disorders

Many patients suffer from chronic pain that remains undiagnosed. Although not all CNP can be associated with a disorder, several disorders commonly cause CNP, including:

- fibromyalgia syndrome
- herpes zoster
- low back pain
- migraine headache
- myofascial pain syndrome
- osteoarthritis
- peripheral neuropathy
- phantom limb pain
- postherpetic neuralgia
- reflex sympathetic dystrophy
- rheumatoid arthritis
- sickle cell anemia
- trigeminal neuralgia.

Fibromyalgia syndrome

Fibromyalgia syndrome (FMS) is characterized by tender spots or muscle aching in several areas of the body as well as disturbed sleep patterns. Nearly 5 million people in the United States suffer from FMS. It typically affects women more than men, and women primarily in their 40s. Because the symptoms are vague, this condition is likely to be perceived as "all in the patient's head" by family members and some health care providers.

Finding a pattern

Research has shown that a pattern of aching exists in these patients, where tender spots are identified in consistent locations on digital examination.

No whys or wherefores

There's no known cause of FMS. Because anxiety and depression commonly coexist with this type of pain, it was thought that they might be at least part of the cause. However, more recent clinical findings suggest that anxiety and depression are more likely the effect of the vicious cycle of chronic pain.

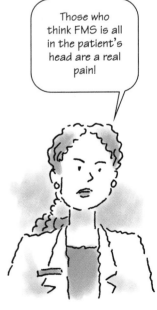

Those who think FMS is all in the patient's head are a real pain!

Here's a thought...

There are many newer theories about the cause of FMS. One suggests poor muscle metabolism might be responsible. Dysfunctional metabolism of toxins releases them into the tissues, causing a metabolic defect or hypoxia in the muscle. This theory answers the problem of joint pain; however, it doesn't successfully address the organ pain (such as in the bladder and stomach) that many patients with FMS experience.

No moanin' with serotonin

A more promising theory suggests that a defect in the central nervous system affects pain perception; patients with FMS have lower serotonin levels than patients without pain. Serotonin levels are inversely proportionate to pain perception; higher levels cause lower pain perception and vice versa. Some interesting research also indicates that FMS may have a neurogenic cause; the concentration of substance P, a peripheral pain neurotransmitter, is several times higher in the CSF of patients with FMS.

What to look for

FMS pain is commonly described as aching, exhausting, or nagging. It doesn't decrease with activity (unlike rheumatoid arthritis pain). Stiffness is common and is relieved by walking around. Patients sometimes experience cramping and spasms as well. The pain is located in discrete areas, most commonly the occiput, neck, back, shoulders, chest wall, elbows, hips, and knees. It tends to worsen in the evening.

> Hang three? FMS patients have shorter periods of delta wave activity during sleep.

Catch the delta wave

Sleep disturbance is characterized by a lack of restfulness upon waking, although the patient may have appeared to sleep soundly through the night. Research has shown that, in the non-REM sleep phases, the EEG of the patient with FMS shows shorter periods of delta-wave activity than those of a normal person. The disruption in this deep sleep phase affects the pain experience when awake.

Assessing FMS

The American College of Rheumatology developed guidelines for identifying FMS pain:
• pain above and below the waist

Fibromyalgia tender points

The patient with fibromyalgia syndrome may complain of specific areas of tenderness, which are indicated in the illustrations below.

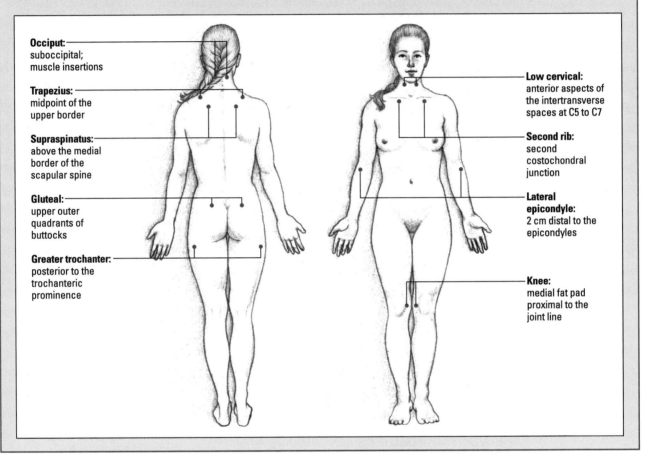

Occiput: suboccipital; muscle insertions

Trapezius: midpoint of the upper border

Supraspinatus: above the medial border of the scapular spine

Gluteal: upper outer quadrants of buttocks

Greater trochanter: posterior to the trochanteric prominence

Low cervical: anterior aspects of the intertransverse spaces at C5 to C7

Second rib: second costochondral junction

Lateral epicondyle: 2 cm distal to the epicondyles

Knee: medial fat pad proximal to the joint line

- pain on both sides of the body
- axial pain (cervical spine, anterior chest, thoracic spine, or low back)
- pain that affects sleep patterns
- pain on digital examination in 11 of 18 tender point sites. (See *Fibromyalgia tender points.*)

Educating the patient with FMS

Fibromyalgia syndrome (FMS) is a chronic pain disorder that involves physiological and psychological issues for the patient. Because a person's quality of life is deeply affected by FMS, the health care provider must use a holistic approach when educating the patient and caregiver. Here are three steps to follow in that process:

Initiate patient and family education by explaining that the pain is real but not life-threatening. Depending on the patient, a psychological evaluation and therapy may be warranted.

Tell the patient that FMS requires lifestyle changes, such as balancing activity with rest and sleep. Explain that this may mean taking a less demanding job and taking more frequent breaks at work and at home. Unfortunately, this can cause stress as well.

Explain the various pharmacologic treatments to the patient, including their rate of effectiveness and any adverse effects. Tell the patient that tricyclic antidepressants (TCAs) and muscle relaxants have been used, but aren't always effective and have the unfortunate adverse effect of sedation. However, a combination of a serotonin uptake inhibitor, such as paroxetine (Paxil) or fluoxetine (Prozac), and the TCA amitriptyline (Elavil) have been effective. In addition, explain that using opioids to treat flare-ups is controversial, but some providers feel its use is warranted when other medications don't work.

Managing FMS

Because there's no known physical pathology involved in FMS, treatment varies. Usually, a rheumatologist is the primary health care provider. Be sure to provide thorough patient education on various FMS treatments. (See *Educating the patient with FMS*.)

Herpes zoster

Herpes zoster (HZ) is believed to result from a reactivation of dormant varicella viruses left over from chickenpox infection. Although this syndrome is commonly seen in immunocompromised patients, it also appears in otherwise healthy

Just when you think it's safe, we can wake up and cause trouble. Heh, heh, heh...

varicella
varicella
varicella

people. The triggering mechanism for the lesions and pain is unknown.

What to look for

The usual pattern of pain in herpes zoster begins with a period of itching, tingling, or aching along a dermatome that lasts for several days, followed by the appearance of vesicles on the skin in a line that follows a nerve pathway. (See *Tracing the path of herpes zoster*.) The vesicles eventually fill with pus, then break open and crust over. The lesions are highly contagious during this time. The pain is typically severe, with deep soreness and sharp, stabbing pain. These symptoms may be accompanied by headache, malaise, nausea, and a low-grade fever. The pain often takes weeks or months to subside after the lesions heal.

Assessing herpes zoster pain

Pain assessment scales are used to understand the severity and character of the pain. Greater intensity of pain with the initial infection increases the likelihood of developing postherpetic neuralgia (PHN). (See "Postherpetic neuralgia," page 191.)

Managing herpes zoster pain

The first step in managing herpes zoster pain is aggressive administration of opioid analgesics, antiviral agents, and nerve blocks, if necessary. This aggressive drug therapy has been effective in decreasing the duration and severity of the disease, the pain caused by it, and the incidence of subsequent PHN.

Short-acting opioids, such as oxycodone, are best for preventing light-headedness and balance problems commonly experienced by elderly patients. They should be used starting with a low dose, as tolerated. The patient should be aware that driving is prohibited while taking these drugs and that balance problems may result from their sedative effect.

Talk about walking a tightrope! Short-acting opioids given to prevent balance problems can sometimes cause them.

Low back pain

Low back pain, a very common CNP disorder, is a big challenge for health care providers. Almost 75% of the population will have back pain at some point in their lives. In many cases, the pain will subside in a few weeks. However, in some cases, the pain doesn't subside. In fact, low back pain is the third most common cause of disability in the United States.

Tracing the path of herpes zoster

The herpes zoster virus infects the nerves that innervate the skin, eyes, and ears. Each nerve (tagged for its corresponding vertebral source) emanates from the spine, banding and branching around the body to innervate a skin area called a dermatome. The herpes zoster rash erupts along the course of the affected nerve fibers, covering the skin in one or more dermatomes (as shown below).

The thoracic (T) and lumbar (L) dermatomes are the most commonly affected, but others, such as those covering the cervical (C) and sacral (S) areas, may also be affected. Dermatome levels may vary and overlap.

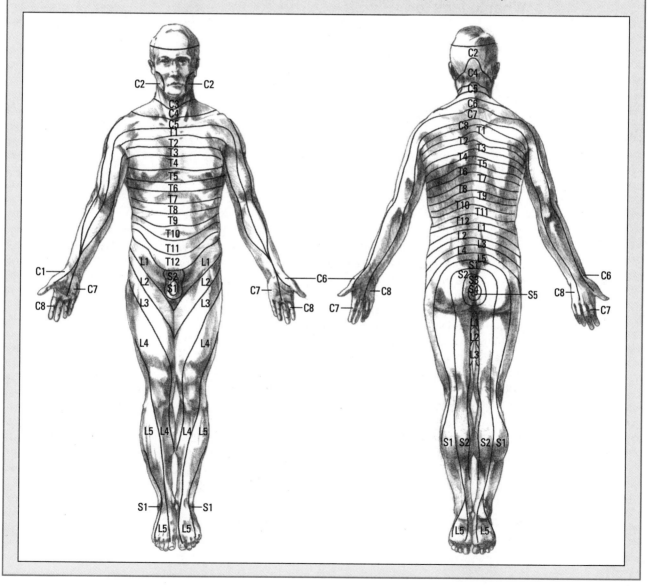

Lift, drive, smoke, and suffer

Usually, no specific event can be linked to the onset of low back pain. However, certain activities, such as heavy lifting or driving long hours, have a higher occurrence rate. Chronic coughing is also associated with low back pain, and it may be the reason why low back pain occurs more frequently in people who smoke cigarettes.

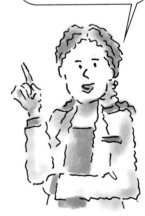

Low back pain is the 3rd most common cause of disability in the United States.

What to look for

Low back pain can be localized to a specific area but may also radiate to the buttocks, perineal area, legs, and feet. There are 2 types of low back pain:

- muscle and tendon injury
- radicular pain.

Tender tendon

Muscle and tendon injury is usually felt as soreness and tenderness. The pain rarely radiates beyond the point of soreness.

Radical radicular

Radicular pain is caused by irritation of the nerves entering and exiting the spinal cord between the vertebral discs or the nerves inside the spinal cord itself. It's commonly a burning, aching pain that radiates into the buttocks and down the back or leg. Treatment of radicular pain is especially challenging because of the many possible causes and the lack of correlation between the type of pain experienced and a logical source.

In many cases, this difficulty has caused providers to be suspicious of the patient's reported experience of pain. However, as always with CNP, it's important to remember that the lack of a clear organic cause (tissue damage) doesn't mean the patient isn't experiencing genuine pain.

Remember, lack of a clear cause for pain doesn't mean the patient isn't in genuine pain.

Assessing low back pain

It's always important to look for possible organic causes of low back pain — even long-standing pain, especially if it has changed in the previous few months. Such conditions as leaking abdominal aortic aneurysm and tumor, which require immediate medical intervention, have been discovered when assessing chronic low back pain.

The unabridged edition

Obtain a complete health history, including records of past diagnostic testing and treatment, as well as a thorough physical examination.

Let's get physical

A thorough physical examination is vital to ensure accurate assessment and diagnosis of the cause of low back pain. It can also reveal problems with the muscles, nerves, spine, and connective tissues. Physical examination of the patient with low back pain should focus on:

- body deformities
- impairments in range of motion
- tender areas
- muscle spasms
- pain on movement of the back
- motor function impairment, such as local muscle weakness or muscle atrophy
- decreased or absent reflexes
- sensory impairments such as loss of sensation in a dermatomal area.

The best way to reveal the cause of low back pain is to conduct a thorough physical exam.

Showing your best moves

Specific maneuvers the practitioner may implement during the examination include:

- adduction of the hips to test symmetric weakness, which suggests myopathy or muscle disorder or, if in a distal muscle, polyneuropathy or peripheral nerve disorder
- palpation over the sacroiliac joint (identified by the dimple overlying the posterior superior iliac spine) to detect tenderness that can pinpoint a common cause of low back pain
- palpation of the sciatic nerve (L4, L5, S1, S2, and S3) to detect tenderness, which may suggest a mass lesion
- lateral bending with the pelvis stabilized by a hand placed on the patient's hip to detect pain or tenderness, especially with radiation to the leg, that suggests underlying cord or nerve root compression (although arthritis, hip infection, rectal infection, or pelvic infection may cause these symptoms in the lumbar spine as well)
- straight leg raises to identify nerve root pain (radicular pain) from a herniated disc.

MRI and CT scanning can detect underlying pathologies that might contribute to low back pain.

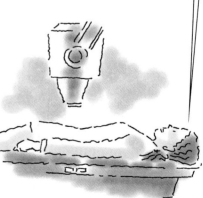

Testing, 1, 2, 3...

Diagnostic testing, especially magnetic resonance imaging and computed tomography scanning, detects underlying abnormalities as well as the extent of any pathologic processes. Sometimes urinalysis and blood studies, including complete blood count and erythrocyte sedimentation rate, are conducted to rule out other pathologic sources of back pain, such as cancer and infection.

Managing low back pain

Patients with acute low back pain and chronic low back pain require different treatment approaches. Management of chronic low back pain involves oral analgesia, physical therapy, injected analgesia, and surgery. Some patients benefit from the use of opioid therapy and can function well on long-term use of opioids. Physical therapies, such as thermotherapy, TENS, and massage, can help ease pain. Stretching and strengthening exercises can help prevent future low back injuries. In all therapies, it's important to emphasize proper body posture and alignment.

Injecting a bit of controversy

Injection therapy, a controversial treatment for chronic low back pain, involves local or regional injection of a local anesthetic and steroids. Injections can be made in soft tissue, trigger points along the muscle, and ligaments that support the muscle in the lumbar spine. For patients who have undergone conservative treatments without success, steroids may be injected into the epidural space at the location of the pain to decrease inflammation and relieve pain. This approach may provide pain relief; however, it doesn't help confirm the source of pain. Thus, it doesn't account for referred pain, which can be a symptom of a possibly serious underlying condition that requires immediate intervention.

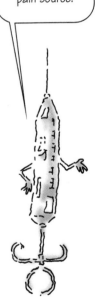

Injection therapy relieves pain, but it's controversial because it doesn't help identify the pain source.

It's complicated

More invasive therapies, such as epidural injection of local anesthetics and steroids, sometimes provide relief and have been used for many years, although there's no scientific evidence yet that these methods are more effective than conservative treatments. They also have a higher risk of complications, including complete motor block causing respiratory arrest and puncture of the dura causing prolonged headaches.

When all else fails, try surgery

Surgical interventions are reserved for patients whose pain hasn't responded to other interventions. Only 1% to 2% of patients with low back pain requires surgical intervention. These interventions include:
• nerve root decompression, in which a small portion of the bone over the nerve root or disc material from under the nerve root is

removed to give the nerve root more space and provide a better healing environment
• spinal fusion, in which specific vertebrae are immobilized by insertion of a wedge-shaped piece of bone or bone chips between the vertebrae to immobilize and stabilize the vertebral column weakened by degenerative disc disease or injury.

Out of fashion

Surgical procedures have been a popular treatment in the past, especially for pain associated with a prolapsed intervertebral disc. However, many individuals who have prolapses of the disc don't have symptoms, and many with prolapsed discs have pain that subsides on its own without surgery. Surgery also has a risk of complications and hasn't been shown to be more effective than conservative measures. Thus, surgery has become less popular in recent years, although some patients for whom other interventions have failed may find relief with surgery.

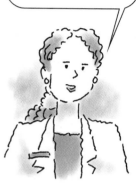

Surgery is almost as out of fashion as nurses' caps, but some patients may find relief with surgery when other methods have failed.

Migraine headache

Migraine headaches affect millions of Americans and three times as many women as men. It's a recurrent disorder and is typically found in the same family (genetic link). The cause of migraine is unknown; however, it's believed to stem from a disorder of the brain's neurotransmitter system (especially serotonin). Migraine can be caused by:
• endogenous triggers, such as depression and menstruation
• environmental triggers, such as stress and emotional distress
• exogenous triggers, such as skipping meals and eating certain foods such as chocolate
• genetic predisposition
• light patterns such as strobe lights.
    There are two types of migraine headache:

Classic—about 20% of migraine headaches, which are preceded by an aura, last 10 to 20 minutes, and usually involve some kind of visual disturbance, such as flashing sparks, weakness, or dizziness.

Common—similar to the classic type but without an aura preceding the onset of pain.

    In both cases, the pain is unilateral, pulsating, and moderately to severely painful. The intensity of the pain is made worse by activity, light, and noise. The headache lasts 4 to 72 hours and is commonly accompanied by nausea and even vomiting.

Classic migraine is preceded by an aura and usually accompanied by visual disturbances.

Assessing migraine headache

It's important to obtain a complete description of the headaches, including family history, age of onset, frequency, triggers, and affected areas. When assessing a patient, be aware that migraine headaches have at least four of the following characteristics:
- severe pain greater than 5 on a scale of 1 to 10
- pain experienced only on one side of the head
- pain intensified by exposure to light
- pulsating, or throbbing, pain
- pain worsened when performing ADLs
- pain accompanied by nausea
- pain aggravated by noise.

Managing migraine headache

The goal of pain management for migraine headache is to relieve pain during attacks and prevent recurrences.

Pain, pain, go away...

Several drugs are used to relieve pain during a migraine "attack."
- *Sumatriptan* (Imitrex) is a serotonin-receptor agonist that causes brief, selective vasoconstriction. This decreases blood flow, thus blocking neurogenic inflammation of the trigeminal nerve and inhibiting sensory nerve output around cerebral blood vessels of the brainstem. This treatment is effective for about 70% of migraine sufferers.
- *Antiemetics* are used to increase gastric motility and allow absorption of analgesic medication more quickly. Some research results suggest that combining metoclopramide and aspirin is as effective as administering sumatriptan (and much less costly).
- *Ergotamine* has been used for years to treat migraine headache. It stimulates smooth muscle and causes vasoconstriction, which helps counteract the painful dilation stage of the headache. It also decreases neurogenic inflammation. It may be given orally as well as rectally (a distinct advantage for patients suffering from nausea). It's typically given with caffeine, which enhances absorption. Disadvantages of the drug are nausea and vomiting (which can be avoided with concomitant use of antiemetics) and rebound headaches (which can occur even when the drug is taken only twice per week).
- *I.V. steroids, dihydroergotamine (Migranal), and metoclopramide (Reglan)*, along with hospitalization, may be required in severe cases of intractable migraine (lasting more than 72 hours).

Memory jogger

To remember the characteristics of migraine headache, remember the pneumonic **SULTANS:**

S = severe (pain greater than 5 on a scale of 10)

U = unilateral (on one side of the head)

L = light sensitivity (photophobia)

T = throbbing

A = activity (worsens with activity)

N = nausea

S = sound sensitivity.

The goal of migraine treatment is to make the pain go away and keep it from coming back.

...and stay away another day

Prophylactic therapy for migraine headache allows the patient to prevent chronic recurrence. Two classes of drugs are effective in preventing chronic migraine headache:

• *Beta-adrenergic blockers*, specifically propranolol (Inderol), are the most widely used treatment for prophylactic migraine therapy. These drugs are thought to inhibit vasodilation of the carotid artery and are effective migraine prophylaxis for about 50% to 60% of patients. Because of the adverse effects of these drugs, such as hypotension, fatigue, bronchospasm, rash, fever, and impotence, their use isn't always advisable. In addition, abrupt withdrawal could lead to cardiac complications.

• *Anticonvulsants*. Valproic acid has been recently approved by the Federal Drug Administration for prophylactic treatment of migraines. Although the mechanism of action of these drugs on migraine isn't entirely understood, researchers think it may involve gamma-aminobutyric acid, an inhibitory receptor in the brain. Valproic acid should be used only as a second-line treatment because of its association with neural tube defects in babies of women taking it during their 1st trimester of pregnancy.

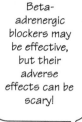

Beta-adrenergic blockers may be effective, but their adverse effects can be scary!

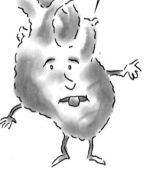

Myofascial pain syndrome

Myofascial pain syndrome (MPS) is highly localized. It occurs most commonly in the postural muscles of the neck, the shoulder girdle, and the lower back. It's characterized by the presence of trigger points, which are small hypersensitive areas within tight muscle bands. It can occur as a result of an acute or chronic muscle strain. It's sometimes associated with other CNP disorders, such as FMS and arthritis.

What to look for

Onset of MPS can be acute or gradual and tends to be related to an overworked muscle group. The pain in MPS is localized over the trigger point and can sometimes be felt by the patient upon palpation of the area. The pain can be deep and aching and alternately dull or burning. The pain is commonly adjacent to the trigger point itself.

MPS is usually related to an overworked — hmph — muscle — ach — group.

Assessing MPS

Manual palpation is commonly used to identify the exact trigger point of MPS.

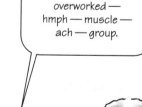

Meet the meters

Algometers (handheld pressure gauges) can measure the amount of pressure needed to induce pain, which aids in the detection of MPS trigger points. Tissue compliance meters measure the relative hardness of tissue by measuring the pressure needed to indent an area of skin. These tools are useful for quantifying for patients the difference between normal tissue and tissue at trigger points and demonstrating the effectiveness of treatment. These quantified results also provide valuable documentation for legal purposes. There are no other laboratory or imaging studies that identify affected tissues.

Managing MPS

Treatment of MPS focuses on eliminating trigger points and enabling the patient to return to full function. Pharmacologic interventions, such as nonopioid (NSAIDs) and opioid therapies, are effective for limited periods to alleviate pain but shouldn't be considered long-term options.

Spray is okay but ice is nice

Sometimes the muscle is anesthetized with local anesthetic or sprayed with a cooling solution such as Fluori-Methane. Because Fluori-Methane is a fluorocarbon contributing to pollution, new techniques use ice stroking instead. Ice stroking involves wrapping ice in thin plastic to prevent overcooling, stroking the muscle with ice, and then passively stretching the muscle.

Don't repeat this...

In addition, identifying and reducing repetitive activities that overwork the muscle can aid in pain reduction. Local anesthetic injections at trigger points reduce pain, increase range of motion, and can last for months. Nonpharmacologic approaches, such as massage, acupuncture, ultrasound, and sustained digital pressure, have also been used with some success.

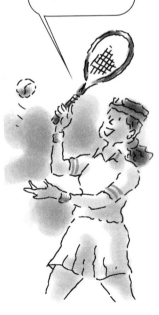

Reducing repetitive activities that overwork a muscle can help reduce pain, but it won't help my game much!

Osteoarthritis

Osteoarthritis, or degenerative joint disease, is the most common form of arthritis, with nearly 60 million persons affected in the United States. It's also the leading cause of disability in elderly patients. The disease results from cartilage breakdown in weight-bearing and finger joints. Many factors influence the development of osteoarthritis, including family history and previous damage to the joint from injury or surgery. (See *What happens in osteoarthritis*.)

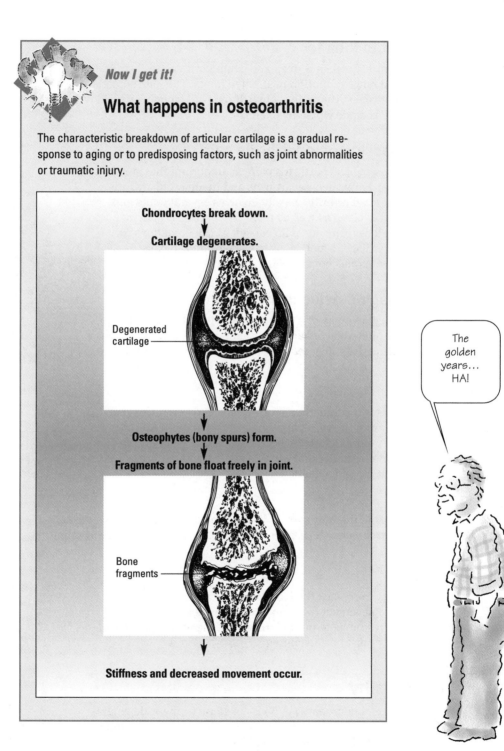

Now I get it!

What happens in osteoarthritis

The characteristic breakdown of articular cartilage is a gradual response to aging or to predisposing factors, such as joint abnormalities or traumatic injury.

Chondrocytes break down.

Cartilage degenerates.

Degenerated cartilage

Osteophytes (bony spurs) form.

Fragments of bone float freely in joint.

Bone fragments

Stiffness and decreased movement occur.

The golden years... HA!

What to look for

Osteoarthritis pain is deep and aching, with related stiffness and limited range of motion in affected joints. The pain sometimes extends to nearby muscle groups. It tends to worsen as the day goes on and is made worse by exercise.

Assessing osteoarthritis pain

In assessing osteoarthritis pain, an important first step is to distinguish between osteoarthritis and rheumatoid arthritis. Rheumatoid arthritis usually involves several joints and causes swelling as well as pain. Osteoarthritis pain involves a deep, aching pain caused by the breakdown of joint cartilage, which leads to bone rubbing against bone. The symptoms worsen as the disease progresses.

Managing osteoarthritis pain

Although overuse of a joint makes osteoarthritis pain worse, underuse results in further stiffness and limitation. Gentle activity may reduce pain if preceded by heat application to relax muscles and followed by cold packs.

Easy does it

Exercises to strengthen muscles are also helpful as long as they don't result in more pain. Other effective physical therapies include hydrotherapy, thermotherapy, use of a firm mattress, and use of a neck or lumbar brace at night for spinal pain.

Drugs that deliver

Nonopioid therapy, such as aspirin and acetaminophen, can usually control pain. NSAIDs are also effective and may reduce swelling as well.

The replacements

Surgery to replace the joint is used in severe cases. Total joint replacement (hip and knee) provides pain relief and improves range of motion. However, the universal risks of surgery must be considered.

> Apply heat to relax muscles before gentle exercise and apply cold to muscles when you're finished.

> Total joint replacement relieves pain and improves range of motion.

> But I've grown quite attached to this hip!

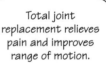

Peripheral neuropathy

Peripheral neuropathy (PN) is a general term for degeneration of nerve function in the extremities. The most common causes of PN are diabetes mellitus, peripheral vascular disease, and drug toxicity as well as a number of rare causes, including human immunodeficiency virus, multiple sclerosis, and connective tissue disorders. It can also occur in people with none of these conditions.

What to look for

There's usually a period of months to a few years after PN develops before it becomes painful. PN pain can be one of three types:
- continuous, deep, burning, aching, or bruising pain
- sudden, "electric shock" pain
- bad sunburn or a crawling feeling on the skin.

The pain is often experienced in a "stocking-glove" distribution, the pain being worst at the tips of the toes and fingers and more proximal areas being numb and tingling.

Assessing PN pain

The exact type of pain and its distribution indicate which type of pain medication to use. Neuralgic pain, or pain that is burning, freezing, or shooting, is more likely to respond to antidepressant and anticonvulsant therapy.

It's electric

Electromyography (EMG) can be done to study nerve conduction. However, EMG doesn't necessarily measure damage to the smaller nerve fibers that are typically affected in PN. In addition, a normal EMG doesn't rule out disease.

Pinpoint assessment

PN pain is usually described as continual, deep, burning, and aching. Sudden stabbing or shooting pain also may occur. Reports of skin sensitivity, such as the feeling of a sunburn, increase. Paresthesia also may occur with proximal pain in the distal sites of the patient's extremities, which can be described as pins and needles. PN pain starts in the toes and feet and progresses to the legs. In the upper body, similar pain occurs.

Managing PN pain

TCAs provide varying degrees of pain relief for most patients with PN. They're particularly effective in relieving neuralgic pain, such as burning and tingling. Doses are usually lower than those used for treating depression, which reduces the occurrence of adverse effects. If one drug in this class doesn't work, usually another will, so the provider should attempt to use several different anti-

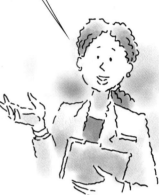

Some types of PN pain, such as neuralgic pain, respond best to antidepressants and anticonvulsants.

Even if the first antidepressant doesn't work, another one probably will.

depressants before considering other pharmacologic treatment. Anticonvulsants are also used and are most effective with lancinating pain.

Bring in the opioids

Opioids have been used with some success in patients who haven't responded to antidepressants or anticonvulsants. However, it's important to try various TCAs and anticonvulsants for at least 2 weeks each time before turning to opioid treatment.

The topic is topical

Topical therapy, such as capsaicin cream (Capsin), is sometimes helpful, although it can cause unbearable burning. Topical lidocaine (Xylocaine) is currently under review as a possible treatment for PN pain.

Phantom limb pain

Almost all amputees have some form of phantom sensation. That is, they feel a sensation of the absent limb being present. Nearly 85% also experience pain in the absent limb, especially if there was pain in the limb before amputation. The phantom sensations may slowly disappear over time, commonly with the sensation of telescoping of the limb as it seems to become shorter. However, for many patients the sensations persist.

What to look for

Phantom limb pain is commonly described as crushing or tearing. However, some patients experience burning, cramping, and shocking or shooting pains.

Assessing phantom limb pain

Patients are commonly reluctant to admit to these sensations out of fear that they were "all in the head" or that they would be told this by unsympathetic clinicians. Thus, it's important to ask about phantom limb pain and inform the patient of the common nature of this kind of pain in amputees.

Managing phantom limb pain

Because there's no actual tissue to treat in most cases, managing phantom limb pain isn't easy. Patient education involves helping them adjust to the probability that the pain may never be completely gone.

It isn't in your head. Nearly 85% of patients who've undergone amputation experience some sensation of the missing limb.

New techniques, better results

Recent treatment techniques before amputation have shown the most encouraging results for reducing phantom limb pain. Preoperative infusion of epidural opioids, when combined with local anesthetics for 1 to 3 days before surgery, prevents or minimizes postoperative and phantom limb pain.

Mixed measures, effective treatments

Pharmacologic treatments combined with nonpharmacologic measures such as biofeedback have been effective as well:
• Muscle relaxants combined with muscle tension biofeedback help treat cramping pain.
• Vasodilators with temperature biofeedback inhibit burning pain.

No more surgery, thank you

Surgical techniques aren't effective in reducing or relieving phantom limb pain. Removal of more of the stump, rhizotomy, cordotomy, or sympathectomy usually results in temporary relief only, with longer-term complications that may be more harmful.

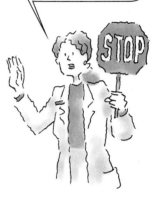

Surgery for phantom limb pain provides only temporary relief and may lead to long-term complications.

How nervy

Nerve blocks, injections of local anesthetic and steroids into the nerve stump, can be effective. If this treatment reduces pain, phenol or cryotherapy is sometimes used to eradicate the neuroma stump, which can be the cause of the pain.

Count to TENS

TENS therapy applied to the stump or the spinal cord has shown positive results and is less invasive than nerve blocks and surgical procedures.

The skin of patients with PHN is typically sensitive to even a light touch.

Postherpetic neuralgia

Postherpetic neuralgia (PHN) is pain that lingers past the normal healing time for the lesions of a herpes zoster outbreak. It develops in about 10% to 15% of cases of herpes zoster, and is most likely to occur in elderly patients. In fact, 80% of patients over age 80 will develop PHN after a bout of herpes zoster.

What to look for

With PHN, the severe pain of herpes zoster gradually becomes a more continuous, deep, burning, aching pain. It sometimes feels more like electric shocks or sharp stabs. The skin is typically highly sensitive to even light touch. While the pain usually follows the area of the lesions, it occasionally spreads to unrelated areas.

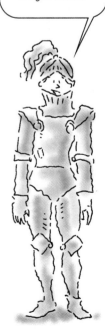

Assessing PHN pain

When assessing PHN pain, note its location and duration, whether it radiates, the quality (burning, lancinating, dull), what aggravates it (movement), and what relieves it (analgesics). Also note if the patient feels a decrease in sensation.

Managing PHN pain

TCAs, especially desipramine (Norpramin), are the first choice for relief from PHN. However, because these drugs have many adverse effects, such as sedation, dizziness, constipation, and dry mouth, some health care providers avoid their use in elderly patients. Even so, if the dose is initially low and gradually increased as needed, many adverse effects can be avoided. Some patients require an anticonvulsant for relief of lancinating pain, but an antidepressant alone typically controls this type of pain as well.

The skinny on topicals

Topical therapy is sometimes helpful for allodynia and itching. Lidoderm gel and patches, topical forms of lidocaine, are applied to the nerve endings in the skin to alleviate pressure- and movement-induced pain and itching. Aspirin in chloroform and capsaicin cream are also effective topical treatments, although the latter causes burning that may be as unpleasant to the patient as the original pain.

Start low and slow

Opioids are the focus of new attention in the treatment of CNP, and some research finds them to be effective for relief of PHN. Adverse effects are a concern with these drugs as well, so low starting doses with gradual increases are also recommended.

If at first you don't succeed, try clonidine

Clonidine (Catapres) and mexiletine (Mexitil) have been used with varying success for pain unrelieved by antidepressants, topicals, and opioids. Nerve blocks are commonly performed, although there's little research to prove it's more effective than these other medicines.

Surgery, smurgery

Surgical procedures, such as nerve resectioning and ablation, haven't been shown to be more effective than pharmacologic treatments.

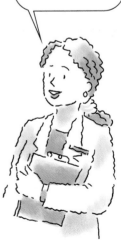

As with any drug, treatment with antidepressants should take into account their possible adverse effects as well as possible benefits.

Sit back and relax

Biofeedback and relaxation therapies are also effective if the patient is willing to learn and practice them. Simpler interventions, such as ice packs, can help to relieve pain and itching.

Relaxation is an effective tool for relieving PHN.

Reflex sympathetic dystrophy

Reflex sympathetic dystrophy (RSD) is one of a group of disorders that fall in the category of complex regional pain syndrome (CRPS). There are two types of CRPS:
• CRPS I is RSD, arising from damage to bone and surrounding soft tissue
• CRPS II is causalgia, arising from direct damage to a nerve.

RSD is a chronic nerve disorder that involves pathologic changes in the bone and skin. Profuse sweating, tissue swelling, and sensitivity to touch are hallmark signs of RSD. The disorder can occur at the site of injury but may also occur without the presence of injury.

The cause of RSD isn't clearly understood. It's now believed that sympathetic nervous system overstimulation is part of the syndrome rather than the cause. A patient may exhibit sympathetic dependent pain or sympathetic independent pain.

A single laboratory test isn't available to diagnose RSD. Therefore, the practitioner must assess and document subjective complaints from the health history and, if present, the objective findings from the physical examination to support the diagnosis.

Fractures and surgery and lesions, oh my!

Because this syndrome is commonly caused by trauma to the extremities, other conditions that may cause RSD include fractures, sprains, surgery, nerve damage, blood vessel damage, and brain lesions. It affects the skin, nerves, blood vessels, muscles, and bones simultaneously. The syndrome can affect patients at any age but is more common between ages 40 and 60.

RSD can occur at the site of injury but may also occur without an accompanying injury.

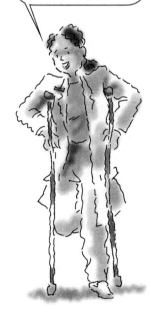

What to look for

The pain of RSD is severe. Pain is experienced near the area of injury with symptoms of muscle spasm, local swelling, burning pain, bone softening, joint stiffness or tenderness, limited range of motion, and skin and nail changes. As the injury heals, the pain doesn't subside but becomes diffuse.

How long has this been going on?

The pain is described as a deep, burning pain that's sometimes throbbing, pressing, or shooting. It doesn't follow the course of any particular nerve. A small percentage of patients have developed generalized RSD affecting the entire body. The duration of RSD varies. In mild cases, it may last for weeks followed by remission. However, in many cases the pain continues for years.

Please don't touch

Normal movement exacerbates the pain, and the pain commonly worsens when the limb is lowered. This makes it difficult to walk and carry out ADLs. There's also hypersensitivity of the skin (allodynia) to touch. Emotional responses develop as a result of anticipation of pain. The level of pain fluctuates and tends to be worse at night. Some patients have pain-free periods that can last for several days or weeks, but the pain returns.

Count 'em — three

Each stage of RSD encompasses changes in skin, nails, joints, ligaments, muscles, and bones. There are 3 stages of RSD:

✌️ *Stage 1* — 1 to 3 months of severe burning at the injury site, muscle spasm, limited range of motion, rapid nail and hair growth, and vasospasm, which affects skin surface temperature and color (warm, red, and dry changing to cold, cyanotic, and sweaty)

✌️ *Stage 2* — 3 to 6 months of intensifying, increasingly diffuse pain; spreading swelling that changes from soft to hard (brawny); cracked nails; decreased hair and nail growth; severe, increasingly diffuse osteoporosis; further muscle atrophy

✌️ *Stage 3* — worsening pain resistant to treatment (retractable) and can involve an entire limb; continued bone, skin, nail, hair, and muscle changes that become irreversible; flexor tendon contractures; deformed appearance; inability to use limbs; and continued bone softening.

Assessing RSD

The patient with RSD usually reports unexplained swelling, burning pain, and temperature changes in the lower part of the arm or leg. To confirm the condition, a three-phase bone scan is used to assess osteoporotic changes that sometimes occur with RSD. In addition, sympathetic nerve blocks are administered using phentolamine. Pain relief following this procedure strongly suggests RSD. However, neither of these diagnostic procedures provides absolute confirmation.

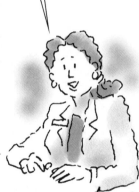

RSD pain is severe and becomes diffuse when the initial injury heals.

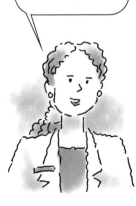

Think of RSD when your patient mentions unexplained swelling, burning pain, and temperature changes.

Because of the severity of RSD pain, patients with RSD are commonly anxious and agitated. Health care providers commonly mistake this behavior as a sign of neurosis rather than RSD.

Managing RSD pain

The key to successful RSD pain management is early detection. Unfortunately, the gradual onset of this syndrome makes early detection extremely difficult. The longer the patient has these symptoms, the less promising the prognosis. Treatment goals include pain relief and restoration of normal function. However, because the limb is often dystrophic, the latter can be difficult to achieve.

Initial treatment is multifaceted and includes pharmacologic and nonpharmacologic therapies. Invasive measures are used only if initial therapy with noninvasive treatments are unsuccessful.

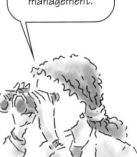

Early detection is the key to successful RSD pain management.

Down on the pharm

Medications commonly prescribed for RSD pain include:
• nonopioids, such as NSAIDs, for pain associated with inflammation and tramadol hydrochloride for continuous pain not caused by inflammation
• TCAs for constant pain or sleep disturbances
• opioids for severe pain
• clonidine patch to decrease pain by decreasing sympathetic nervous system transmission
• muscle relaxants, such as baclofen, for muscle cramping
• local anesthetics, such as lidocaine, injected into the paravertebral area to anesthetize sympathetic ganglia in the spinal cord
• sympathetic blocks administered at 2-week intervals (to determine effectiveness) to relieve pain and determine location of sympathetic nervous system dysfunction so that sympathectomy may be performed to achieve permanent RSD remission.

Practice PT carefully

Nonpharmacologic therapies for RSD pain include TENS to block pain by closing off neurotransmissions to the spinal cord, elevation of the affected extremity to decrease swelling, and physical therapy to help with range of motion (carried out with extreme caution to avoid stressing the muscles).

Rheumatoid arthritis

Rheumatoid arthritis affects small and large joints, causing enlargement and sometimes crippling deformity. It's two times more common in women than in men. Onset can begin in early adulthood but is most common during middle age.

What to look for

Rheumatoid arthritis pain is usually described as aching and burning. It tends to be worse first thing in the morning or after a period of inactivity. Typically, there are periods of inflammation and pain alternating with pain-free periods. During flare-ups, fatigue, lack of appetite, and low-grade fever are also common.

Assessing rheumatoid arthritis pain

Distinguishing between osteoarthritis and rheumatoid arthritis is important. Rheumatoid arthritis usually involves more than one joint and small joints as well as the large, weight-bearing joints affected by osteoarthritis. Over time, rheumatoid arthritis sufferers will develop deformities of the hands and feet and, possibly, rheumatoid nodules.

> Rheumatoid arthritis is two times more common in women than in men.

> Phew!

> Uh oh.

It's in the blood

Blood testing for rheumatoid factor is a standard diagnostic test, although approximately 20% of those with rheumatoid arthritis will test negative for rheumatoid factor. Increased erythrocyte sedimentation rate, anemia, and thrombocytosis are also common in patients with rheumatoid arthritis.

Managing rheumatoid arthritis pain

The same pain management methods used for osteoarthritis pain, such as gentle activity preceded by heat and followed by cold, hydrotherapy, and thermotherapy, are effective relief for rheumatoid arthritis pain.

Many meds

Nonopioids, such as aspirin, acetaminophen, and NSAIDs, are used in the initial treatment of rheumatoid arthritis pain. As rheumatoid arthritis worsens, various drugs may be used to achieve relief:
• Corticosteroids, given orally or by injection to the affected area, are first-line drugs used for short flare-ups to decrease inflammation. Adverse effects of these drugs (osteoporosis, moon face, buffalo hump) prohibit long-term use.

> Unlike osteoarthritis, rheumatoid arthritis involves small joints as well.

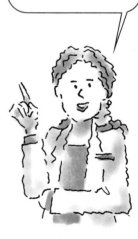

• Hydroxychloroquine (Plaquenil) and sulfasalazine (Azulfidine), both oral medications, are used as second-line agents if pain isn't relieved by NSAIDs.
• Gold salts are injected into a joint to control swelling. This treatment is 50% effective in the first 5 years of use, but the success rate then falls to 5% to 15%.
• D-penicillamine is used to decrease rheumatoid factor.
• Immunosuppressive drugs, such as methotrexate (MTX) and azathioprine (Imuran), are used to reduce swelling.
• Opioids are used only when other medications are no longer effective.

Last resort

Surgical interventions, such as cervical spine fusion, tendon repairs, and joint replacements (hip and knee), can help, especially in restoring function. However, because of the higher risks associated with any surgical procedure, surgery is reserved for cases where other treatment methods have failed to relieve pain.

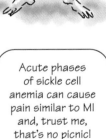

Because of the risks associated with surgery, it's reserved for patients whose pain isn't relieved by more conservative treatment.

Sickle cell anemia

Sickle cell anemia is an inherited disorder of the red blood cells (RBCs) and typically affects African Americans and Hispanics. When blood oxygen levels are low, RBCs flatten into a sickle shape and become sticky, forming clumps and blocking small blood vessels. There's no cure for this disease, which eventually causes organ failure and death. (See *Distinguishing between sickled cells and normal cells*, page 198.)

What to look for

In acute phases, blockage of normal blood flow causes ischemic pain similar to that of myocardial infarction (MI). Pain commonly involves the low back and other joints and may last several hours to several days. Visceral pain is sometimes involved due to vaso-occlusion in the spleen, liver, and lungs. A sickle cell crisis may be set off by fever, dehydration, infection, or overexertion.

A chronic complaint

CNP experienced by patients with sickle cell anemia is related to organ and connective tissue damage. Chronic leg ulcers may develop as well as osteonecrosis of the femoral head or vertebra.

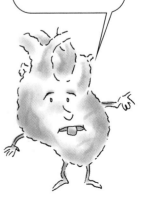

Acute phases of sickle cell anemia can cause pain similar to MI and, trust me, that's no picnic!

Distinguishing between sickled cells and normal cells

Normal red blood cells (RBCs) and sickled cells vary in more ways than shape. They can also differ in life span, oxygen-carrying ability, and the rate at which they're destroyed (see below).

Normal RBCs

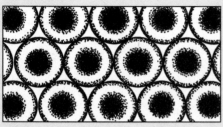

Sickled cells

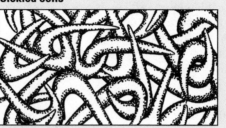

* 120-day life span
* hemoglobin has normal oxygen-carrying capacity
* 12 to 14 g of hemoglobin per milliliter
* RBCs destroyed at normal rate

* 30- to 40-day life span
* hemoglobin has decreased oxygen-carrying capacity
* 6 to 9 g of hemoglobin per milliliter
* RBCs destroyed at accelerated rate

Assessing sickle cell anemia pain

In addition to a thorough health history and physical examination, two assessment points are important for sickle cell anemia pain:
• Always ask the patient if the pain is at the usual level experienced because it's possible that a different condition is causing the pain, including complications of the disease, such as bowel obstruction, or an unrelated illness, such as appendicitis.
• Patients in severe pain may not have the usual behaviors associated with severe pain, such as blood pressure changes, guarding, and sweating, because they have learned to control their physiologic response to pain.

Managing sickle cell anemia pain

Opioid therapy is an important element in combating sickle cell anemia pain. Withholding or limiting opioid medication isn't recommended. The patient with sickle cell anemia may tolerate higher doses of opioids than, say, a postoperative patient (up to 50 mg/hr I.V.). Morphine is usually the preferred analgesic, given I.V. or in a subcutaneous infusion if venous access is difficult.

Don't underestimate the pain experienced by patients with sickle cell anemia. Many have simply learned to control their responses to pain.

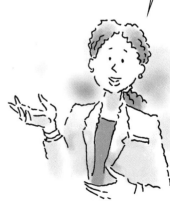

Give them what they need

There are several points to remember in managing sickle cell anemia pain:

• Don't withhold opioid medication because of a fear of addiction. Opioids are an important element of sickle cell anemia pain relief.

• Placebo use is ineffective in the long run and destroys any hope of trust between the patient and health care provider.

• Meperidine (Demerol) should be avoided due to the inactive metabolite normeperidine, which is toxic and has a long half-life. Morphine or hydromorphone (Dilaudid) are effective alternatives.

• I.V. administration of medication is preferable to the I.M. route because of possible pain and irritation at the I.M. injection site.

• As pain decreases, analgesics may be administered orally. However, because sickle cell anemia pain is so severe, administration should proceed slowly and with the willing cooperation of the patient.

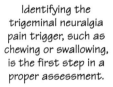

Don't gamble with your patient's trust. Placebos aren't effective treatment for sickle cell anemia pain.

Trigeminal neuralgia

Otherwise known as tic douloureux, trigeminal neuralgia is a disorder of the fifth cranial nerve (trigeminal nerve). Areas of pain occur on the scalp, eyes, nose, lips, forehead, and upper and lower jaw.

What to look for

Trigeminal neuralgia pain is described as a brief burst of "electric shock" pain across the face. It tends to occur in clusters; between clusters, there's no pain or discomfort. One side of the face or the other can be affected at different times; however, it's rare for both sides of the face to be affected at once. The slightest tactile stimulus can trigger a burst of pain.

Assessing trigeminal neuralgia pain

First, the pain trigger should be identified (talking, brushing teeth, chewing, swallowing, touching the face) to identify the nerve branch involved. Pain may last for several weeks or months, followed by a period of remission, which can last for days or years. Due to pain and anxiety about it, the patient may have difficulty performing ADLs.

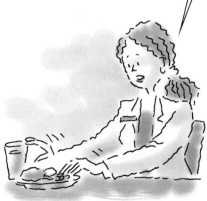

Identifying the trigeminal neuralgia pain trigger, such as chewing or swallowing, is the first step in a proper assessment.

Managing trigeminal neuralgia pain

Carbamazepine (Tegretol) is the drug of choice for treating the pain of trigeminal neuralgia, beginning with a low dose and increasing gradually up to 1,200 mg over 24 hours to prevent further episodes.

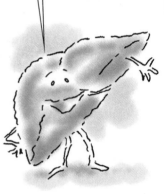

Sodium valproate? Yeah, I know him. Sometimes he really pushes my enzyme levels.

Dizzy, sleepy, and more

Common adverse effects are dizziness, ataxia, sedation, and nausea. In some patients, these adverse effects are so strong that they can't tolerate therapeutic doses. Sometimes, if relief has been obtained, it's possible to stop the medication for a day and restart at lower doses. Tolerance to the drug also develops, which limits administration to periods of pain only. Bone marrow suppression may occur, so blood cell counts should be done on a regular basis.

First runner-up

Sodium valproate is also used to treat trigeminal neuralgia pain. It tends to be better tolerated and is just as effective. Even so, adverse effects are still possible, and occasionally alopecia (hair loss) will occur. All effects are reversible when the drug is stopped. Hepatic function can be affected, and liver enzyme levels should be checked regularly.

Second runners-up

Other common pharmacologic treatments for trigeminal neuralgia pain are:
• Phenytoin, which can be given I.V. to treat severe pain, relieves pain in more than 50% of patients and is an effective adjunct to carbamazepine.
• Gabapentin is an effective adjunct to carbamazepine and is well-tolerated by most patients.
• Baclofen isn't as effective as carbamazepine or phenytoin but may be used in combination with these medications. Its short action requires frequent dosing (every 3 to 4 hours) and it loses its effect over time.
• Local anesthetic injections into the trigger area or pain site are used for temporary relief when drug therapy isn't successful.

Miss congeniality

Nonpharmacologic and surgical interventions to treat trigeminal neuralgia pain include:
• acupuncture
• microvascular decompression to relieve pulsatile compression of the trigeminal nerve
• radio-frequency electrocoagulation, which uses heat to destroy selected portions of the ganglion suspected to be the cause of pain

and provides relief in most patients (with 20% to 30% of patients experiencing a recurrence of pain)

• peripheral neurectomy or neurolysis to surgically or chemically destroy the peripheral branches of the trigeminal nerve, producing dense numbness and pain relief that rarely lasts more than 1 year.

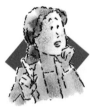

Quick quiz

1. CNP is pain that lasts:
   A.   for at least 6 months.
   B.   12 months.
   C.   2 to 6 weeks.
   D.   less than 1 month.

Answer: A. To be considered CNP, the pain experience must last for at least 6 months.

2. CNP is the result of:
   A.   nociceptive pain.
   B.   neuropathic pain.
   C.   nociceptive or neuropathic pain.
   D.   psychological dysfunction.

Answer: C. CNP can result from nociceptive pain of an external stimulus, such as a laceration, or from neuropathic pain of chronically activated tissues, such as a damaged blood vessel.

3. Assessment of the patient with CNP should always include:
   A.   identification of trigger points.
   B.   psychological evaluation.
   C.   determination of neuropathic vs. nociceptive pain.
   D.   psychological referral.

Answer: B. Because of the emotionally debilitating effects of chronic pain, CNP sufferers are at greater risk for suicide. Thus, a psychological evaluation is essential to determine if immediate action is necessary.

4. The most common anticonvulsant drug used to treat CNP is:
   A.   carbamazepine.
   B.   phenytoin.
   C.   sodium valproate.
   D.   oxycodone.

Answer: A. Carbamazepine is used most commonly to treat CNP pain, despite some serious adverse effects, such as dizziness, nausea, and sedation.

5. Patients undergoing cordotomy will experience what adverse effect from the procedure?
   A.   paralysis.
   B.   worsening pain in peripheral areas.
   C.   loss of motor function.
   D.   loss of temperature sensation.

Answer: D. Cordotomy unilaterally or bilaterally severs the nerve fibers in the spinal cord. Because pain and temperature sensation travel the same pathway, patients who undergo this procedure will experience temperature sensation impairment as well as pain relief.

6. Thermotherapy is a nonpharmacologic treatment for CNP that:
   A.   closes the gate to painful stimuli.
   B.   increases collagen extensibility and blood flow.
   C.   restores tone and strength to muscles.
   D.   induces hypothermia, resulting in decreased spasticity.

Answer: B. Thermotherapy increases collagen extensibility and blood flow and decreases inflammation and joint stiffness.

Scoring

✩✩✩   If you answered all six questions correctly, gadzooks! You've got what it takes to drain the pain!

✩✩   If you answered four or five correctly, yahoo! You're well on your way to blocking those nosy nociceptors!

✩   If you answered fewer than four correctly, don't sweat it! Review the chapter and give yourself a local information injection!

7

Cancer pain

Just the facts

In this chapter, you'll learn:

♦ types of pain experienced by patients with cancer

♦ how to use the World Health Organization analgesic ladder to manage cancer-related pain

♦ pharmacologic and nonpharmacologic methods to control cancer-related pain.

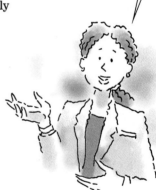

Having cancer doesn't always mean having pain.

A look at cancer pain

Cancer pain management techniques have advanced significantly in the past few years. Thanks to new technology and drugs, most patients with cancer can participate in daily activities as fully as their disease allows them. Many pain management techniques are relatively straightforward, while others may require the expertise of a pain management specialist.

And now for the good news

Pain management is one of many challenges faced by the patient with cancer. According to current research, of all the symptoms that cancer patients may experience, pain is the symptom they fear most. The good news is that most people with cancer pain (approximately 90%) can be effectively treated using pharmacologic and nonpharmacologic therapies.

Causes of cancer pain

Cancer patients may experience pain for many reasons, not just from the cancer itself. Because cancer patients are vulnerable to so many potential causes of pain, accurate assessment and treatment are vital. Some causes of cancer-related pain include:

• invasion, obstruction, distention, or compression of tissue by a tumor
• cancer treatments, such as chemotherapy and radiation
• surgery to reduce or resolve symptoms
• diagnostic procedures, such as blood sampling, biopsies, and lumbar puncture
• infection, inflammation, and ischemia.

Notorious P.A.I.N.

Some cancers are more likely to cause pain than others. Cancers that invade bone tissue, such as metastatic breast cancer, prostate cancer, and osteosarcoma, are notoriously painful. The same is true of cancers that attack abdominal organs, such as pancreatic and uterine cancer. Cancers that are much less likely to cause pain include those that involve the blood, such as leukemia.

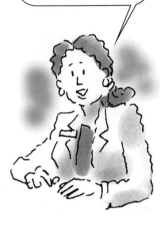

The patient with cancer may experience pain from a variety of sources.

Types of cancer pain

The patient with cancer may experience nociceptive pain, neuropathic pain, or both. Because nociceptive and neuropathic pain are activated by different mechanisms, accurate pain assessment is vital to formulating an effective pain management plan. Nociceptive and neuropathic pain can occur at the same time and in several different locations concurrently and may be referred to other areas of the body as well. (See *Understanding referred pain.*)

Nociceptive pain

Nociceptive pain occurs when a noxious stimulus activates nociceptors associated with primary afferent neurons. Activation of these receptors is the body's way of warning us to withdraw from something harmful and to protect the injured area so that it can heal. Nociceptive stimuli may be chemical, thermal, or pressure sources. Nociceptive pain receptors are located in most tissues of the body.

Somatic pain

Somatic pain occurs when nociceptors are activated in the skin, bones, muscle, deep tissues, and joints. Somatic pain is localized and commonly described as continuous, sharp, throbbing, or achy. Somatic cancer pain might result from bone cancer or invasion of the body wall by a tumor, for example.

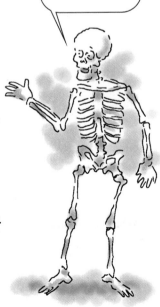

Cancers that invade bone tissue are some of the most painful. Gulp!

Now I get it!

Understanding referred pain

Referred pain occurs when the patient experiences pain in an area of his body away from the cause of the pain. For instance, the patient with metastatic hip lesions may report knee pain and the patient with pancreatic or liver cancer may experience back or shoulder pain.

Scientists have several theories to explain referred pain. The most popular explanation is called the "convergence-projection" theory, which focuses on the very busy converging visceral and somatic afferent neurons in the spinal cord. Visceral afferent nerves carrying messages from the damaged area converge at the same point where the somatic afferent nerves also enter the spinal cord. Researchers believe that the incoming messages from the viscera are shared with the same projection neurons (those nerves that take the pain messages from the spinal cord to the brain) used by the somatic neurons. Thus, the brain confuses where the messages originated.

Because many cancer syndromes have a component of referred pain, pain assessment and treatment of the cancer patient can be a challenge. The list below identifies common cancer sites and associated areas of referred pain for each.

Cancer site	Potential area of referred pain
Cervical vertebrae	Posterior skull
Abdomen	Shoulder, groin, back
Retroperitoneum	Intercostal area along nerve root
Lung	Shoulder, down arm
Hip	Knee
Pancreas	Shoulder, back

Visceral pain occurs when an organ is stretched or distended. Ach!

Visceral pain

Visceral pain occurs when the afferent nociceptive fibers in and around organs are activated. Causes of visceral cancer pain include inflammation of a solid organ, such as the liver, or an obstruction caused by a tumor. The patient with visceral pain usually reports a deep, gnawing, or crampy pain, especially when caused by an obstruction. Visceral pain that originates in the mesentery or capsules of an organ may be described as sharp or throbbing.

Neuropathic pain

Neuropathic pain occurs when the sensory nervous system is injured and sends pain impulses to the brain, despite absence of tissue injury. Unlike nociceptive pain, neuropathic pain isn't protective. This type of pain may occur intermittently or continuously and may be described as squeezing, shooting, shocklike, burning, or pins and needles. Causes of neuropathic cancer pain might include damage to the peripheral nerve by tumor invasion or compression of other tissue by a tumor.

Assessing cancer pain

Careful pain assessment on a regular basis is the key to effective pain management. Keep in mind that complaints of pain commonly precede the initial diagnosis of cancer or tumor recurrence.

Assess the onset, location, intensity, quality, and duration of the pain. What aggravates and relieves the pain? Ask what medications the patient is taking, including nonprescription drugs and those not related to the cancer or pain treatment. Also, be sure to ask about the use of nonpharmacologic therapies or experimental medications acquired in other countries to ensure safety and avoid adverse interactions with prescribed therapies.

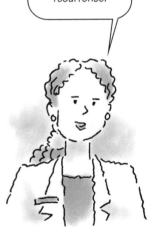

Complaints of pain commonly precede the initial diagnosis of cancer or tumor recurrence.

Neurologic examination

A thorough neurologic examination should be performed. A subtle change in sensation or strength can be the first sign of new disease or disease progression. One pain management center reported that more than 60% of the cancer patients sent for evaluation were found to have previously undetected lesions that were ultimately identified by neurologic examination. (See *Spinal cord compression: An emergency in cancer pain management.*)

Managing cancer pain

To raise awareness about cancer pain management and offer a universal system of treatment, the World Health Organization (WHO) created the three-step analgesic ladder. Among other measures, the plan promotes the use of basic, easily accessible, inexpensive drugs. (See *The WHO analgesic ladder*, page 208.)

Spinal cord compression: An emergency in cancer pain management

Spinal cord compression (SCC) is an oncologic emergency. Prompt recognition and treatment of SCC can prevent serious disability such as quadriplegia. Patients with bone metastases from breast, prostate, lung, and colon cancers are at risk for SCC. In some patients, SCC may be the first sign of a malignancy.

What to look for
SCC occurs when a tumor in the area of the spinal cord compresses the cord. The first symptom is commonly new back pain, which the patient may be able to pinpoint to a partic-ular vertebra. The pain is usually made worse by lying down, coughing, sneezing, or bearing down. Typically, the patient reports pain before sensory or motor changes occur. Immediately assess any new report of back pain because SCC is a rapidly deteriorating condition. Other signs of SCC include sensory changes, tender-ness on percussion of the spine, urine reten-tion, constipation, bladder and bowel dysfunc-tion (usually a late sign), and ataxia.

How it's treated
Treatment for SCC includes high-dose corti-costeroids, radiation to the affected spinal area, and analgesics. Surgical decompression may be performed if further radiation isn't an option, if symptoms progress despite radiation therapy, or if bony fragments are involved.

What can happen
The patient whose treatment begins while he's still able to walk has a 75% chance of remain-ing ambulatory. That percentage drops to 30% to 50% if treatment is started when the patient has partial or incomplete paralysis and down to 10% to 20% if he's already paralyzed. Un-treated, about one-third of patients will devel-op paralysis within 7 days of the first sign of weakness.

New pain in a cancer patient may be the sign of a new lesion.

CAUTION!

Ladder principles

Keep the following principles in mind when using the WHO anal-gesic ladder to manage cancer pain:
• Give the patient drugs orally, if possible.
• Administer analgesic medications around the clock and add breakthrough medication as needed.
• Evaluate the patient's quality of life and tailor the pain manage-ment plan to his needs. Be on the lookout for interruptions in the patient's normal activities, especially decreased social interaction and eating and sleeping difficulties.

But wait, there's more

Some pain management specialists suggest that epidural and in-trathecal drugs and spinal cord stimulators represent a fourth rung in the ladder. In addition, the specialists include invasive interven-tions, such as pituitary ablation and cordotomy, as a fifth rung.

The WHO analgesic ladder

The World Health Organization (WHO) developed a three-step ladder (shown below) to guide pain-relief efforts for patients with cancer. Analgesics are selected based on the intensity of the patient's pain. The ladder includes three categories of drugs: nonopioids, opioids, and adjuvant drugs. Adjuvant drugs can be used on any step of the ladder.

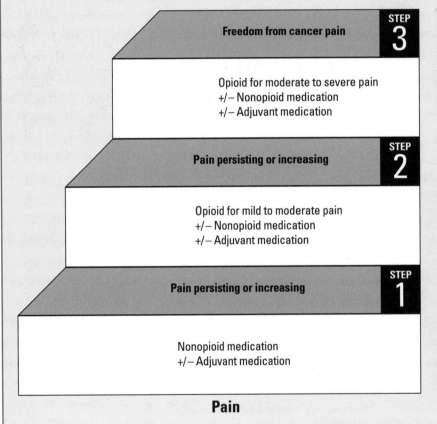

Freedom from cancer pain

STEP 3

Opioid for moderate to severe pain
+/− Nonopioid medication
+/− Adjuvant medication

When the patient's pain reaches the moderate to severe level, administer more potent opioid drugs, including morphine, oxycodone, hydromorphone, fentanyl, and methadone. Nonopioid drugs may be continued.

Pain persisting or increasing

STEP 2

Opioid for mild to moderate pain
+/− Nonopioid medication
+/− Adjuvant medication

Add opioid drugs, such as codeine or hydrocodone, for the patient with mild to moderate pain that isn't relieved by a nonopioid. If the patient is already taking NSAIDs, continue to use them as they add to the analgesic effect.

Pain persisting or increasing

STEP 1

Nonopioid medication
+/− Adjuvant medication

Pain

Administer nonopioid analgesics, such as acetaminophen, aspirin, and nonsteroidal anti-inflammatory drugs (NSAIDs), to the patient just beginning to experience discomfort and mild pain. Although the patient's pain might not be adequately controlled with nonopioid drugs, their use may reduce the overall amount of opioids needed to achieve pain control.

Primarily palliative

Two primary cancer treatments, chemotherapy and radiation, may be used as palliative treatments to relieve pain in the terminally ill cancer patient. In many circumstances, these therapies improve quality of life.

• *Chemotherapy*—Palliative chemotherapy can reduce tumor size, thus relieving pain caused by pressure from the tumor. However, because chemotherapy can produce many adverse effects, the patient and his health care providers should weigh the benefits of chemotherapy against its potential adverse effects. Make sure the patient understands that palliative chemotherapy isn't being given to cure his cancer or prolong his life. Two chemotherapeutic drugs have been approved by the Food and Drug Administration for palliative symptom relief: gemcitabine for relief of pancreatic cancer pain and mitoxantrone (Novantrone) for prostate cancer pain.

• *Radiation* — Palliative radiation therapy provides fast and lasting relief from pain caused by metastases or local disease. In addition, radiation therapy commonly enhances other pain relief measures, such as analgesic therapy, because it treats the cause of pain. It can also help manage pain from spinal cord compression, nerve infiltration, blockage of hollow organs, and other pain caused by space-occupying tumors (especially in the brain).

> Radiation therapy can relieve pain caused by bone metastases.

Pharmacologic management of cancer pain

Because of the variability in adverse effects and patient response to drugs used for cancer pain, trial periods may be necessary to find the best drug and method of administration. Alleviate the patient's fears by explaining that switching drugs and doses is a normal part of the pain management process and doesn't mean his pain can't be controlled. Pharmacologic therapies used to treat cancer pain include nonopioid analgesics, opioid analgesics, and adjuvant therapies, such as anticonvulsants, antidepressants, and corticosteroids.

Nonopioid analgesics

Nonopioid analgesics used to treat cancer pain have a dosing limit called a ceiling effect, which means that increasing the dose doesn't benefit the patient and increases the risk of toxicity. Unlike with opioids, the patient taking nonopioid analgesics doesn't develop tolerance, physical dependence, or addiction. These drugs produce an antipyretic effect, and most inhibit the formation of prostaglandins by interfering with the inflammatory response. Nonopioid analgesics used to treat cancer pain include aspirin, acetaminophen, and nonsteroidal anti-inflammatory drugs (NSAIDs).

> The ceiling's the limit when using nonopioid analgesics.

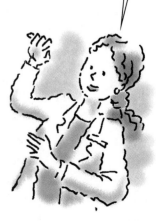

Aspirin

Aspirin, a common over-the-counter drug, is useful for mild pain. However, it has many potential adverse effects, including GI distress, prolonged bleeding time, decreased platelet aggregation, Reye's syndrome in children with viral illnesses, and hypersensitivity reactions.

Acetaminophen

Acetaminophen produces analgesic and antipyretic effects but has little effect on the inflammatory response, GI tract, or platelet function. It's commonly used in drug combinations, such as Tylenol #3, Darvocet, or Percocet. Be sure to account for all sources of acetaminophen to ensure that the patient doesn't receive toxic levels. The maximum daily dose of 4,000 mg/day is tolerated well by most people.

NSAIDs

NSAID use may require initial trials to find the best drug and dose. Patients with a history of GI bleeding or the elderly should be treated prophylactically with omeprazole (Prilosec), ranitidine (Zantac), or misoprostol (Cytotec) to protect the gastric mucosa. Use NSAIDs cautiously in patients with renal insufficiency. The use of NSAIDs may be contraindicated in patients with a history of ulcers or prolonged bleeding time. These patients may need to start on a low-dose opioid at step 1 of the WHO ladder.

Parenterally speaking

Currently, ketorolac (Toradol) is the only NSAID that can be administered parenterally in the United States. Ketorolac may be used for up to 5 days to control mild to moderate cancer pain. Major adverse effects include gastric distress and bleeding tendencies.

Opioid analgesics

Despite some patient and practitioner fears about opioids, they're the foundation for pharmacologic treatment of cancer pain. (See *Opioid fears.*) Most cancer patients obtain pain relief with these drugs. While morphine is the "gold standard" opioid for treating cancer pain, many natural and synthetic opioids are also available. (See *Opioid strength.*)

Administration routes

Opioids can be given by various routes. Although the oral route is preferable, your patient may need to switch to a different route of administration as his cancer progresses. In addition to

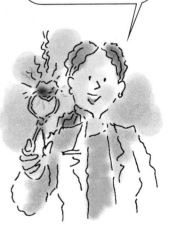

Morphine is the gold standard for treating cancer pain, but there are lots of other opioids that can help, too.

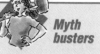

Myth busters

Opioid strength

Myth: Some opioids are weak and others strong. Therefore, different opioids must be used to treat different levels of pain.

Fact: Most opioids can be titrated to treat mild, moderate, or severe pain, although some may be considered "mild" because the dose is limited by adverse effects. Although there *is* a difference in potency between different opioids (where 1 mg of one opioid may provide more pain relief than 1 mg of another), these numbers don't ultimately matter because the amount can be varied according to need.

Myth busters

Opioid fears

Myth: Cancer patients are in danger of becoming addicted to opioid analgesics. What's more, using opioids near the end of life will hasten death.

Fact: Research doesn't demonstrate an increased risk of addiction in patients taking opioids for pain. In addition, research has suggested that using opioids at the end of life can actually prolong life and improve the quality of those final days.

oral administration, opioids may be administered rectally, topically, I.M., subcutaneously (S.C.), I.V., epidurally, and intrathecally.

Oral's laurels

Oral administration should be considered before other routes because it's inexpensive, noninvasive, and capable of producing a steady analgesic state. It also allows flexibility in dosing and can provide relief for different pain levels, ranging from mild to severe. The most common reason for failure to achieve pain relief by this route is insufficient dosing by the prescriber.

Quarrels with orals

Disadvantages of oral administration include:
• extensive metabolism of drug in the liver (first-pass metabolism), which can lessen the degree of effectiveness
• slow onset
• delayed peak time (90 to 120 minutes in a controlled-release tablet)
• short dosing intervals (usually 4 hours) when using short-acting opioids, which can interfere with activities, such as sleeping
• not possible for patients with swallowing difficulties or impaired GI functioning or those on nothing-by-mouth status
• absorption altered by food, gastric emptying time, and GI motility.
   Patient compliance is also a factor in oral opioid effectiveness. Because of frequent dosing, the patient may forget to take some doses. The new controlled-release opioid medications are convenient because they allow the patient to dose once or twice daily. It allows uniform absorption for 12 to 24 hours, making these drugs effective for management of continuous cancer pain. Morphine

(MS Contin) and oxycodone (OxyContin) are the most commonly used oral opioids.

Rectal rationales

Rectal administration may be used for patients who are unwilling or unable to take analgesics orally. Dosing amounts and onset of rectal drugs differ from oral administration because of irregular or incomplete drug absorption. However, many opioids may be prepared by the pharmacy for rectal administration or given in an aqueous solution (except controlled-release formulations), an unmodified tablet, or crushed (except controlled-release tablets) and placed in a gelatin capsule. Just as with oral dosing, the most common reason for inadequate analgesic effect from rectal opioid administration is insufficient dosing.

Totally topical

Fentanyl patches (Duragesic), which deliver sustained-release 3-day therapy, are ideal for the patient with stable pain who can't take or tolerate oral drugs or finds frequent dosing inconvenient. The patient using fentanyl should have a breakthrough pain drug available. Disadvantages of using fentanyl patches include skin irritation from the adhesive, possible altered absorption in the cachectic patient, and a delay in pain relief when increasing or decreasing a dose.

Bypassing the I.M. route

Although the I.M route is commonly used for administering opioids, it isn't recommended in pain management. In fact, there are no advantages to this route for achieving pain management goals. However, there are many disadvantages:

- painful administration
- variable absorption time (30 to 60 minutes to peak in the blood)
- rapid drop in action compared to oral administration due to variability of muscle mass or poor blood supply to muscle
- risk of improper technique, which can cause accidental injection of the drug into the patient's bloodstream, greatly increasing the risk of overdose or adverse reaction (respiratory depression)
- abscess at the muscle site and fibrosis of the muscle caused by continuous administration
- lack of pain relief for elderly patients, who have decreased muscle mass
- undue pain for children, who may endure severe pain to avoid a feared needle.

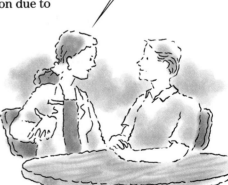

Fentanyl patches provide 3-day pain relief.

The skinny on sub-Q delivery

Opioids delivered S.C. may provide pain relief if the patient has adequate local perfusion and absorption. Even so, serum levels are more stable with I.V. administration than with S.C. administration. Opioids given S.C. should be administered at volumes less than 10 ml/hr to avoid irritation and absorption problems. Many opioids can be concentrated to keep infusion rates within this limit.

I.V. on the Q.T.

Patient-controlled analgesia (PCA) is ideal for the patient who desires increased control and flexibility over his pain relief. PCA can be delivered continuously and on demand via a pump that can be carried in a fanny pack or small backpack. Drugs commonly used to treat cancer pain by PCA include morphine and hydromorphone. Fentanyl and methadone may also be delivered in this way.

Continuous I.V. infusion doesn't mean more work for me anymore. PCA allows patients to control their medication without inhibiting their lifestyle. And I get to do more reading!

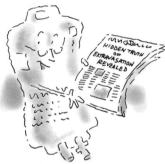

Intrathecal decrease

Opioids may also be administered intrathecally or epidurally through catheters placed in the intrathecal or epidural spaces. This method of drug delivery greatly reduces the dose of opioids the patient requires for pain relief. (See *Neuraxial opioid therapy*, page 214.)

Dosing methods

Dosing in all pharmacologic pain management should be evaluated regularly and adjusted as needed. Dosing methods for opioids differ based on whether short- or long-acting opioids are prescribed.

Get Shorty

Short-acting opioids may be prescribed for the patient with sporadic pain that can be managed by "as needed," or p.r.n., dosing. These drugs, such as immediate-release morphine sulfate, oxycodone, and hydromorphone, are taken only when pain occurs or shortly before pain is likely to occur. These drugs may also be used for breakthrough pain during use of a longer-acting opioid. (See *Understanding breakthrough pain*, page 214.)

Hey, who are you calling short?! I prefer "vertically challenged."

Make it last

When pain is constant, scheduled administration of a long-acting opioid, such as morphine (MS Contin), oxycodone (OxyContin), and methadone (Dolophine), provides regular, con-

Neuraxial opioid therapy

In neuraxial opioid therapy, the patient receives opioids through epidural or intrathecal catheters. A major advantage of this delivery system is that the patient obtains pain relief at much lower doses than those needed with oral or I.V. use. The patient receiving an opioid through an epidural device requires about one-tenth the I.V. dose to achieve the same level of comfort. With intrathecal delivery, the dose is reduced to one one-hundredth the dose needed for I.V. delivery. Lower drug doses dramatically reduce potential adverse effects. Other drugs, such as bupivacaine and clonidine, can also be delivered through these catheters.

The patient undergoing neuraxial therapy may have external catheters connected to an external injection port or pump or he may have a completely internal system. An internal pump must be refilled about every 30 days, depending on the type of pump and dosing parameters. The pump is refilled through a special port with a needle and syringe.

Understanding breakthrough pain

When the patient with stable pain occasionally experiences an exacerbation, this is called breakthrough pain. From 50% to 65% of patients with cancer can expect to experience breakthrough pain. The exacerbation may be associated with activity, movement, physiologic changes, or even the time of day.

What you can do
Anticipate breakthrough pain that's predictable (such as procedure-related pain), and medicate the patient with a short-acting opioid beforehand.

sistent pain relief. When starting the patient on a long-acting opioid, begin with a low dose and provide short-acting opioids. In addition to relieving breakthrough pain, the short-acting drug can help gauge necessary increases in dosing of the long-acting opioid.

Adverse effects

Opioid analgesics can produce adverse effects, many of which go away over time. Some adverse effects can be diminished by slowly increasing doses; others must be managed at all times. Constipation and sedation are particularly troublesome adverse effects in cancer patients. To reduce the risk of constipation, place the patient on a bowel program that includes adequate fluids and stimulating laxatives. In addition, if the patient believes that sedation is negatively impacting his quality of life, consider adding a stimulant drug (such as methylphenidate [Ritalin]) or maximizing nonopioid analgesics and nonpharmacologic therapies.

Adjuvant drug therapies

Adjuvant drugs are drugs approved for uses other than pain management that may also relieve or reduce some cancer pain. Many classes of drugs fit into this category. Some adjuvant drugs work directly on pain messaging mechanisms while others work on other life disturbances, such as the adverse effects of pain therapies or psychological stressors (anxiety, depression, and insomnia).

Several drugs from different classes may be used in adjuvant pharmacologic therapy for cancer pain. Some of the most common adjuvant therapies include anticonvulsants, antidepressants, and corticosteroids.

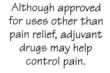

Although approved for uses other than pain relief, adjuvant drugs may help control pain.

Anticonvulsants

Typically, anticonvulsants stabilize neuronal membrane activity, making them particularly useful in treating neuropathic pain. Anticonvulsants used to treat cancer pain include gabapentin (Neurontin) and carbamazepine (Tegretol).

Antidepressants

Tricyclic antidepressants (TCAs) are the most common antidepressants used in cancer pain management. They work by inhibiting the reuptake of serotonin and norepinephrine, which are involved in the descending analgesic system. The patient may receive a TCA to control neuropathic pain from cancer treatment. The most common TCAs used to treat cancer pain are amitriptyline (Elavil), desipramine (Norpramin), and nortriptyline (Pamelor).

Corticosteroids

Corticosteroids are used for different types of cancer pain, such as neuropathic pain from tumor compression and bone pain. Corticosteroids inhibit most of the pathways involved in inflammation. This action makes them a potent pain reliever whenever inflammation is involved. For this reason, the patient may experience an increase in pain when corticosteroids taken for other indications are tapered or stopped.

Do they have a good benefits package?

Sometimes, short-term administration of a corticosteroid, such as methylprednisolone (Medrol dose pack), can relieve sudden pain escalation, such as the increased pain associated with a new pathologic fracture resulting from bone cancer. As an added benefit for the cancer patient, corticosteroids may increase appetite and produce euphoria. Some indications for corticosteroid use include spinal cord compression, bone pain, and headaches caused by increased intracranial pressure.

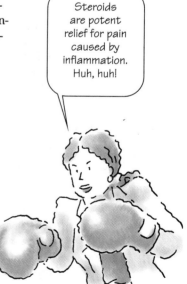

Steroids are potent relief for pain caused by inflammation. Huh, huh!

Other adjuvant therapies

Other common adjuvant therapies used to treat cancer pain include the ones listed here:

- Caffeine, when used with NSAIDs, can improve analgesia in some conditions, such as headache and mouth pain resulting from cancer or chemotherapy. Some research suggests that children with cancer pain can benefit from single caffeine doses.
- Clonidine (Catapres) is used primarily to treat neuropathic pain. Recently its use in epidural and intrathecal infusions has increased, with positive results.
- Radiopharmaceutical infusions, such as strontium-89, may reduce bone pain caused by metastasis. Radiopharmaceuticals can reduce the progression of the cancer, the number of new pain sites, and the need for analgesic drugs. Although pain relief can last from 3 to 6 months, warn the patient that maximum benefit may not be achieved for 2 to 3 weeks. Other less common radiopharmaceuticals include rhenium-186 and samarium-153.
- Bisphosphonates, such as pamidronate (Aredia), may be useful in treating bone pain caused by osteoclast-induced bone resorption by the cancer (for example, breast metastases). These drugs are also used to treat life-threatening hypercalcemia in such disorders as lung or breast cancer and multiple myeloma.

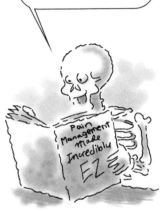

Radiopharmaceuticals can provide pain relief for up to 6 months. Yippee!

Calcitonin stops the moanin'

- Calcitonin inhibits bone resorption. Because bone resorption can lead to increased pain through sensitization and activation of pain-messaging fibers in and around the periosteum of the bones, calcitonin action has an analgesic effect. However, although the patient may initially obtain pain relief with calcitonin, its effectiveness appears to decrease with prolonged use.
- Octreotide (Sandostatin) treats severe pain of bowel obstruction by dramatically reducing gastric secretions and motility. As a result, nausea, vomiting, and refractory diarrhea can be controlled.
- Benzodiazepines, such as diazepam (Valium) and lorazepam (Ativan), may be used to treat painful muscle spasms and anxiety, which can heighten a person's overall distress. On their own, these drugs don't provide analgesia.

Psychostimulants help counteract somnolence caused by opioids and may improve a person's appetite. Bon appetit!

Party of one? Your table is ready.

- Psychostimulants, such as methylphenidate (Ritalin) and dextroamphetamine (Dexedrine), help counteract adverse effects of somnolence or confusion that some opioids can cause. Stimulants may also improve the patient's appetite.
- Local anesthetics, such as lidocaine and bupivacaine, block pain primarily by inhibiting sodium channel activity along neurons, stopping nerve conduction. Although the effect is temporary, analgesic response after a nerve block has been shown to last much longer than the known pharmacologic life of the drug. They can also be used to prevent the development of long-lasting pain syndromes such as

phantom limb pain following surgical removal of a limb with a tumor. In addition, targeted injections can help pinpoint a specific neuronal source of pain, differentiating whether the pain is from a somatic, visceral, or sympathetic source.

Chip off the old block

• Neurolytic blocks used in the patient with cancer are the celiac plexus block and the superior hypogastric block. The celiac plexus block is commonly used to reduce the pain associated with pancreatic cancer. It may take several days for the patient to notice an improvement in pain, but relief may last for several months. The superior hypogastric plexus block is sometimes used and may treat pain arising from the pelvic wall, which might occur in prostate, rectal, bladder, or cervical cancer.

Surgical intervention

Surgical intervention for pain management is typically considered only when pharmacologic therapies fail. More and more, however, these techniques are being used earlier with excellent effect. When considering surgical intervention to treat cancer pain, the patient and health care provider should examine the patient's therapy goals and lifestyle as well as possible risks weighed against potential benefits.

Cut it out or just stop it

Surgery can reduce tumor bulk to relieve pressure on body structures, thus reducing pain and other complications. In contrast, some surgical interventions access a particular nerve or pain source to deactivate it. Terminally ill cancer patients may undergo palliative surgery when less invasive measures haven't provided adequate relief or resulted in unbearable adverse effects. Surgical procedures used to treat cancer pain include neurectomy, rhizotomy, cordotomy, hypophysectomy, orthopedic surgery, cryoanalgesia, and radio-frequency lesioning.

More and more, surgery is used as an earlier treatment for pain relief.

Neurectomy

Neurectomy involves the resection or partial or total excision of a spinal or cranial nerve. It may be done for chest wall pain or when a patient has a paraspinal tumor (multilevel neurectomy). This procedure is relatively quick and only requires local or regional anesthesia. Unfortunately, loss of motor sensation is a possible adverse effect and pain relief may be only temporary. Peripheral neurectomy is considered when all standard pain management therapies have failed.

Rhizotomy

Rhizotomy involves cutting a nerve to relieve pain. Rhizotomy of the dorsal nerve root may produce analgesia for localized severe pain, such as on the trunk, abdomen, or limb. Motor function is usually unaffected if one dorsal nerve root for the area is left intact.

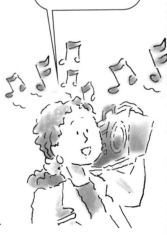

Rhizotomy takes some nerve! Fortunately, it usually doesn't affect motor function.

Cordotomy

Cordotomy can be performed as an open surgery or percutaneously. A unilateral cordotomy is performed to relieve somatic pain on one side of the body. A bilateral cordotomy is performed to relieve visceral pain on both sides of the body.

Hypophysectomy

Hypophysectomy destroys the pituitary gland. Hypophysectomy may be performed to treat severe pain from metastatic bone cancer that doesn't respond to less invasive therapies. It provides pain relief in 40% to 70% of patients.

Orthopedic surgery

Orthopedic surgery is mainly used as a prophylactic pain treatment for the patient with bone metastases. It aims to lessen the risk of pathologic fractures and, consequently, the associated risks of thromboemboli and nerve compression due to immobility. The guidelines for prophylactic orthopedic surgical intervention include more than 50% of cortical bone destroyed, a lesion in the proximal femur larger than 2.5 cm, and the continuation of stress pain despite radiation treatment to the bone. After a bone has fractured, stabilization surgery may be necessary, improving life expectancy and relieving pain. In addition, the patient with a collapsed vertebral body due to vertebral metastases may require resection of the vertebral body and spine stabilization.

I wonder if radio-frequency lesioning would affect my new Radiohead CD.

Cryoanalgesia

Cryoanalgesia deactivates a nerve using a cooled probe that causes temporary nerve injury. Nerve function returns over time and the procedure can be repeated. Cryoanalgesia can provide effective pain relief for the patient with pain from a surgical scar, a neuroma trapped in scar tissue, and occipital neuralgia.

Radio-frequency lesioning

Radio-frequency lesioning may affect the nerve from the heat generated, the magnetic field created by the radio waves, or both.

Nerve function is stopped for a prolonged period. If it does return, the procedure can be repeated. The most frequent use of this technology is to treat pain related to the facet joint and lumbar sympathetic and peripheral nerves. Because it's a very focused therapy, it's used when specific nerves can be targeted.

Complementary and alternative therapies

Many complementary and alternative therapies can reduce cancer pain or help the patient with cancer cope with pain. A pain management plan commonly combines one or more of these therapies with drug therapy. Some complementary and alternative therapies used to treat cancer pain include:

- hypnosis
- psychotherapy
- relaxation
- biofeedback
- thermotherapy
- cryotherapy
- transcutaneous electrical nerve stimulation (TENS)
- acupuncture.

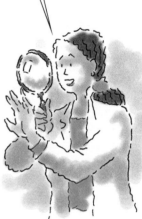

Hypnosis increases awareness and concentration so a person can alter cognitive perceptions.

Hypnosis

Hypnosis produces a state of increased awareness and concentration, allowing patients to alter their cognitive perceptions. Some cancer patients are able to use this technique to help them reduce or cope with pain.

Psychotherapy

Receiving a diagnosis of cancer or news that cancer has spread can create a sudden emotional crisis. Short-term psychotherapy can help a person cope with this type of crisis. Evidence-based research shows that the cancer patient who receives structured, active support from therapists lives longer and reports less pain.

Relaxation

Relaxation techniques can reduce elevated heart rate, relax tense muscles, distract a patient from his pain, and enhance coping. Progressive muscle relaxation, deep breathing, and imagery can enhance relaxation.

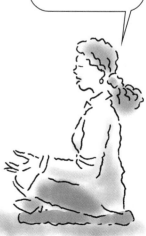

Relaxation can reduce heart rate, relax muscles, and distract a patient from his pain.

Biofeedback

Biofeedback is a method of promoting relaxation by consciously controlling body functions, such as blood pressure, heart and respiratory rates, temperature, and perspiration. To use biofeedback, the patient uses equipment that allows him to track changes in these body functions. This technique has been found to reduce cancer pain through the patient's learned conscious control of these body responses.

Cryotherapy

Cryotherapy, or cold application, can reduce inflammation, slow transmission along nerve fibers, reduce edema, decrease muscle spasms, deactivate trigger points, and numb the skin before a procedure. Cryotherapy shouldn't be used on a patient who is confused or cognitively impaired or has decreased consciousness.

TENS

TENS alters the patient's perception of pain by blocking painful stimuli traveling over nerve fibers. It may be effective in the treatment of cancer pain by reducing muscle spasm, decreasing edema, and raising the pain threshold. Moreover, TENS provides the patient with an increased sense of control. The therapy appears to be most effective in treating neuropathic pain, such as postthoracotomy pain, radicular lower-extremity pain after radical pelvic tumor dissection and, in some cases, intractable pain following pelvic extenuation due to radiation necrosis.

Acupuncture

Acupuncture is a form of traditional Chinese medicine that uses thin needles inserted at designated points on the body to restore health. The needles are believed to work by enhancing the flow of energy *(qi)* in the body. Acupuncture may control nausea and vomiting from chemotherapy and appears to reduce pain in some patients. A recent study from Duke University reports that women who had breast surgery and used acupuncture as an adjunct reported less postoperative nausea, vomiting, and pain.

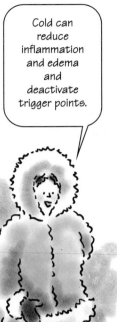

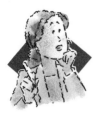

Quick quiz

1. Cancer pain can be caused by:
A.   surgical removal of a tumor.
B.   radiation damage to tissues.
C.   adverse effects of chemotherapy.
D.   all of the above.

Answer: D. The cancer patient can develop pain from surgery, radiation, and chemotherapy as well as many other causes. Surgery causes nociceptive pain. Radiation can cause delayed neuropathic pain but can also cause short-term nociceptive skin irritation. Some chemotherapy agents can produce an immediate burning sensation while being infused, and others can cause neuropathic pain over the course of therapy.

2. One of the first signs or symptoms of spinal cord compression is:
A.   nausea and vomiting.
B.   new back pain.
C.   bladder dysfunction.
D.   pathologic bone fractures.

Answer: B. As spinal cord compression begins, new back pain is most commonly the first symptom.

3. Which alternative therapy is most beneficial in treating the patient experiencing neuropathic pain?
A.   Cryotherapy
B.   Biofeedback
C.   Herbal therapy
D.   TENS

Answer: D. TENS therapy is most effective in treating neuropathic pain because it alters the patient's pain perception by blocking painful stimuli traveling within the nerve fibers.

4. According to the WHO analgesic ladder, which of the following drugs would most likely be used first to treat mild pain?
A.   Opioids
B.   Antidepressants
C.   NSAIDs
D.   Local anesthetics

Answer: C. According to the WHO analgesic ladder, the patient with mild pain should start with nonopioid analgesics such as NSAIDs.

5. Which of the following drugs should be given with NSAIDs to reduce the risk of adverse GI effects?

    A.   Misoprostol
    B.   Methadone
    C.   Aspirin
    D.   Naloxone

Answer: A. Such drugs as misoprostol, ranitidine, and omeprazole can reduce the risk of adverse GI effects in the patient taking NSAIDs.

Scoring

 If you answered all five questions correctly, zowee! You've certainly shown that you're a person WHO knows about cancer pain!

If you answered three or four questions correctly, super! You have cancer pain on the run!

If you answered fewer than three questions correctly, don't despair. Increase your dose of information by reading the chapter again!

HIV-AIDS pain

Just the facts

In this chapter, you'll learn:

♦ the types of pain experienced by patients with HIV-AIDS

♦ pharmacologic and nonpharmacologic methods to control HIV-AIDS pain

♦ polypharmacy in HIV-AIDS treatment

♦ pain syndromes associated with HIV-AIDS.

A look at HIV-AIDS pain

Human immunodeficiency virus (HIV) disease is a chronic infection that occurs after infection with HIV. After the virus spreads throughout the bloodstream (up to 2 weeks after infection), the patient may be asymptomatic from months to more than 10 years. During this latent period, the virus is continually replicating and attacking the immune system. Eventually, a state of profound immunodeficiency occurs, known as acquired immunodeficiency syndrome (AIDS). Without antiviral treatment, the immune system declines until the body is no longer able to mount normal protective defenses, typically resulting in many opportunistic infections and related malignancies.

HIV attacks and weakens the immune system.

Technology to the rescue

Recent advances in the treatment of HIV-AIDS have significantly altered the course of the disease and prolonged life. Highly active antiretroviral therapy (HAART), a combination drug therapy, and prophylactic therapy for opportunistic infections are largely responsible for the dramatic decline in death rates from AIDS since

1996 as well as for the decreased number of complications of advanced AIDS. HIV has changed from an almost universally deadly disease to a chronic, medically managed illness.

Now the bad news

Even so, pain in patients with HIV-AIDS is common and usually undertreated. Surveys show that 50% to 80% of adult patients with HIV-AIDS report having pain. In addition, a recent survey discovered that analgesic therapy was prescribed for only 32% of patients with AIDS who reported pain and only 28% of patients who reported pain greater than 4 on a 0-to-10 scale. (See *Pain control challenges in HIV-AIDS.*)

> Thanks to combination drug therapy, life expectancies from AIDS are increasing. Now, back to the Hall of Justice!

Causes of HIV-AIDS pain

Despite the encouraging advances in treatment, the patient with HIV-AIDS continues to suffer pain that's frequently severe. Moreover, the patient commonly has multiple sources of pain. In fact, he may experience an average of seven simultaneous pain symptoms. In addition, emotional distress, anxiety, and depression typi-

> Pain control in the patient with HIV-AIDS may be complicated by many types of pain, advanced cancer, I.V. drug abuse, methadone treatment, and opioid tolerance and addiction.

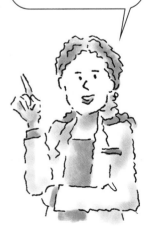

Pain control challenges in HIV-AIDS

The patient with HIV-AIDS may have acute and chronic pain as well as procedural-related pain. This combination presents a considerable challenge in pain control.

Worse than cancer
Although HIV-AIDS-related pain is sometimes compared to cancer pain, there are some unique features. Compared to the nonimmuno-compromised cancer patient, the patient with HIV-AIDS commonly has cancer in a more advanced stage that follows a more aggressive course.

Abuse isn't an excuse
Additionally, because many patients with AIDS have a history of I.V. drug abuse and may be on methadone, concerns about tolerance and addiction may complicate opioid treatment decisions. Particularly in the terminally ill, it's important that concerns about addiction don't prevent or limit appropriate opioid treatment.

cally accompany the pain. Sources of pain in the patient with HIV-AIDS include:

• direct effects of HIV on the nervous system such as peripheral neuropathy
• opportunistic infections such as oral and esophageal lesions caused by herpes simplex
• immunosuppression-related tumors such as Kaposi's sarcoma
• abdominal pain resulting from an infectious process, diarrhea, or organomegaly
• therapeutic interventions such as pharmacologic treatments with chemotherapy or antiviral medications
• musculoskeletal pain (arthralgia).

Types of HIV-AIDS pain

The patient with HIV-AIDS may experience nociceptive pain, neuropathic pain, or both. In addition, the pain may be acute or chronic.

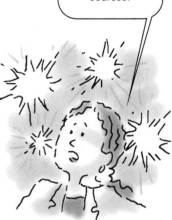

The HIV-AIDS patient can simultaneously experience many types of pain from many sources.

Nociceptive pain

Nociceptive pain occurs when a noxious stimulus activates primary afferent nerve endings called nociceptors. Nociceptive pain receptors may be located in somatic or visceral tissue. Here are some causes of nociceptive pain in the patient with HIV-AIDS:

• *somatic* — Reiter's syndrome, myalgia, osteopenia resulting in osteoporosis, and arthritis.
• *visceral* — Kaposi's sarcoma and other oral cavity lesions, GI infections, tumors, and drug treatment adverse effects.

Neuropathic pain

Neuropathic pain occurs when sensory nerves are damaged and become irritable and hyperexcitable and continually send pain messages. The pain may occur without identifiable tissue injury. It can be intermittent or continuous and may be described as deep-aching, freezing-cold, itching, shooting, shocklike, burning, or pins and needles. Neuropathic pain in HIV-AIDS might involve the central or peripheral nervous system or both. Here are some causes of neuropathic pain in the patient with HIV-AIDS:

• *central* — neurosyphilis, some malignancies, and brain abscesses.
• *peripheral* — peripheral neuropathy, herpes zoster, and postherpetic neuralgia.

Assessing HIV-AIDS pain

Correct assessment of HIV-AIDS pain depends on successfully identifying underlying disorders that cause pain. Pain may be related to malignancies, infection, or the treatments themselves. Careful assessment is a must to detect and treat all sources of pain because the complications of HIV-AIDS are unpredictable.

At present, there are no individualized pain assessment tools devised specifically for the patient with HIV-AIDS. Be sure to ask the patient if he's using any nonpharmacologic therapies, herbal products, or experimental medications to ensure safety and to avoid the adverse interactions with prescribed medical interventions.

Opportunity hard knocks

It's especially important to be aware of opportunistic infections that occur with this disease because such symptoms as fever, diarrhea, and anorexia can cause pain. It's also important to know other medications that the patient is taking and to evaluate if he has a substance abuse problem. Knowing these facts will assist the health care provider in developing an effective pain management plan.

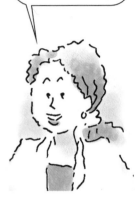

Be sure to ask the HIV-AIDS patient about nonpharmacologic therapies, herbal products, or experimental drugs he may be using.

Managing HIV-AIDS pain

The major treatment approach for HIV-AIDS pain is administration of drugs, such as antibiotics, antifungals, and antivirals, to treat a correctable cause of pain. Opioids and nonopioid analgesics are administered to control the pain itself. Nonpharmacologic therapies are also used as an adjunct to pharmacologic therapies to enhance the drug's effects or the patient's ability to control pain.

Pharmacologic management of HIV-AIDS pain

Pharmacologic management of HIV-AIDS pain should be based primarily on the guidelines set forth in the World Health Organization (WHO) analgesic ladder. These guidelines suggest a three-step "ladder," with gradually increased drug strength and dosing to achieve pain relief based on the intensity of the patient's pain. The ladder includes three categories of drugs: nonopioids, opioids, and adjuvant drugs. Adjuvant drugs can be used on any step of the ladder. Some sources add a fourth step to the ladder for interventional (invasive) pain management approaches, such as regional blocks, epidural and intrathecal medications, electrical stimulation, and neurodestruction techniques.

Abuse alert

It's important to remember as well that one-third of AIDS cases are the result of I.V. substance abuse. Therefore, in addition to adjusting treatment to the patient's pain level, it's commonly necessary to adjust analgesic medications upward to account for opioid tolerance from substance abuse. Finally, because HIV-AIDS treatment requires concurrent administration of several drugs (polypharmacy) and the patient with advanced HIV-AIDS is susceptible to cognitive impairments, close monitoring of drug therapy and potential interactions is a must.

> For managing HIV-AIDS pain, check out the WHO ladder plus one.

Nonopioids

On the first step of the analgesic ladder, mild pain is treated with nonopioids, such as acetaminophen or nonsteroidal anti-inflammatory drugs (NSAIDs), with or without adjuvant drugs.

Acetaminophen adversity

While acetaminophen can provide relief for mild to moderate pain, keep these precautions in mind for the patient with HIV-AIDS:
• Acetaminophen, even in therapeutic doses, can have hepatotoxic effects in the HIV-AIDS patient with liver disease, malnourishment, or alcoholism. Use acetaminophen cautiously or avoid its use altogether in this high-risk case.
• Be aware that combination drugs, such as Vicodin and Percocet, contain acetaminophen.
• Educate HIV-AIDS patients about the potential risks associated with taking acetaminophen. Because it's available over the counter, many people are unaware of possible adverse effects.

> Many combination pain relievers contain acetaminophen, which can be hepatotoxic. You wouldn't do that to me, would you? Nah!

Something old, something new

NSAIDS have anti-inflammatory and analgesic effects, which may be a benefit over acetaminophen in conditions involving inflammatory response. However, achieving an anti-inflammatory effect requires higher dosing than what's necessary for analgesic effect. NSAIDs are also associated with some adverse effects:
• Common adverse effects of NSAIDs are GI irritation and ulceration. Although the risk of developing these problems is no greater from NSAIDs than HIV disease itself, HIV-AIDS patients with past or current GI ulcers, with infectious or inflammatory GI

illnesses (cytomegalovirus, colitis), or using corticosteroids are at higher risk for ulceration. NSAIDs should be used cautiously or avoided altogether in these patients.

- Newer COX-2 inhibitor NSAIDs, such as rofecoxib (Vioxx), celecoxib (Celebrex), and valdecoxib (Bextra), are good alternatives to standard NSAIDs because they cause significantly less GI irritation and ulceration.
- HIV-AIDS patients with liver dysfunction are at risk for bleeding and coagulation problems. Standard NSAIDs interfere with platelet activity and increase the risk of bleeding. The COX-2 inhibitor drugs have no effect on platelets, although rofecoxib does cause a small increase in the International Normalized Ratio (INR).

Unlike other NSAIDs, COX-2 inhibitors don't interfere with platelets.

Why risk it?

- Chronic use of NSAIDs at high doses can cause renal dysfunction, particularly in high-risk groups. HIV-AIDS patients at higher risk include those with preexisting renal impairment (such as HIV-associated nephropathy), liver dysfunction, heart failure, concurrent use of ACE inhibitors or diuretics, and use of potentially nephrotoxic drugs. To prevent renal damage, start NSAIDs at low doses, closely monitor kidney function, and ensure adequate hydration before initiating therapy. Consider using aspirin because of its lower incidence of adverse renal effects. Avoid indomethacin (Indocin), if possible, because of its association with increased adverse renal effects.

Opioids

With increasing pain levels, the second and third steps of the WHO analgesic ladder call for the use of opioids, with or without nonopioid and adjuvant drug use. However, adding a nonopioid drug can usually significantly increase pain control. Detecting and managing adverse drug effects in the patient with HIV-AIDS can be a challenge. In addition, keep these cautions in mind:

Hold the morphine

- If the patient has renal disease, choose opioids without active metabolites, such as hydromorphone (Dilaudid), oxycodone (OxyContin), and fentanyl (Sublimaze). In contrast, morphine has metabolites that have active analgesic and adverse effects and can accumulate after continuous dosing in the patient with renal disease, leading to opioid overdose and respiratory depression.
- The patient with HIV-AIDS who has a history of substance abuse may have developed opioid tolerance, requiring higher opioid doses for pain control. This patient is at risk for undertreatment of pain, as evidenced by a number of studies reporting high-

Now I get it!

Opioid tolerance and substance abuse

The patient with AIDS who has a history of substance abuse may need higher opioid doses for pain control. One study showed that patients with AIDS who had a history of substance abuse required more than twice the dosage of morphine to control pain than patients with AIDS who didn't have a history of abuse. This was true whether the patient abused opioid or nonopioid drugs—for example, heroin, cocaine, amphetamines, or marijuana. Moreover, patients with past addictions, whether they were on methadone or drug-free, had a lower pain threshold and a shorter tolerance of pain than patients without addiction.

Block the NMDA

Some recent evidence links the development of opioid tolerance to N-methyl-D-aspartate (NMDA) receptors in the central nervous system. Drugs that block NMDA receptors, such as ketamine (Ketalar) and dextromethorphan (Pertussin), may decrease the degree of tolerance. Methadone may also contain some NMDA-blocking action and may provide added benefit in managing pain in patients with opioid tolerance.

er levels of pain in the patient with a history of substance abuse than in other patients with AIDS. (See *Opioid tolerance and substance abuse*.)

• The patient with HIV-AIDS may receive methadone (Dolophine) for substance abuse recovery or pain control. Unlike most other opioids, methadone is metabolized by a group of liver enzymes known as the cytochrome P-450 (CYP-450) enzymes. Drugs that increase or decrease CYP-450 enzymes alter the metabolism of substances such as methadone that are metabolized by these enzymes. Many HIV medications induce or inhibit (such as protease inhibitors) the CYP-450 enzyme.

Pitch the patch

• Because the release rate of transdermal fentanyl increases when the patch is exposed to elevated temperatures, the febrile HIV-AIDS patient may receive higher doses, putting him at risk for opioid overdose and respiratory depression. To reduce the risk of these complications, remove the patch when the patient is febrile and switch to an oral or parenteral opioid. Likewise, warn him not to apply heat to the patch, such as heating pads, heat lamps, and heated waterbeds.

• Although constipation can be a problem in many patients taking opioids, in HIV-AIDS patients, who commonly suffer from diarrhea, this adverse effect may be of benefit.

• Cognitive impairment can occur with opioids as well as HIV-AIDS-related conditions, such as HIV encephalopathy and dementia and central nervous system (CNS) infections. Keep in mind that HIV encephalopathy develops gradually over months and doesn't cause significant changes in levels of alertness. In contrast, declining alertness and increasing sedation caused by opioids always precede the more serious adverse effect of respiratory depression. The use of opioids with sedatives and other CNS depressant drugs increases the patient's risk of severe respiratory depression.

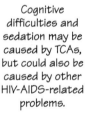

Release of transdermal fentanyl increases when the patch is exposed to elevated temperatures, including fever.

Adjuvant therapies

The WHO analgesic ladder recommends the use of adjuvant drugs be considered at any time during treatment. Use caution when administering adjuvant therapies, however; many interact with drug therapies commonly used to treat HIV-AIDS, causing altered serum drug levels and potential toxic effects. Some common adjuvant drugs used to treat HIV-AIDS pain are tricyclic antidepressants (TCAs), anticonvulsants, antispasmodics, and topical analgesics. In addition, according to ongoing research, human nerve growth factor (NGF) appears to provide excellent pain relief as well.

Tricyclics statistics

The dose of TCAs needed for analgesia is lower than the dose required for treating depression. While all TCAs are similar in their analgesic effect, there are differences in their adverse effects. For example, nortriptyline (Pamelor) has fewer cardiac effects than amitriptyline (Elavil) and may be preferable for patients with cardiac arrhythmias. TCAs may interact with such drugs as methadone, selective serotonin reuptake inhibitors, and quinidine (Quinaglute), causing an increase in TCA drug levels that may lead to toxicity.

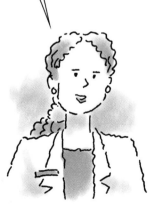

Cognitive difficulties and sedation may be caused by TCAs, but could also be caused by other HIV-AIDS-related problems.

You're getting sleepy...

All TCAs cause some degree of sedation and are usually given at bedtime to help combat insomnia. However, remember to consider other possible sources of these symptoms in the patient with HIV-AIDS, such as CNS infections, HIV dementia and encephalopathy, and other sedating drugs or drug interactions.

Up the anti

The anticonvulsant gabapentin (Neurontin) is usually the first choice among anticonvulsants for relieving neuropathic pain, including peripheral neuropathy, postherpetic neuralgia (PHN), and chronic radicular pain. Gabapentin has almost no drug interactions with HIV drugs. Other anticonvulsants may interact with drugs commonly taken by patients with HIV, such as isoniazid (Nydrazid) and protease inhibitors, and can also cause sedation. In addition, the anticonvulsant zonisamide (Zonegran) causes mild appetite suppression, which can be a drawback for some patients with HIV-AIDS. Combining a TCA and an anticonvulsant (for example, amitriptyline and gabapentin) can increase analgesia, but requires monitoring for drug toxicities and interactions.

As with antidepressant administration, don't forget to explore other possible causes for these types of symptoms, such as CNS infections, HIV dementia and encephalopathy, and other sedating drugs or drug interactions.

Back lovers love baclofen

Baclofen (Lioresal) is an antispasmodic drug that decreases hyperexcitability in neuropathic pain and promotes spinal cord inhibition of pain. However, when discontinuing baclofen after prolonged use at high doses, particularly if used intrathecally, taper the drug over 10 to 14 days to prevent a rare but potentially fatal withdrawal syndrome of rebound spasticity, rhabdomyolysis, multiple organ failure, and death.

Spicy topicals

Topical analgesics used for neuropathic pain include capsaicin (Zostrix) and lidocaine (Lidoderm). Capsaicin, the active ingredient in hot peppers, causes the release of substance P from peripheral nerve endings, which in turn causes a burning sensation (followed by analgesia in 20 to 30 minutes). Because of the initial burning sensation, some patients find capsaicin intolerable. The lidocaine patch has recently been approved for use in PHN with intact skin. Up to three patches can be applied on top of the painful area for 12 hours every 24 hours. However, toxic effects may occur if used concurrently with a Class I antiarrhythmic such as mexiletine (Mexitil). (See *Applying the Lidoderm patch safely*, page 232.)

Lidocaine patches can relieve the pain of PHN.

Will they grow back?

Human NGF is currently being studied and shows promise for pain relief in diffuse neuropathies, such as HIV-associated distal sensory neuropathies. NGF appears to modify nerve activity, especially in the small, sensory nerve fibers

Peak technique

Applying the Lidoderm patch safely

The Lidoderm patch contains 5% lidocaine to help the patient achieve relief from neuropathic pain such as postherpetic neuralgia. When administering the patch, first check the health care provider's order for the proper dose, such as half a patch, a full patch, or even up to three patches. Apply all patches at the same time to intact skin only, over the area of pain. Allow the patch to remain in place for 12 hours, then take it off for 12 hours. Fold the used patch onto itself and discard it safely. The drug could be fatal if the patch is chewed by a child or an animal. Be sure to wash your hands before and after applying the patch. Monitor the patient receiving class I antiarrhythmics carefully for additive effects and toxicity. Observe the patient for allergic reactions.

affected by distal sensory neuropathies. It isn't clear, however, if it's successful in stimulating new nerve growth. Even so, many patients taking human NGF experience significant pain relief while continuing to use antiretroviral drugs known to cause peripheral neuropathy. Patients reporting the most severe pain before treatment show the most improvement. This therapy does, however, require twice weekly injections.

Polypharmacy

For many patients with HIV-AIDS, polypharmacy (the use of multiple drugs at the same time) is necessary to control the disease and its complications. Unfortunately, it also increases the risk of adverse effects and interactions. Many patients will be concurrently taking some or all of the following drugs or therapies:
• 3 or more HAART drugs
• drugs to prevent or treat opportunistic infections, associated cancers, and adverse drug effects, such as diarrhea and sedation
• illegal substances (due to substance abuse problems)
• herbal preparations, vitamins, and supplements
• alternative therapies and experimental drugs
• pain management drugs.

> Patients with HIV-AIDS may be taking many drugs simultaneously. This is called polypharmacy.

How to react when they interact

Many antiretrovirals, so vital to the survival of the patient with HIV-AIDS, interact with the drugs prescribed to treat pain. For example, ritonavir (Norvir) may produce life-threatening drug interactions when taken with meperidine (Demerol), propoxyphene (Darvon), and midazolam (Versed). To reduce the risk of drug interactions, review the patient's drugs with the doctor and pharmacist. If possible, reduce the number of drugs the patient takes and eliminate those that aren't necessary. Be sure to ask about herbal remedies, over-the-counter drugs, and vitamin and nutritional supplements when taking a drug history. (See *Common analgesic and HIV drug interactions*, pages 234 to 236.)

Nonpharmacologic therapies

There are many nonpharmacologic therapies that can help reduce HIV-AIDS pain or help the patient better cope with his pain. These therapies include:
• thermotherapy to increase blood flow and decrease inflammation
• cryotherapy to decrease muscle spasticity
• vibration to relieve muscle aches, headache, and neuropathic pain
• transcutaneous electrical nerve stimulation (TENS) to block painful stimuli, altering the patient's pain perception
• strengthening and exercise to restore muscle tone and strength
• massage to enhance immune system response and decrease anxiety and depression
• acupuncture to alter circulation of energy *(qi)* in the body, reducing pain
• relaxation to help reduce stress and pain severity
• hypnosis to increase concentration and better cope with pain.

HIV-AIDS pain disorders

Because HIV-AIDS is an immunodeficiency disorder, many associated pain disorders stem from infection. Others are the result of adverse effects of medication, inflammation, and effects of the disease on body systems. Some common disorders associated with HIV-AIDS pain are:
• oral and esophageal ulcers
• other GI tract disorders, such as diarrhea, hepatosplenomegaly, pancreatitis, and AIDS-related cholangitis, causing abdominal pain
• musculoskeletal disorders, such as Reiter's syndrome, reactive arthritis, fibromyalgia, and vasculitis
• herpes zoster
• other neuropathic syndromes, including various peripheral neuropathies.

(Text continues on page 236.)

Common analgesic and HIV drug interactions

Because of the polypharmacy common in HIV-AIDS treatment, it's important to know how pain medications interact with drugs used to treat HIV-AIDS. The chart below lists common pain medications, corresponding HIV drugs, their effects on the analgesics, and actions to consider.

Analgesic	Drug used to treat HIV or co-infection	Interaction	Special considerations
Opioids			
Methadone	Nevirapine Efavirenz Amprenavir Lopinavir/Ritonavir Rifampin	Substantial decrease in methadone level	• Monitor for signs and symptoms of opiate withdrawal. • Consider increasing the methadone dose to provide analgesia or decrease withdrawal symptoms.
	Nelfinavir Ritonavir	Moderate decrease in methadone level	• Increase methadone dose as appropriate.
	Fluconazole	Increase in methadone level	• Monitor for methadone toxicity. • Consider decreasing methadone dose.
	Delavirdine	May increase methadone level	• Monitor for methadone toxicity. • Consider decreasing methadone dose.
	Abacavir	May decrease methadone level and increase abacavir level	• Monitor for signs and symptoms of opiate withdrawal. • Consider small increase in methadone dose if needed. • Monitor for abacavir toxicity.
	Diadanosine	May decrease diadonosine levels (with tablets only)	• Consider increasing diadonosine dose.
Morphine	Rifampin	May decrease morphine level	• Monitor for signs and symptoms of opiate withdrawal. • Consider increasing morphine dose or use alternative opioid.
Meperidine	Ritonavir	Increased normeperidine (toxic metabolite) level and decreased meperidine level	• Contraindicated for concurrent use. • Monitor for normeperidine toxicity (CNS irritability, tremor, seizure). • Monitor for signs and symptoms of decreased analgesia. • Switch to a different opioid.

Common analgesic and HIV drug interactions (continued)

Analgesic	Drug used to treat HIV or co-infection	Interaction	Special considerations
Opioids (continued)			
Propoxyphene	Ritonavir	Increased propoxyphene level	• Contraindicated for concurrent use. • Monitor for signs and symptoms of propoxyphene toxicity.
NSAIDs			
Celecoxib	Fluconazole	Increased celecoxib level (up to two times normal)	• Use lowest recommended dose or use a different NSAID. • Monitor for signs and symptoms of celecoxid toxicity.
Rofecoxib	Methotrexate	Possible increased methotrexate level with higher doses of rofecoxib	• Monitor for methotrexate toxicity.
Benzodiazepines			
Flurazepam Diazepam Midazolam Triazolam	Delavirdine Efavirenz Indinavir Saquinavir Nelfinavir Amprenavir Lopinavir/ritonavir Fluconazole Itraconazole	Increased flurazepam, diazepam, midazolam, or triazolam level and prolonged effects	• Not recommended for concurrent use. • Monitor for signs and symptoms of benzodiazepine toxicity (increased sedation and respiratory depression). • Decrease benzodiazepine dose. • Use an alternative benzodiazepine, such as temazepam or lorazepam.
	Ritonavir	Increased flurazepam, diazepam, midazolam, or triazolam level and prolonged effects	• Contraindicated for concurrent use. • Monitor for signs and symptoms of benzodiazepine toxicity.
	Rifampin Nevirapine	Decreased flurazepam, diazepam, midazolam, or triazolam level	• Increase benzodiazepine dose cautiously. • Use an alternative benzodiazepine such as temazepam or lorazepam.

(continued)

Common analgesic and HIV drug interactions *(continued)*			
Analgesic	**Drug used to treat HIV or co-infection**	**Interaction**	**Special considerations**
Anticonvulsants			
Carbamazepine Phenytoin Phenobarbital	Indinavir Saquinavir Nelfinavir Amprenavir Lopinavir/ritonavir	Decreased carbamazepine, phenytoin, or phenobarbital level; may decrease indinavir, saquinavir, nelfinavir, amprenavir, or lopinavir/ritonavir level	• Monitor drug levels. • Consider increasing anticonvulsant dose. • Consider using an alternative anticonvulsant such as gabapentin.
Carbamazepine	Ritonavir Clarithromycin	Increased carbamazepine level	• Consider lowering the carbamazepine dose. • Consider using an alternative anticonvulsant such as gabapentin.

Oral and esophageal ulcers

Oral and esophageal ulcers are a common cause of GI tract pain experienced by the patient with HIV-AIDS. Prompt identification and treatment of oral lesions are important because they can impair nutrition and result in wasting. Causes of oral and esophageal pain are:

• *fungal.* Oral candidiasis is one of the most common oral diseases in the patient with HIV-AIDS. It may appear as painless white spots or painful discrete lesions and fissures at the corners of the mouth. Pain is commonly described as burning accompanied by dysphagia (difficulty swallowing) and odynophagia (pain upon swallowing) if the lesions extend into the esophagus.

• *viral.* Cytomegalovirus (CMV) and herpes simplex may cause painful oral lesions in HIV disease.

• *bacterial.* Necrotizing ulcerative gingivitis, necrotizing ulcerative periodontitis, and necrotizing ulcerative stomatitis caused by bacteria destroy the mucosa and tooth-supporting bone structures. These ulcerative lesions may be necrotic and painful and may expose underlying bone, producing deep-seated pain as well as tooth loss. Pain from epiglottiditis may result in throat soreness, odynophagia, and laryngeal tenderness. The condition mandates close observation for airway compromise.

It's important to treat oral lesions right away to avoid nutrition problems.

• *oncologic.* Kaposi's sarcoma commonly causes neoplasms in the mouth. Small, flat lesions may be painless, but bigger, bulkier lesions may produce painful ulcers. Non-Hodgkin's lymphoma may produce oral ulcers or diffuse lymphatic swelling, causing pressure and pain on surrounding tissues.

• *idiopathic.* Oral aphthous ulcers are of unknown origin; they may cause severe pain and extend into the esophagus.

Managing oral and esophageal ulcer pain

The first step in reducing pain caused by oral lesions is treating them with appropriate antimicrobials and other drugs, depending on the cause. Various combinations of topical mixtures, or "cocktails," may be administered to soothe oral and esophageal ulcer pain.

Teetotalling topical cocktails

One example is a mixture of viscous lidocaine, diphenhydramine (Benadryl), and Maalox to "swish and swallow or spit." Lidocaine produces local anesthesia, diphenhydramine promotes an anti-inflammatory effect, and Maalox coats the mucosa and helps the mixture cling to the ulcers. Administration of topical steroids such as triamcinolone acetonide (Kenalog in Orabase) may be helpful for aphthous ulcers. Be sure to use alcohol-free preparations to avoid stinging open ulcerations. Although these drug mixtures are commonly helpful in decreasing mucosal pain, their effect is often short-lived. Thalidomide (Thalomid) is occasionally used to treat recalcitrant mucosal ulcers.

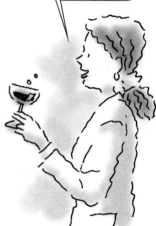

Topical cocktails aren't your normal cocktails, but they're a lot more effective at relieving pain!

Other GI tract disorders

Many other GI tract disorders associated with HIV-AIDS cause general abdominal pain. Diarrhea is the most frequent GI complaint in the patient with HIV-AIDS. Pain from diarrhea is usually felt as abdominal cramping when the small intestine is affected or as left lower quadrant pain and tenesmus (painful rectal spasm with involuntary but ineffectual straining at stool) with colonic disorders.

Some other causes of abdominal pain are:

• *hepatosplenomegaly.* Patients with disseminated *Mycobacterium avium* complex with infiltrations into the liver and spleen commonly report episodes of severe, sharp, stabbing pain in the left upper quadrant, flank, and back. Hepatitis B is the most common form of hepatitis found in patients with HIV-AIDS. About 90% of patients infected with hepatitis B will experience acute infection and then develop protective immunity to the disease. In con-

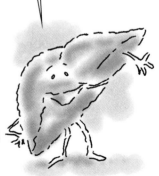

Ninety percent of patients who contract hepatitis B will develop protective immunity. Phew!

trast, about 85% of patients infected with hepatitis C (HCV) will develop chronic HCV.

• *pancreatitis.* Painful pancreatitis with severe epigastric or left upper quadrant pain may be caused by opportunistic infections or neoplasms. However, the cause is usually related to medications (such as didanosine [Videx], stavudine [Zerit], zalcitabine [Hivid], and co-trimoxazole [Bactrim]) or due to drug or alcohol use. Biliary tract infection with microsporidia or cryptosporidia can also cause pancreatitis. Gallstones and biliary strictures can also precipitate the disorder.

• *AIDS-related cholangitis.* Multiple pathogens cause inflammation and injury to the bile ducts, ultimately resulting in cholangitis, or thickening, narrowing, and obstruction in the biliary tree. Patients report sharp pain in the right upper quadrant that may radiate to the back, typically accompanied by nausea and vomiting. Unfortunately, for most patients, AIDS-related cholangitis worsens despite antimicrobial therapy and has a mortality of 86% within 1 year of diagnosis. Therefore, pain control and patient comfort measures become paramount in treating this disorder.

Managing abdominal pain

Opioid analgesics, such as morphine, hydromorphone, or fentanyl, may be necessary to control the severe, visceral pain that typically occurs with biliary and pancreatic disease. In addition to pain control, opioid therapy decreases bowel motility and may help to slow diarrhea as well. (See *Meperidine and biliary spasm.*)

A celiac plexus block of the sympathetic nerves supplying the organs may relieve pain caused by cholangitis or pancreatitis. Endoscopic sphincterotomy may provide significant and lasting pain relief for patients with cholangitis.

Musculoskeletal disorders

Many patients with HIV-AIDS experience arthralgia (joint pain), some of which is significant enough to interfere with daily activities. Some common musculoskeletal disorders include:

• *Reiter's syndrome.* An inflammatory arthritis, Reiter's syndrome may occur in the general population after a genitourinary or GI infection. It occurs, however, at a higher rate in HIV-AIDS patients even though an infectious cause isn't always identified. The patient with Reiter's syndrome commonly reports painful knee, ankle, foot, and sacroiliac joints. Other manifestations may include urethritis, conjunctivitis, and painless skin and mucous membrane lesions. Reactive arthritis causes the same joint pain as Reiter's syndrome, but without the other associated symptoms.

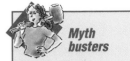

Myth busters

Meperidine and biliary spasm

Myth: Meperidine causes fewer biliary or sphincter spasms than other opioids. In the past, it was the drug of choice because of its rapid onset of action and short duration in the body.

Fact: Meperidine doesn't cause fewer biliary or sphincter spasms than other opioids. Moreover, it offers no advantage in treating biliary and pancreatic pain. Given meperidine's toxic potential, short duration of analgesia, and tendency to cause tachycardia, other less toxic and more effective opioids should be used to control pain caused by biliary spasm.

• *HIV–AIDS-associated arthropathy.* Joint pain, mostly in the knees and ankles, develops slowly over 1 to 6 weeks and lasts for 6 weeks to 6 months in HIV–AIDS-associated arthropathy. It has no known cause.

• *painful articular syndrome.* Like HIV–AIDS-associated arthropathy, painful articular syndrome has no known cause. It occurs in about 10% of patients with AIDS. Symptoms include severe joint pain, typically in the knees, elbows, and shoulders, lasting from a few hours to a few days.

• *myalgia.* Myalgia (muscle pain) can occur in patients with HIV-AIDS as a result of drug therapy, particularly with zidovudine (commonly called toxic myopathy), or from HIV-related muscle inflammation and necrosis (polymyositis). Pain can be severe and may be accompanied by muscle weakness, elevated muscle enzymes, and electromyogram changes.

• *fibromyalgia.* A poorly understood condition of widespread pain with multiple, defined musculoskeletal "tender points," fibromyalgia is diagnosed at a higher rate in patients with HIV-AIDS than in the general population.

• *generalized arthralgias.* HCV infection may accompany generalized arthralgias. Severe polyarthralgias may also occur during treatment with HIV drug therapies, possibly due to increased CD4+ T-cell counts and an improved immune response. This is thought to be part of "immune reactivation syndromes" in which AIDS-related illness may reappear or increase in severity as a result of improved immune markers responding to anti-HIV drug regimens.

• *vasculitis.* Blood vessel inflammation, or vasculitis, should also be considered in the patient with HIV-AIDS who has unexplained arthritis or myopathy.

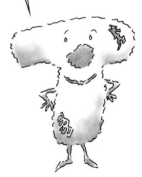

Sometimes more of me can lead to immune reactivation syndromes. Talk about a Catch-22!

Managing musculoskeletal pain

The underlying cause of muscle or joint pain should be treated, if it can be identified. If the patient's arthralgia is thought to be drug-related, stop the offending drug. After stopping zidovudine, muscle strength, enzymes, and pain levels usually return to normal within 4 to 8 weeks. Corticosteroids may be indicated in some conditions. NSAIDS and opioids may be given to control pain.

Herpes zoster

Herpes zoster is an opportunistic infection more commonly experienced by immunosuppressed patients, including patients with HIV-AIDS, than the general patient population. Herpes zoster can occur at any stage of HIV-AIDS, and may be the first indication of declining immune function. Herpes zoster also has a higher rate of recurrence in immunosuppressed patients, including patients with HIV-AIDS.

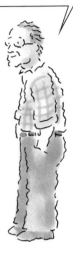

A zoster by any other name

Also called shingles, herpes zoster occurs when the varicella zoster virus is reactivated after being dormant within nerve roots since a previous episode of chickenpox. Herpes zoster occurs mainly in people over age 50 and in people with immunosuppressed states that allow the virus to "wake up."

Peripheral target

The reactivated virus travels along a peripheral nerve, causing skin eruptions and painful nerve irritation. Occasionally, the disease can be disseminated throughout the body and even into the viscera. On average, it occurs 5 years after HIV infection.

Herpes zoster causes skin vesicles and pain, usually distributed in specific patterns along dermatomes innervated by the affected nerves. The pain is commonly described as sharp, stabbing, or lancinating with intense, deep soreness that commonly requires hospitalization for pain control.

Shingles tingles

The patient may experience unilateral pain, itching, and tingling 1 to 4 days before the skin rash occurs. After the pain starts, small, red, nodular skin lesions erupt in the painful areas and spread unilaterally around the chest or vertically over the arms or legs. They change rapidly to pus- or fluid-filled vesicles. About 10 to 21 days after the rash appears, the vesicles dry and form scabs. The patient with HIV-AIDS is at higher risk for disseminated herpes zoster lesions that cover large areas of multiple dermatomes and occasionally the entire body.

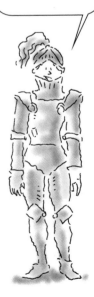

Then, PHN

PHN is generally diagnosed when the pain of herpes zoster persists beyond 3 months. PHN is a chronic neuropathic pain syndrome felt along the same areas as the herpes zoster rash. The patient with PHN experiences constant pain described as burning, tingling, throbbing, and aching or sometimes itching. Intermittently, sharp and shooting pain with allodynia (pain occurring with ordinarily painless stimulation such as light touch) may be present as well. Risk factors for the development of PHN in the patient with HIV-AIDS include the severity of pain during the herpes zoster outbreak as well as the severity, extent, and duration of lesions.

Managing herpes zoster pain

Prompt pain control within the first 48 to 72 hours after the appearance of the herpes zoster rash may prevent PHN and delay the onset of AIDS. Antiviral drugs, such as acyclovir (Zovirax), valacyclovir (Valtrex), and famciclovir (Famvir), limit viral reproduction and complications of herpes zoster as well as decrease pain and promote rash healing. Analgesics, such as acetaminophen, NSAIDS, and opioids may be administered to reduce pain. Adjuvant drugs to treat neuropathic pain may be helpful, including TCAs, such as amitryptiline, and anticonvulsants such as gabapentin.

Inject, patch, or stimulate

A series of local anesthetic injections with or without steroids, including local infiltration of skin lesions, peripheral nerve blocks, and sympathetic nerve blocks, may contribute to pain relief. An epidural infusion with a local anesthetic solution may also provide excellent pain control during herpes outbreaks. If the skin is intact, a topical lidocaine patch may relieve postherpetic pain. TENS has also been successful in reducing pain from PHN.

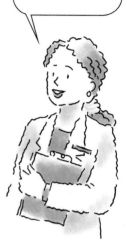

PHN is herpes zoster pain that lasts longer than 3 months.

Other neuropathic syndromes

Neuropathic pain in the patient with HIV-AIDS may occur when nerves are damaged, compressed, or infiltrated by organisms, disease, malignancies, or toxic therapies. Many HIV drugs, chemotherapeutic agents, and radiation therapy can cause nerve damage. Common nonmalignant neuropathic syndromes affecting the patient with HIV-AIDS include various forms of peripheral neuropathy.

Peripheral neuropathies

Peripheral neuropathies afflict approximately 20% to 50% of patients with HIV-AIDS. They affect peripheral sensory nerves, primarily in the feet, lower legs, and hands, producing altered sensation and reflexes. They can occur at any stage of HIV infection, but become more common as the disease advances. What's more, certain drug therapies for HIV, such as didanosine, zalcitabine, and isoniazid, can cause peripheral neuropathy. The presence of risk factors for peripheral neuropathies, such as diabetes, alcoholism, and vitamin B_{12} and folate deficiencies, tend to cause an earlier onset and increased severity of peripheral neuropathies. (See *Peripheral neuropathies in HIV-AIDS*, page 242.)

Peripheral neuropathies in HIV-AIDS

Type	Incidence	Onset in HIV	Cause
Distal sensory or symmetrical polyneuropathy	10% to 35%	Late	• Drug toxicities from such drugs as zalcitabine, didanosine, and stavudine 3 to 8 months after drug is started • HIV
Inflammatory demyelinating polyneuropathy	4%	Early or late	• Unknown • HIV-immune activation
Mononeuropathies (Mononeuritis multiples)	0.6% to 3%	Early or late	• HIV • Cytomegalovirus (CMV) • Karposi''s sarcoma • Early lymphona
Radiculomyelopathy (progressive polyradiculopathy)	<2%	Late	• CMV or herpes zoster

Managing peripheral neuropathy pain

Currently, no medical treatment can reverse or stop peripheral neuropathy. Effective management of peripheral neuropathy pain requires quick identification and treatment of the cause (HIV disease or the treatment modalities). Distal neuropathy pain is best treated with a combination of analgesics and adjuvant drugs, which relieve symptoms but don't heal underlying nerve damage. NSAIDs, opioids, gabapentin, TCAs, and baclofen are usually used. Inflammatory demyelinating polymyopathy, a less frequent but more severe form of neuropathy, causes pain that may respond to corticosteroids as well as NSAIDs and opioids (fentanyl, morphine, and oxycodone). Mononeuropathy pain, which is treated similarly to that of distal sensory neuropathy, may also respond to nerve blocks. Radiculomyelopathy (or CMV-related neuropathy) pain develops rapidly and is treated with antiviral agents,

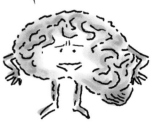

Peripheral neuropathies affect peripheral sensory nerves, producing altered sensation and reflexes. What's a brain to do?

Signs and symptoms	Treatment
• Symmetrical pain and paresthesias in extremities (legs more affected than arms) • Boot pattern numbness • Decreased ankle reflexes • Distal sensory loss • Minor or no weakness	• *Early treatment:* Stop offending drug for improvement in 4 to 8 weeks • *Analgesics:* NSAIDS, opioids • *Adjuvant:* TCAs, gabapentin, baclofen, zonisamide, clonidine, tizanidine, lidocaine patch, mexiletine, nerve growth factor
• Ascending weakness (from toes to head) • Paresthesias and pain • Decreased reflexes • Mild sensory loss	• *Early treatment:* Immunotherapy with corticosteroids, plasmapheresis, immunoglobulin • *Late treatment:* treatment of CMV • *Analgesics:* NSAIDS, opioids
• Multiple cranial and peripheral nerve dysfunction and pain, depending on location of nerve affected (such as arm pain, facial weakness, foot or wrist drop)	• *Early treatment:* Treatment of underlying cause (may resolve spontaneously) • *Analgesics:* NSAIDS, opioids • *Adjuvants:* gabapentin, baclofen, zonisamide, clonidine, tizanidine, lidocaine patch, mexiletine, nerve growth factor, local anesthetic block • *Early onset:* immunotherapy • *Late onset:* CMV treatment likely
• Lumbosacral pain radiating to the leg • Leg weakness and numbness • Sacral and saddle anesthesia • Bowel and bladder dysfunction • Decreased ankle and knee reflexes	• CMV treatment • *Analgesics:* NSAIDS, opioids • *Adjuvants:* gabapentin, baclofen, zonisamide, clonidine, lidocaine patch, mexiletine, nerve growth factor, local anesthetic block (treat promptly to preserve spinal cord and limb function)

analgesics, adjuvants, and local anesthetic blocks. Patients with this type of pain have a limited prognosis.

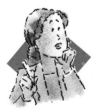

Quick quiz

1. HIV-AIDS is currently viewed as:
   A. an acute illness that's almost always fatal.
   B. a terminal disease with the focus on end-of-life care.
   C. a chronic disease requiring medical management.
   D. a highly communicable disease that can be cured.

Answer: C. Due to advances in HIV-AIDS treatment, particularly related to the use of HAART, patients with HIV are living longer, and HIV-AIDS is changing from a universally fatal disease to a chronic disease requiring long-term medical management.

2. Which statement best describes AIDS-related pain?
   A. Patients with AIDS-related pain receive adequate pain control.
   B. AIDS-related pain is almost always nociceptive.
   C. AIDS-related pain is rarely accompanied by emotional distress or anxiety.
   D. Patients with AIDS commonly have multiple sources of pain.

Answer: D. Patients with HIV-AIDS commonly have multiple sources of pain. In fact, they may experience an average of seven simultaneous pain symptoms.

3. Which of the following is a risk factor for herpes zoster?
   A. Immunosuppression
   B. Peripheral neuropathy
   C. Being under age 50
   D. Having open skin lesions

Answer: A. Herpes zoster occurs mainly in people over age 50 or in people with immunosuppressed states that allow the virus to "wake up."

4. When administering a TCA to the patient with HIV-AIDS to treat neuropathic pain, which of the following statements should the nurse keep in mind?
   A. The dose of TCA used for analgesia is lower than that used for depression.
   B. Nortriptyline has the most cardiac adverse effects.
   C. TCAs don't cause sedation.
   D. Drug interactions involving TCAs are rare.

Answer: A. The TCA dose needed for analgesia is lower than the dose required for treating depression.

Scoring

✮✮✮ If you answered all four questions correctly, great job! You're an HIV-AIDS pain management maven!

✮✮ If you answered three questions correctly, good going! You're on your way to making HIV-AIDS pain pretty puny!

✮ If you answered fewer than three questions correctly, chin up! Just review the chapter and try again!

Pain in pediatric patients

Just the facts

In this chapter, you'll learn:

♦ common misconceptions about pain in young patients

♦ barriers to effective pain management

♦ useful tools to assess pain in infants and young children

♦ effective strategies for treating pain in children.

A look at pediatric pain

Pain is a subjective experience, and for infants and children, it's possibly the most bewildering and frightening occurrence in their young lives. Until age 3 or so, children can't grasp abstract concepts, such as time, cause and effect, and quantification. Consequently, it's impossible for them to understand why pain occurs or that relief is just around the corner. They know only that something hurts right now.

What makes the experience particularly distressing is that infants and young children lack the language skills needed to tell someone that they're in pain, where it hurts and how much, or to ask for help. In this respect, infants and children are uniquely dependent on the ability of their parents and health care providers to recognize and relieve their pain. Similarly, children could reasonably expect these same caregivers to anticipate and prevent or minimize painful experiences whenever possible. Unfortunately, our health care system all too often fails to meet this expectation.

We know now what we didn't know then

Until the 1970s, there was little research into pain and pain management. Since that time, we've learned a great deal about pain in adults, but have made only limited headway in understanding and treating pain in the very young. We have learned, however, that infants and children experience pain in much the same way as older

> I'm trusting you to keep me from pain. Are you cool with that?

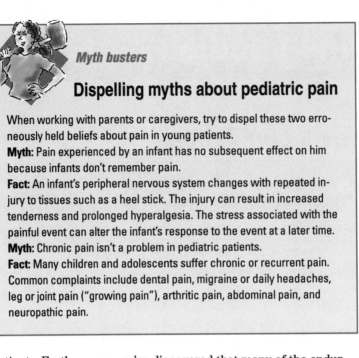

Dispelling myths about pediatric pain

When working with parents or caregivers, try to dispel these two erroneously held beliefs about pain in young patients.

Myth: Pain experienced by an infant has no subsequent effect on him because infants don't remember pain.

Fact: An infant's peripheral nervous system changes with repeated injury to tissues such as a heel stick. The injury can result in increased tenderness and prolonged hyperalgesia. The stress associated with the painful event can alter the infant's response to the event at a later time.

Myth: Chronic pain isn't a problem in pediatric patients.

Fact: Many children and adolescents suffer chronic or recurrent pain. Common complaints include dental pain, migraine or daily headaches, leg or joint pain ("growing pain"), arthritic pain, abdominal pain, and neuropathic pain.

patients. Furthermore, we've discovered that many of the enduring beliefs about pain in children and treatment options for them have turned out to be wrong. (See *Dispelling myths about pediatric pain.*) As a result, pain in infants and children has commonly gone untreated or undertreated.

Tell us where it hurts

The problem isn't a lack of compassion on the part of practitioners; instead, it's a matter of their working with inaccurate or incomplete knowledge of pain in children and viable treatment options. At this juncture, we're still learning about the physiology of the developing nervous system, the ways in which very young children react to pain, and the most effective pharmacologic and nonpharmacologic methods of treating pain in this population. If we are truly intent on improving the way we manage pain in young patients, health care providers must stay abreast of developments.

When it comes to pain and pain relief, infants and children will always need to rely on their parents and health care providers to recognize and react to the physiologic and behavioral signs of pain. To meet this challenge, it's important that we:

• continue research into pain in this population
• improve assessment skills by learning as much as we can about pain in children and how to anticipate, recognize, and relieve it
• learn about the pharmacodynamics (the dosage-effect relationship) and pharmacokinetics (drug movement in the body over

My doctors and nurses have to read all this pain research. I get to stand on it!

time) of infants and young children to overcome our resistance to using analgesics (especially opioid analgesics) in treatment
• provide parents with more accurate teaching about the nature and treatment of their child's pain
• refine and use pain assessment tools designed for this age-group
• improve opportunities for multidisciplinary care in all health care settings.

Misconceptions and other barriers

The first step toward better pain management for infants and children is letting go of common misconceptions that hamper treatment. Let's look at some of the most common and damaging misconceptions and what we now know to be true.

Misconceptions about pain in young patients

• *Misconception:* An infant's nervous system is still developing and therefore he doesn't feel pain, or he feels pain less acutely than an older child or adult.
• *Present understanding:* The central nervous system (CNS) is capable of pain transmission by 20 weeks' gestation. In other words, infants have virtually the same ability to sense pain as adults. This misconception may stem from the fact that infants don't always express or respond to pain in the same way as older patients. Health care providers may have overlooked or misconstrued signs of pain due to a poor understanding of how infants express pain. Also, for many years we believed that myelination of nerve fibers was necessary for transmission of pain stimuli. (In infants, myelination is still underway.) We now know that myelinated and unmyelinated nerve fibers are capable of transmitting pain.
• *Misconception:* Infants can't remember pain, so there can be no long-term affects from pain suffered at this early stage of life.
• *Present understanding:* Research indicates that infants perceive, respond to, and remember pain. Untreated and undertreated pain in infants can lead to sleep and eating disturbances, disruption of maternal-infant bonding, and a heightened response in the future to painful stimuli. Pain from procedures such as heel lancing and circumcision commonly causes a greater reaction to painful procedures, such as immunizations, long after the initial painful experience.

> Contrary to common belief, an infant's nervous system is capable of transmitting pain.

The language of the very young

- *Misconception:* It isn't possible to accurately assess pain in infants and children.
- *Present understanding:* While they may not be able to talk about their pain, infants and children express their pain very clearly—but you have to know how to interpret the signs. Young patients exhibit behaviors in response to pain that are consistent with stress and pain responses in older patients. These behaviors may include crying, withdrawing from the stimulus, grimacing, holding their breath, clenching their fists, shielding an injured limb, looking fearful, or becoming agitated, to mention a few. (For a more comprehensive discussion of behaviors associated with pain, see chapter 2, Assessing pain.) In infants, these signs may be subdued or exaggerated depending on the stage of CNS development, but the signs *are* there and there are a number of good, age-specific assessment tools that can help you interpret these signs.

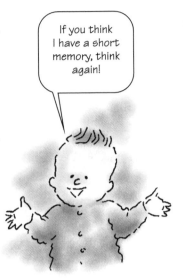

If you think I have a short memory, think again!

Just say "Yes!"

- *Misconception:* Analgesics (especially opioid analgesics) and other pain medications aren't safe for infants and children because of the risk of respiratory depression and possible addiction.
- *Present understanding:* Research into the pharmacodynamics and pharmacokinetics in very young children indicates that, if properly prescribed and carefully monitored, there's no reason to avoid these very beneficial pain control options for young patients. Possible adverse affects are dosage-related, so careful monitoring is appropriate at any age. Many parents and practitioners alike use the terms *addiction* and *dependence* interchangeably. They are two very different concepts, however. Although there's always some risk of a patient developing a dependence on a drug, this possibility is foreseeable and manageable. On the other hand, proper dosage and monitoring makes addiction extremely unlikely.

Other potential barriers to pain management

The next step toward improved pain management for infants and children is developing the ability to overcome barriers as they present themselves, and there are many. Some of the barriers are erected on the clinical side of the care equation. Others relate to the patient and his family.

Clinical barriers

Most of the clinical barriers to effective treatment stem from outdated knowledge or supposition regarding pain in children and its treatment. Much of what we now know to be true in this regard we learned in the past 20 years or so. Most medical and nursing educators, and many health care providers, received their training in an era when pediatric pain was poorly understood and afforded only limited attention in medical and nursing curricula. An aggressive campaign to educate all health care providers regarding pain in children would work wonders in moving the health care community over the remaining clinical barriers to effective pain management. These barriers include:

* outdated or insufficient pain assessment skills
* incomplete knowledge of the physiologic and behavioral signs of pain in infants and young children
* overlooking pain related to chronic conditions, procedures, or therapies (I.M. injections, for example)
* a poor understanding of the consequences of undertreated or untreated pain in infants and young children
* incomplete or inaccurate knowledge regarding the use of analgesics with young patients
* unfounded or exaggerated concerns about risks associated with opioid therapy
* a poor understanding of effective nonpharmacologic interventions for pain relief
* a lack of a multidisciplinary approach
* the low priority given to pain management.

You only hurt the ones you love

The most common cause of acute pain in young children is medical procedures and treatments. Not abuse or accidents, but health care! Circumcision, heel sticks, catheterization, and I.M. injections are just a few of the painful procedures sick infants and children must endure. Yet practitioners continue to forego preventive measures and routinely undertreat these types of pain, typically because they have lingering concerns about the use of analgesics and anesthetics in children.

A doctor or nurse who, without stopping to think, will explore the pain of an adult during an assessment commonly will ignore the topic completely when assessing an infant with an underlying disorder. Even when the child has a chronic condition *known* to cause

Classroom study can be a pain, but it's a great place to learn the latest developments in pain management!

pain, such as sickle cell anemia, juvenile rheumatoid arthritis, complex regional pain syndromes, or fibromyalgia.

Pain should be one of the first items assessed in children, and pain relief should be one of the first items of business when treating children. In addition, health care providers need to anticipate painful procedures and consider less painful options or the use of preventive analgesia.

Get the whole gang involved

One way to ensure that pain isn't overlooked is to adopt a multidisciplinary approach to pain management in infants and children. Health care teams comprised of doctors, nurses, pharmacists, pain specialists and physical and behavioral therapists, and other areas of specialization bring a unique synergy to pain management and lessen the impact of individual biases regarding treatment options. In many smaller facilities, it can be difficult to form such teams; however, any movement toward multidisciplinary treatment is a step in the right direction. (See *Creating a pain management program from scratch.*)

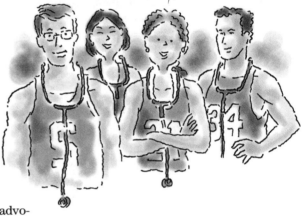

We need to work together as a team for the sake of the kids!

When it comes to opioid therapy for children, the facts are clear: opioids and other analgesics can be administered to very young children without excessive risk of adverse effects. For more than a decade, the World Health Organization (WHO) has advocated the use of opioid analgesics to manage moderate to severe pain. Yet many providers remain reluctant to use opioids, fearing that they may cause respiratory depression or promote dependence. Also, due to years of media coverage focused on addiction and the improper use of opioids, many parents have an exaggerated fear of these analgesics. Working to overcome parental fears just compounds the problem for health care providers.

Patient-related barriers

The patient and his parents can create significant barriers to treatment as well. Most are related to the child's stage of development and his parents' beliefs. Potential problems can stem from the:
- child's previous experience with pain
- parents' previous experience with pain or that of their child
- child's limited ability to communicate
- parents' fears of injury, disability, or death of their child
- methods of administering medications

Creating a pain management program from scratch

There's no time like the present to start an infant pain management program. If your facility doesn't have one, here are the steps you can take to get the ball rolling.

• Enlist doctors, nurses, pain specialists, pharmacists, physical and behavioral therapists, social workers, and management.
• Have each individual research the latest developments in his or her discipline.
• Develop a comprehensive protocol that's based on evidence rather than opinion.

• Study existing assessment tools and select the best ones for your team and patients.
• Educate all staff about the latest findings regarding infant physiology, how they experience and respond to pain, and the value and safety of analgesic therapy.
• Develop teaching tools for parents.

> When prescribed and monitored carefully, opioid analgesics are safe for young patients.

• parents' concerns about drug therapies, especially opioid analgesics.

Getting to know you

Like adults, infants and children experience stress and anxiety when in pain. Unlike adults, children can't find solace in knowing that relief will come because they lack the language skills necessary to discuss their pain with parents and practitioners. Instead, children know only that they hurt, and their level of stress and anxiety remains high. Unrelieved stress and anxiety can be just as devastating to children as unrelieved pain. It's important to understand how stress and pain work together in children.

I don't feel a thing

As a child approaches school age, he develops a sense of time and of cause and effect. This makes it possible to talk about pain in very basic terms, but it also can be a stumbling block. For example, a child may mask pain or fail to tell you that he hurts because he believes that doing so will result in even more pain—an I.M. injection, catheterization, or an uncomfortable exam.

The parents' beliefs, religious and cultural customs, and personal experience with pain will influence treatment. If a parent believes that shots hurt a lot or, conversely, that pain builds character, these beliefs will influence his decisions about the care of his child. Cultural attitudes, such as the belief that a boy should endure pain while a girl shouldn't or that suffering is a part of life, also affect treatment decisions. Language may be a problem as well if the parents' primary language isn't English.

Teaching becomes an important component of working with parents. They have much to learn about the mechanisms of pain and the safety and effectiveness of treatment alternatives. Providing the parents with teaching helps reduce their stress and encourages their willing and active participation in treatment.

> Parents know best when it comes to their child's experience with pain.

Talk to the parental units

Parents remain the best source of information about their children. They are the experts when it comes to understanding their child's normal behavior and response to pain. Be aware that many parents, when confronted with the hospitalization of their child, assume that doctors and nurses know best and will automatically treat their child's pain. Conversely, health care professionals commonly assume parents will speak up if they have something of value to contribute. Talking with the parents early and often can prevent this type of standoff. Ask questions about the child, and assess the parents' need for information. Parents are an invaluable resource in pain management; make sure they understand their important role.

Fear and anxiety and stress...Oh my!

Young children don't know why pain occurs or how long it will last or even that relief is possible. Neither parents nor provider can explain treatment or that the pain will go away. Consequently, pain for children involves fear, anxiety, and stress. Untreated stress can exacerbate pain in young patients and, if prolonged, can have detrimental physical and psychological effects as well.

The body responds to injury and pain by releasing "stress hormones" (catecholamines, corticosteroids, growth hormones, and glucagons). These hormones break down carbohydrates, fats, and protein in the body to help prevent additional injury. Stress hormones help reduce blood loss, maintain vital organs, promote healing, and prevent infection. Prolonged stress, however, causes hypermetabolic states that can lead to complications. Managing stress hormones in infants and children is more difficult than in adults because of ongoing physiologic development.

The older patient can talk about his pain and treatment and can anticipate relief, all of which helps reduce stress. The young child doesn't have this advantage, and stress tends to remain elevated until his pain is relieved. Consequently, managing the child's stress and anxiety is a key element in controlling his pain.

Assessing pain in infants and children

A growing number of health professionals who work with children talk about pain as a fifth vital sign, and one that should be assessed early and often to ensure prompt, effective relief. Assessing pain in infants and young children requires the cooperation of the parents and the use of age-specific assessment tools. If the child can communicate verbally, he can also aid the process.

Health history and physical examination

Normal clinical assessment involves taking a health history that includes a description of any pain and palliative measures and a comprehensive physical examination. When assessing infants and children, you must rely on parents for the health history and background on experience with pain.

Wanna play 20 questions?

To help you better understand the child's pain, ask the parents these questions:
• What kinds of pain has your child had in the past?
• How does your child usually respond to pain?
• How do you know your child is in pain?
• What do you do when he's hurting?
• What does your child do when he's hurting?
• What works best to relieve your child's pain?
• Is there anything special you'd like me to know about your child and pain?

No wonder they call 'em vital signs!

The child's vital signs can be pain indicators. Elevated pulse, blood pressure, or respiration can be signs of pain and stress. However, findings here must be viewed in conjunction with other assessment data because nonpainful stimuli can elicit changes in vital signs as well. For example, just touching an infant can speed or calm the child's pulse rate.

Behavioral responses to pain

Behavior is the language infants and children rely on to convey information about their pain. Areas of behavior that change due to pain include body positioning, facial expression, patterns of eating and sleeping, attention level, and vocalization.

Memory jogger

To help you stay focused when assessing pain in the young patient, remember the mnemonic **QUEST**:

Q – Question the child's parents (and the child, too, if he's old enough to respond).

U – Use appropriate pain assessment tools.

E – Evaluate the child's behavior.

S – Secure the parents' active participation in treatment.

T – Take the cause of the pain into consideration.

In an infant, facial expression is the most common and consistent behavioral response to all stimuli, painful or pleasurable, and may be the single best indicator of pain for the provider and parent. Studies indicate that facial expression is a more reliable pain indicator than crying, heart rate, or body position and movement. Facial expressions that tend to indicate that the infant is in pain include:
• mouth stretched open
• eyes tightly shut
• brows and forehead knitted (as they are in a grimace)
• cheeks are raised high enough to form a wrinkle on the nose.

In young children, facial expression is joined by other behaviors to convey pain. In these patients, look for such signs as:
• narrowing of the eyes
• grimace or fearful appearance
• frequent and longer lasting bouts of crying, with a tone that's higher and louder than normal
• less receptive to comforting by parents or other caregiver
• holding or protecting the area of the body that's painful.

Cry me a river

Enlist the parents' help in interpreting the child's crying. Pain may be the cause, but hunger, anger, fear, or a wet diaper can also elicit crying. Commonly, parents can distinguish among the different cries of their child and help narrow down the possible causes.

Crying associated with pain is distinguished by the frequency, duration, pitch, and intensity. Cries of pain are usually short, sharp, higher in pitch, tense, harsh, nonmelodious, and loud. On the other hand, some infants don't cry in response to pain, even pain associated with an invasive procedure. Also, some treatments make crying impossible. Intubated infants, for example, can't cry. However, these infants still exhibit the facial expressions that accompany crying— mouth opened wide and eyes tightly closed, insinuating crying.

No foolin'!

It's a mistake to rely too heavily on observed behavior alone when assessing pain in young patients. Some young patients will suffer pain rather than report it or allow others to see that they're in pain. Others are adept at distracting themselves so that they may appear pain-free. Some children will sleep soundly, not because they have no pain, but because they're physically and emotionally exhausted.

Learning to talk the talk

A child who has mastered the rudiments of language can provide some useful information. However, keep in mind that his language skills are very basic and he may not understand words you use. You may call it pain, but he may think of it as a hurt or boo-boo. Find the words that work best by talking with his parents and during brief talks with the child.

Keep in mind that children who are just learning to talk have a great deal more skill in reading the facial expressions and body language of their parents and caregivers. After all, they've been reading this language since birth. Be sure your expression and body posture is conveying a message consistent with your words. If you or his parents appear concerned, he may feel there's something to fear, and this may color his description of the pain he's feeling.

> You don't have to use baby talk to make a child understand — just choose your words carefully.

Assessment tools

There are a number of proven assessment tools designed for a young patient. Many of these seek to quantify the child's pain, one of the harder things to accomplish during assessment and observation. Using an assessment tool will help, but quantifying pain in the infant or preverbal child will still be difficult.

Pain assessment tools are described as being unidimensional (measuring or assessing one indicator) or multidimensional (measuring or assessing multiple indicators). Composite measures of pain include physiologic, behavioral, sensory, and cognitive indicators. These tools tend to be especially useful when assessing children under age 3 or older children with cognitive deficits.

Painful measures

Due to the complexity of assessing pain in infants, there's no single pain measurement tool that works well for all patients. However, there are three multidimensional tools for measuring pain in infants that have proved to be quite effective. These include the:
• CRIES (**C**rying, **R**equires oxygen to maintain saturation more than 95%, **I**ncreased vital signs, **E**xpression, and **S**leepless) Neonatal Postoperative Pain Measurement Scale
• Neonatal Infant Pain Scale (NIPS)
• Premature Infant Pain Profile (PIPP).

The CRIES inventory is one of the easier tools to use. Five separate factors are scored 0 to 2. Infants with a score of zero would be pain-free. A score of 10 would indicate extreme pain. (See *Measuring pain in infants*, page 256.)

Measuring pain in infants

Assessing pain in infants can be challenging for health care providers. The chart below describes three assessment tools that can help you meet this challenge.

Assessment tool	Factors measured
Neonatal Infant Pain Scale (NIPS)	• Facial expression • Crying • Breathing patterns • State of arousal • Movement of arms and legs
Neonatal Postoperative Pain Measurement Scale (NPPMS)	• Crying • Oxygen saturation • Heart rate and blood pressure • Expression • Sleeplessness
Premature Infant Pain Profile (PIPP)	• Gestational age • Heart rate • Oxygen saturation • Behavioral state • Brow bulge • Eye squeeze • Nasolabial furrow

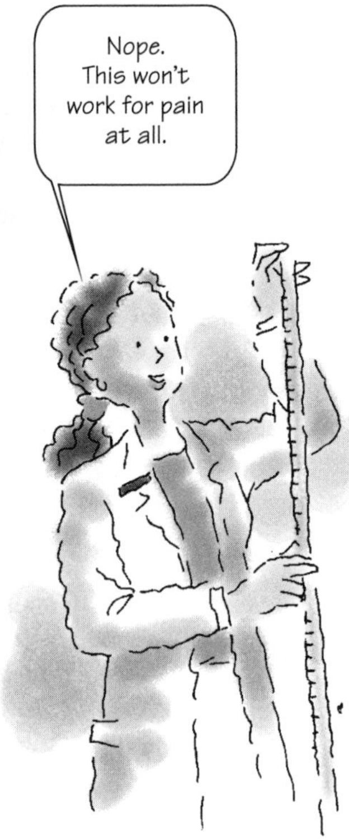

Nope. This won't work for pain at all.

All of the assessment tools for infants were developed to help assess acute pain. Currently, there are no tools to help measure chronic pain in infants. The variability of pain response and pathology of chronic pain in infants and young children makes measurement very difficult.

Hey, speaking of pain

For the child capable of speaking, typically age 3 or so, the task is somewhat easier. There are several simple and effective pain measuring scales that help the child identify a level of pain. These include a:
• faces pain measuring scale
• chip pain measuring tool
• visual analog scale. (See *Measuring pain in young children*.)

Measuring pain in young children

For children who are old enough to speak and understand sufficiently, three useful tools can help them communicate information useful in measuring their pain. Here's how to use each one.

Faces Scale for Measuring Pain

The child age 3 and older can use this scale to rate his pain. When using this tool, make sure he can see, and then point to each face and describe the amount of pain each face is experiencing by reading the text under the picture. Avoid saying anything that might prompt the child to choose a certain face. Then, ask the child to choose the face that shows how he's feeling right now. Record his response in your assessment notes.

| Happy because he doesn't hurt at all! | Hurts just a little bit. | Hurts a little more. | Hurts even more. | Hurts a whole lot. | Hurts the most. |

Chip Tool for Measuring Pain

This tool uses four identical chips to signify levels of pain and can be used for the child who understands the basic concept of adding one thing to another to get more. If available, you can use poker chips. If not, simply cut four uniform circles from a sheet of paper and use these.

Here's how to present the chips

• First say, "I want to talk with you about the hurt you might be having right now."
• Next, align the chips horizontally on the bedside table, a clipboard, or other firm surface where the child can easily see and reach them.

• Point to the chip at the child's far left and say, "this chip is just a little bit of hurt."
• Point to the second chip and say, "this next chip is a little more hurt."
• Point to the third chip and say, "this next chip is a lot of hurt."
• Point to the last chip and say, "this last chip is the most hurt you can have."
• Ask the child, "How many pieces of hurt do you have right now?"
   By the way, you won't need to offer the option of "no hurt at all" because the child will tell you if he doesn't hurt.
• Record the number of chips. If the child's answer isn't clear, talk to him about his answer, then record your findings.

Visual analog scale

A visual analog pain scale is simply a straight line with the phrase, "no pain" at one end and the phrase, "the most pain possible" at the other. Children who understand the concept of a continuum can mark the spot on the line that corresponds to the level of pain they feel.

No pain   The most pain possible

Pain management

Infants and young children may experience acute pain, cancer pain, or chronic pain associated with an underlying disorder. Pain management is most effective when it prevents, limits, or avoids noxious stimuli and involves administering analgesics. Regardless of the underlying cause, pain management for these young patients seeks to:
• identify and relieve existing pain
• anticipate and prevent or minimize pain related to hospitalization, procedures, and treatments
• optimize pharmacologic and nonpharmacologic intervention to reduce stress, increase comfort, and enhance healing.

Pharmacologic intervention

Pharmacologic therapy is the mainstay of pain management for an infant or a child. The selection of medications, dosage, and administration routes depends on the specific needs of the patient.

The use of drug therapy in infants and children is gradually beginning to overcome the lingering concerns of many health care providers, principally because our understanding of the pharmacokinetics and pharmacodynamics of infants and young children has significantly improved in recent years.

Pharmacokinetics and pharmacodynamics

It's important to understand how the unique physiology of a young child affects pharmacokinetics and pharmacodynamics. The metabolism of an infant differs significantly from that of an older patient.

Infants and young children are still developing physiologically, and this affects the way their bodies absorb, distribute, and metabolize drugs. Gastric acidity, for example, doesn't stabilize until age 3 or so. This can affect the absorption and concentration of drugs that require an acid environment to be fully assimilated. Similarly, protein binding, which aids distribution of drugs in the body, is lower in infants and children than in older patients. Compared to adults, infants have proportionately more water weight and extracellular water, less fat, and less muscle tissue. In infants, hepatic (liver) metabolism is slower and renal clearance is delayed. The liver has a key role in metabolizing analgesics, the class of drugs most commonly prescribed in pain management, and delayed renal clearance means that these drugs remain in young patients longer.

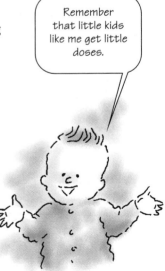

Remember that little kids like me get little doses.

Opioid analgesics

Opioid analgesics are highly effective pain relievers and constitute the core of most pharmacologic interventions to manage acute pain (especially postoperative pain) in infants and children. Morphine (MS Contin) and fentanyl (Duragesic) are the two opioids used most commonly in these patients. While they're thought to be equivalent, morphine may provide better sedation and a lower risk of chest wall rigidity than fentanyl. Opioid analgesics are available in oral, sublingual, rectal, nasal, subcutaneous, transdermal, I.V., and intraspinal forms, which makes it relatively easy to find an acceptable route.

Although we've learned much about the pharmacodynamics and pharmacokinetics of opioids in young children, many practitioners still resist prescribing them.

PCA...Hooray!

Patient-controlled analgesia (PCA) can be useful in the management of pain in the young patient, provided the parents are involved and trained in the theory and proper use of this equipment. PCA allows the patient to maintain a therapeutic level of the prescribed opioid analgesic at all times. PCA has been effective in children age 5 and older. Parent-controlled analgesia is another way for children age 4 and younger or who are developmentally delayed to receive I.V. PCA medication.

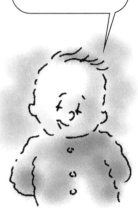

I bet I could handle PCA. Mom says I know exactly which buttons to push.

Nonopioid analgesics

Nonopioid analgesics, which include acetaminophen and nonsteroidal anti-inflammatory drugs (NSAIDs), are prescribed to manage mild to moderate pain. In instances of severe pain, nonopioid analgesics can be used in conjunction with opioid analgesics to reduce the required dosage of opioid analgesic.

Infants and children metabolize nonopioid analgesics in the same manner and at the same rate as adults; consequently, the selection criteria, affects, and possible adverse effects are the same as they are for adults.

Acetaminophen anyone?

Acetaminophen is the drug of choice for treating mild pain. It has the added benefit of helping reduce fever and is very safe, even for neonates. Acetaminophen has few adverse effects or contraindications. However, long-term use can increase the risk of liver damage, and it's possible to reach a point where additional doses no longer provide an analgesic affect. On the plus side, acetaminophen is available in suppository, liquid, and tablet form, making it easy to administer and appropriate for most situations.

Who said NSAIDs?

NSAIDs relieve mild to moderate pain and also act as an anti-inflammatory. Commonly prescribed NSAIDs such as ibuprofen (Advil), naproxen (Naprosyn), tolmetin (Tolectin), indomethacin (Indocin), and ketorolac (Tordol), are approved for use with children as well. Possible adverse effects of NSAIDs include inhibition of platelet aggregation and GI irritation.

Adjuvant therapy

Although there are no studies of the effectiveness of adjuvant therapy in infants and children, doctors prescribe a range of medications as adjuvant therapy, usually when treating cancer pain in infants and children. The response has been such that adjuvant therapy is now gaining acceptance as a constructive facet of pain management in other chronic conditions as well, such as neuropathies, headache, myofascial pain, and recurrent abdominal pain. The types of drugs and therapeutic effects include:
- antianxiety medications, such as lorazepam (Ativan), diazepam (Valium), and midazolam (Versed), which are used to enhance the effect of opioids
- anticonvulsants, such as phenytoin (Dilantin), carbamazepine (Tegretol), and gabapentin (Neurontin), which are used to treat neuropathies caused by certain diseases or trauma
- corticosteroids, which help alleviate severe inflammation and bone pain
- neuroleptic drugs, which are antipsychotic, tranquilizing, sedative, and analgesic and help relieve pain associated with cancer, certain neuralgia, phantom limb, and muscular discomfort
- tricyclic antidepressants, such as amitriptyline (Elavil), which are sometimes used to manage headache and chronic pain
- anesthetics (topical, local), which are given ahead of time to reduce pain caused by procedures such as starting an I.V. catheter.

Nonpharmacologic interventions

For the infant and young child, nonpharmacologic interventions pick up where drug therapies stop by reducing stress and anxiety and increasing comfort and security. Typically, these measures are just as critical to the patient's well-being as pain relief.

Nonpharmacologic interventions cause no adverse effects, require no special equipment, and can be used anytime. This is where parents can really shine.

No side effects! Are you thinking what I'm thinking? Sign us up!

Cognitive-behavioral therapies

Cognitive-behavioral interventions for the infant include positioning, containment or swaddling, distraction, touching, and gentle massage. Placing an infant in a midline, or supine, position has a calming affect, as does wrapping him snugly in a soft blanket. Providing distraction—for example, with a bedside mobile or a safe, colorful toy or stuffed animal—helps the infant focus on something enjoyable rather than his hurt.

For a toddler, distraction, hypnosis, guided imagery, gentle massage, snuggling with mom and dad, and curling up in bed listening to a story are all methods of moving the child's focus away from his pain to more serene, safe, and comforting thoughts.

Physical therapy

Thermotherapy is the most common form of physical therapy used with infants. Applying warm and cold to painful areas can make them feel better. Heat promotes circulation, and cold helps reduce swelling and provides a limited amount of numbing.

Complementary therapies

Complementary therapies, such as music or aromatherapy, are gaining acceptance because of the influence music and smells can have on emotions and state of mind. For the infant or child, soothing music has a calming effect and can help him drift off to sleep at naptime. More lively music can stimulate memories or encourage singing, which distract the child for a time. Smells that remind him of mom, dad, or grandma's house can be comforting as well.

For the infant, nonnutritive sucking using a pacifier, a pacifier dipped in sucrose, or a small bottle of water containing sucrose is effective in reducing pain associated with procedures. Nonnutritive sucking with or without sucrose can be used to calm the infant before the procedure as well as afterward.

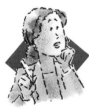

Quick quiz

1. All of the following can be barriers to effective pain management in young children except:

    A.   the child's previous experience with pain.

    B.   the parents' cultural beliefs.

    C.   the child's fine motor skills.

    D.   the child's stage of development.

Answer: C. There are no known barriers to pain management associated with a child's fine motor skills.

2.   When assessing a young child for pain, you should investigate all of the following except:
- A.   the child's previous experience with pain.
- B.   the parents' previous experience with pain.
- C.   behavioral responses.
- D.   physiologic indicators.

Answer: B. A thorough pain assessment focuses on the child's past pain experiences, not the parents' past experiences.

3.   All of the following are examples of nonpharmacologic interventions that help manage pain in young children except:
- A.   sleep.
- B.   distraction.
- C.   containment.
- D.   positioning.

Answer: A. While sleep is usually beneficial, it isn't an example of a nonpharmacologic intervention.

4.   What's the most common cause of acute pain in infants and young children?
- A.   Cancer
- B.   Child abuse
- C.   Rheumatoid arthritis
- D.   Treatment procedures

Answer: D. The most common cause of acute pain in children comes from procedures such as venipunctures.

Scoring

☆☆☆   If you answered all four questions correctly, fantastic! Your insight into infant pain management is incredible!

☆☆   If you answered three questions correctly, nice job! There are no barriers in your path to understanding pain management for children.

☆   If you answered fewer than three questions correctly, don't grimace. A quick review of this chapter won't hurt a bit.

Pain in elderly patients

Just the facts

In this chapter, you'll learn:

♦ common misconceptions about pain in elderly patients and the potential barriers to effective treatment

♦ specific assessment criteria for elderly patients

♦ effective pain management strategies

♦ topics to cover during patient education.

A look at pain in the elderly

The population of the United States is graying at an unprecedented rate. In 1999, approximately 34.5 million Americans, or 13% of the population, were age 65 or older. During the next two decades aging baby boomers will cause an explosion in the population of elderly Americans. By 2030, elderly patients will number 70 million and account for 20% of the population as a whole. In addition, older Americans are living longer, healthier lives thanks to advances in science, medicine, and related health care technologies.

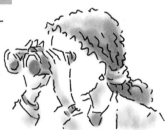

Aging can be a (chronic) pain!

Unfortunately, longer life doesn't mean that we'll be immune to the changes in physiology and cognition that accompany age. As we grow older, we're more susceptible to injury, more likely to suffer from chronic disease, and less capable of healing efficiently. Consequently, pain — especially chronic pain — is common in older adults. As the elderly population grows, so will the number of elderly patients requiring treatment for pain.

Recent studies indicate that 45% to 80% of all nursing home residents suffer some measure of chronic pain. Some of the most common causes of pain in elderly patients include:

- fractures due to falls or osteoporosis
- skin breakdown
- impaired circulation due to chronic disease (atherosclerosis, for example)
- osteoarthritis
- diabetic neuropathy
- stroke
- headaches.

   Untreated or undertreated pain can have a profound effect on the patient's quality of life. Unrelieved pain can precipitate:
- depression
- anxiety
- a decline in social interaction
- problems with sleep and nutrition
- impaired mobility, function, and rehabilitation
- impaired cognition
- a growing dependence on health care systems.

   In 2000, the Joint Commission on Accreditation of Health Care Organizations (JCAHO) issued standards for pain assessment, management, and documentation requiring that all elderly patients be screened for pain upon admission to a JCAHO-accredited facility. Furthermore, the facility's policy must include the use of a standard pain assessment tool. (See *Screening elderly patients for pain.*)

Are you up to the challenge?

To meet the growing challenge of managing pain in elderly patients, all health care providers need a clear understanding of the unique physiologic, social, and psychological make-up of this population of patients. Effective pain management can only occur when we shed common misconceptions about pain in elderly patients and overcome the barriers to treatment.

Misconceptions and barriers

Misconceptions about elderly patients can interfere with effective treatment for pain. Let's look at several common misconceptions and what we've come to understand as the truth.

Pain isn't inevitable

Misconception: Pain is a normal part of the aging process.
Present understanding: Although elderly patients are at greater risk for pain related to injury, disease, or a combination of health problems, pain is *not* an inevitable part of growing older.

Better take my pain pill before things start going from bad to worse.

Screening elderly patients for pain

A screening tool like the one below can give you a better understanding of your elderly patient's pain and perhaps guide effective treatment. Use the Faces scale if your patient can't easily communicate with you.

Date: __3/25/03__   Medical record number: __0040202__

Patient: __Elroy Fine__

Problems: __Peripheral vascular disease__   Medications: __Insulin__
_____Diabetes__

PAIN DESCRIPTION

Pattern: (Constant) Intermittent

Duration: __2 weeks__

Location: __(R) Lower extremity__

Character:
Piercing or stabbing (Burning) Stinging
Radiating   Shooting (Tingling)

Other descriptors: _____

Exacerbating factors: _____

Relieving factors: _____

Pain intensity:

0	1	2	3	(4)	5	6	7	8	9	10
None				Moderate						Severe

Worst pain in last 24 hours:

0	1	2	3	4	5	6	(7)	8	9	10
None					Moderate					Severe

Mood: __Anxious__

Depression screening score: __N/A__

Impaired activities: __Walking__

Sleep quality: __Poor__

Bowel habits: __Regular__

Other comments: _____

Probable cause of pain: __Peripheral neuropathy from diabetes and PVD__

Plan: __Initiate desipramine therapy__

FACES SCALE

| 0 | 1 | 2 | 3 | 4 | 5 |

Sensitive? You bet!

Misconception: Sensitivity to pain and pain perception decrease with age.

Present understanding: Studies of pain sensitivity and tolerance in all age-groups fails to show a significant change in pain perception or sensitivity due to age.

I'll never tell

Misconception: Elderly patients will tell you when they're in pain.

Present understanding: Not so. Elderly patients commonly hesitate to report pain. The reasons are as diverse as the patients themselves. Some of the more typical reasons include:

• fear of addiction to analgesics
• a belief that pain is a sign of weakness
• fear of additional discomfort from diagnostic tests or adverse reactions to medications
• concern about not being "good" patients or being a "bother"
• fear that pain medications will be ineffective if started too soon
• belief that pain is a deserved punishment
• concern about the costs of treatment (medications, hospitalization, disability)
• fear that reporting pain will uncover a new health problem
• lack of knowledge about available pain management options
• fear of losing control and independence
• sensory and cognitive impairment.

Overcoming the barriers

After a lifetime of experience, most elderly patients have firm opinions on just about all topics, but especially their health. Sometimes these beliefs can interfere with pain management. Some examples of potential patient-related barriers to effective pain management include:

• anxiety that treatment will make the discomfort worse or that it will uncover additional health problems
• belief that taking drugs, especially opioids, will lead to addiction
• religious and cultural beliefs about illness, pain, or aging that conflict with the treatment plan
• financial concerns.

   An open discussion of the patient's general health, specific pain, and the treatment plan will help overcome most obstacles. For example, take time to describe proposed treatments in detail and explain how each aspect will contribute to pain relief. Address the question of addiction directly by explaining the great care taken in prescribing any drug, especially opioids, and that the

Don't assume that your patient is pain-free just because he fails to mention pain.

incidence of addiction is less than 1%. Knowledge is the key to diffusing objections.

If the patient has strong religious or cultural beliefs that seem to conflict with the treatment plan, take time to discuss these issues with the patient to determine a satisfactory compromise. Usually, family members can be a helpful addition to these discussions.

Cost can be a particularly frightening aspect of care for an elderly patient on a fixed income. If possible, refer the patient (or family member) to an appropriate counselor within your facility or a local public assistance agency.

The latest and greatest

Health care providers can be guilty of lapses in knowledge that pose barriers to effective treatment. It's critical to regularly update your knowledge of guidelines for elder care, pain assessment techniques, and treatment options. Some examples of common yet erroneous beliefs that affect pain management include:
• older patients are susceptible to addiction
• adverse reactions to opioids are particularly dangerous for elderly patients
• patients with cognitive impairment don't feel pain
• pain sensitivity decreases with age
• pain management is a lower priority in the treatment plan.

Assessing pain in elderly patients

Assessing pain in elderly patients differs markedly from assessment in children and younger adults. In fact, the Agency for Healthcare Research and Quality (AHRQ) recognizes that elderly patients have unique requirements for pain assessment and management.

Typically, the older patient has multiple health problems, making the assessment and management of pain a complex process. For this reason, he requires a more comprehensive approach to assessment than a younger patient. Simply identifying the source (or sources) of pain can be a challenge when the patient has multiple pain-producing ailments.

In addition to the criteria discussed in chapter 2, Assessing pain, assessment of an elderly patient must also consider the age-related changes in cognitive status and in motivational, behavioral, and affective capacities. While the patient's physical condition is important, the choice of interventions will depend on his psychological status and cultural and spiritual beliefs as well.

Focusing on elderly patients

When assessing an elderly patient for pain, follow the guidelines discussed in chapter 2, Assessing pain, and then investigate the following areas for important additional information:
• a health history of all prescriptions, over-the-counter medications, and herbal preparations; surgical procedures; and the patient's response to pain
• physical examination of neuromuscular and musculoskeletal systems
• functional abilities (mobility, gait, balance, self-care proficiency, activity tolerance, any pain-related disabilities)
• psychosocial skills and cultural and spiritual beliefs (with a focus on pain coping skills and strategies)
• cognitive ability (note impairment or depression)
• sensory deficits (auditory, visual, verbal)
• family support systems and social networks.

A sensory impairment, such as a vision or hearing deficit, can complicate the assessment process and require that you adapt your approach. If the patient has a sensory deficit, choose a quiet, well-lit room that's free from distractions. Make sure the patient is wearing his glasses or hearing aid, if appropriate. As you discuss assessment topics, be sure to face the patient and speak slowly and clearly. Facial expressions, body language, and hand gestures will help the patient understand your discussion. Allow the patient enough time to respond at a comfortable pace.

When you interview me about pain, don't forget to ask about my family support systems.

Speak the same language

During your assessment, let the patient choose the words and framework for the discussion. His perception of pain is affected by many factors, including his cultural heritage, religious beliefs, the etiology of the pain, and his previous experience with pain. He may feel more comfortable referring to pain as discomfort, aching, soreness, or hurting—let him. Don't let language get in the way. It's important that he feel comfortable with the discussion and with you, so follow his lead whenever possible.

Specialized assessment tools

There are many assessment tools available to help assess pain, depression, cognitive awareness, and general function in an elderly patient. Most use a standard format and are available in large-print editions or in different languages. Examples of commonly used quantitative assessment tools include:

- Folstein Mini-Mental Exam, which screens for cognitive impairment
- geriatric depression scale
- SF36 (Short Form 36) and SF12 (Short Form 12), which evaluate general function and quality of life, respectively
- Functional Independence Measurement Scale (FIMS), which helps assess activities of daily living.

Psychological assessment

Psychological factors, such as fear, anxiety, depression, and suffering, contribute to pain and can help predict the patient's response to a treatment regimen. Addressing these factors is just as important as providing analgesic medications. A psychological evaluation helps determine the psychosocial, cognitive, and behavioral factors that contribute to or exacerbate the patient's experience of pain.

Depression can intensify a patient's perception of pain, and pain can cause depression.

Effective pain management means addressing depression too!

The pain-depression connection

An important focus in the psychological assessment is the relationship between depression and pain. Elderly patients with diagnosed depression typically report more incidences of pain and pain of greater intensity than patients without depression. However, high levels of pain can also *precipitate* episodes of depression. In elderly patients, depression is usually accompanied by anxiety, difficulty concentrating, and impaired memory. Health care providers need to understand the unique relationship between pain and depression and that either one can intensify the other.

Impaired cognition

Typically, the patient does a reasonable job providing information about this pain. However, when the patient has a cognitive impairment, it may be impossible to gather information in this manner. Impaired cognition can range from simple confusion to transient delirium to profound dementia. (See *Distinguishing delirium from dementia*, page 270.) In most cases, patients with mild to moderate cognitive impairment can describe pain intensity and use specially designed pain rating scales.

Distinguishing delirium from dementia

Dementia is the slow, progressive, and irreversible loss of cognitive function, including memory, judgment, and abstract thinking, and may involve changes in personality as well.

In contrast, delirium has a quick onset and is usually reversible by treating the underlying cause. Delirium is characterized by fluctuating disturbances in cognition, mood, attention, arousal, and self-awareness and can have an acute onset or occur in conjunction with a chronic intellectual impairment. Delirium may be associated with:

- advanced age
- dementia
- use of medications, such as opioids, benzodiazepines, anticholinergics, or psychoactive agents, or the use of multiple medications
- withdrawal from alcohol or sedatives
- fluid or electrolyte imbalance
- severe pain
- hypoxemia
- infection.

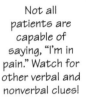

Not all patients are capable of saying, "I'm in pain." Watch for other verbal and nonverbal clues!

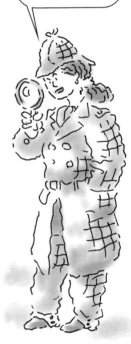

A patient with severe dementia, however, requires another approach. Watch for verbal signs of pain, such as moaning, crying, or screaming, and behaviors that may indicate pain — for example, grimacing, frowning, restlessness or agitation, and rubbing or guarding a part of the body. Be sure to record these observations as part of the assessment.

Family members can help

If members of the patient's family are available, talk with them about the patient's normal behavior patterns and functional abilities. This baseline data will help members of the health care team identify changes in behavior patterns as they occur. Even subtle changes in routine behavior can be key to assessing and treating pain. Some signs to watch for include:

- a drop in the patient's normal level of activity
- loss of appetite
- the sudden onset of agitation or difficulty sleeping
- a reduction in social interaction.

Pharmacologic pain management

Pain management for older patients typically involves a combination of pharmacologic intervention and cognitive-behavioral and physical therapies. However, the changes in physiology that accompany aging present a special set of hurdles for the health care team to overcome as they consider possible drug therapies.

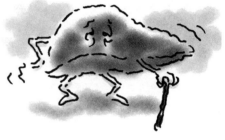

Age brings change. I just don't work as efficiently as I did when I was younger.

Pharmokinetics and aging

Aging triggers changes in the digestive system, liver, and kidneys that affect drug metabolism, absorption, distribution, and excretion. These changes influence drug dosage and administration route and technique. Physiologic changes can also increase the patient's risk of adverse reaction and interfere with therapeutic compliance.

Absorption

Although absorption isn't significantly affected by aging, there are factors associated with aging that can slow the rate at which the body absorbs drugs, for example:
• gastric pH increases as the stomach secretes less hydrochloric acid (an acid environment speeds the absorption of some drugs)
• the stomach takes longer to empty
• contents of the GI tract move more slowly
• blood flow to the intestines is reduced
• structural changes in the villi that line the small intestines slow their function.

Distribution

Aging also affects drug distribution within the body—where and how rapidly a drug is distributed within the tissues and the concentrations achieved. Older adults have more body fat, less muscle mass, and a lower level of water in the body. In addition, age causes a redistribution of subcutaneous tissue. As a result, a given dosage of a water-soluble drug can result in higher blood levels of the drug and thus a greater, and potentially toxic, pharmacologic effect. A barbiturate anesthetic may be distributed more widely due to the increase in fatty tissue, and this tissue may release the drug more slowly, prolonging its effect. Consequently, the health care team must carefully consider the dosage and administration route and technique. (See *Modifying I.M. injections*, page 272.)

Peak technique

Modifying I.M. injections

Before administering an I.M. injection to an elderly patient, consider the physiologic changes that accompany aging and choose your equipment, site, and technique accordingly.

Choosing a needle
Remember that an elderly patient usually has less subcutaneous tissue and less muscle mass than a younger patient—especially in the buttocks and deltoid muscles. As a result, you may need to use a shorter needle than you would for a younger adult.

Selecting a site
An elderly patient typically has more fat around the hips, abdomen, and thigh areas. This makes the vastus lateralis muscle and ventrogluteal area (gluteus medius and minimus but not gluteus maximus muscles) the primary injection sites.

You should be able to palpate the muscle in these areas easily. However, if the patient is extremely thin, gently pinch the muscle to elevate it and avoid putting the needle completely through (which will alter the absorption and distribution of the drug).

Immobile? Move on to another site!
Caution: Never give an I.M. injection in an immobile limb—drug absorption is poor, and there's a risk that a sterile abscess will form at the injection site.

Checking technique
To avoid inserting the needle in a blood vessel, pull back on the plunger and look for blood before injecting the drug. Because of age-related vascular changes, the elderly patient is also at greater risk for hematomas. To avoid bleeding after an I.M. injection, you may need to apply direct pressure over the puncture site for a longer time than usual.

The massage message
Gently massage the injection site to aid drug absorption and distribution. However, avoid site massage with certain drugs given by the Z-track injection technique, such as iron dextran and hydroxyzine hydrochloride.

Metabolism

Liver mass and function declines with age, as does the action of certain liver enzymes. These changes slow the metabolism of drugs, which can lead to higher blood levels and the potential for exaggerated effects. However, the liver's capacity to metabolize drugs doesn't decline consistently for all drugs, so it's imperative to carefully consider each of the drugs selected for the treatment regimen.

Elimination

Declining kidney function, which typically accompanies aging, can increase the effects of a given drug as well as the potential for

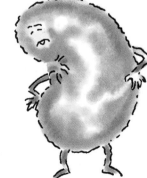

Hey, go easy on me! I'm running at half speed these days.

drug toxicity. Renal function begins to decline around age 30, but the change isn't significant until age 50 or 60. By age 80, however, renal function can be 50% of what it once was, largely due to reduced renal perfusion. As excretion slows, the half-life of administered drugs — and the risk of toxicity — increases.

Pharmacodynamics and aging

Studies reveal that tissue sensitivity to drugs changes with age, enhancing the effects of some drugs. This change may be related to the function or number of tissue and organ receptors, which may contribute to adverse neurologic effects, such as confusion and loss of balance. To compensate, drug dosages are typically lower for elderly patients.

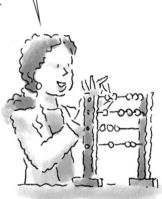

Age-related changes plus multiple health problems plus multiple drugs can equal adverse effects.

Adverse effects

The potential for misdiagnosis or failure to identify adverse affects of a drug are two difficult problems in managing drug therapy for elderly patients. Determining optimal dosage can be difficult because age-related changes in pharmokinetics and pharmacodynamics can vary greatly from one patient to the next. The problem is compounded by the fact that many elderly patients receive medications for multiple health problems. When adverse effects occur, the doctor typically adjusts the dosage or selects an alternative drug.

Fighting adversity

An adverse reaction is a noxious or an unwanted response that occurs at a dosage that's otherwise considered therapeutic. If the patient is on multiple medications, the interaction of the medications may be at the root of an unwanted and unanticipated response. In any event, adverse effects require prompt intervention; careful monitoring is crucial. Common signs of an adverse reaction include:
- confusion
- depression
- anxiety
- forgetfulness
- drowsiness
- urine retention or incontinence
- hives
- impotence
- stomach upset
- rash.

Unless health care providers are well informed, these signs may be erroneously dismissed as typical elderly behavior rather than recognized as adverse drug reactions.

More serious adverse reactions include:

- orthostatic hypotension
- dehydration
- altered mental status
- anorexia
- blood disorders
- tardive dyskinesia.

Even when the drug dosage is correct, elderly patients are still at risk. Ongoing physiologic changes, poor compliance with the drug regimen (typically due to common adverse effects such as nausea), and multiple prescriptions are just some of the factors that contribute to elderly patients experiencing twice as many adverse reactions as younger patients.

> Monitor your elderly patient for confusion, anxiety, and other signs of an adverse drug reaction.

Analgesic therapy

Analgesic therapy is the most common strategy for managing pain in an elderly patient. Careful titration (slowly increasing the amount of drug until the desired effect is reached) in concert with frequent assessment is the safest method of establishing optimal pain relief. Unfortunately, health care providers commonly fail to use analgesic therapy to its full potential. Incomplete or inaccurate knowledge of available drugs and administration guidelines is usually at fault, and unnecessary suffering on the part of the patient is the result. The solution is easy: continuing education for all health care providers who work with elderly patients.

Reach 'em when you teach 'em

Analgesic therapy requires the active participation of the patient. The more the patient learns, the better his compliance with treatment. Be sure to teach the patient about the proper dosage for all medications, possible adverse reactions, how long until the drug takes effect, and the duration of pain relief. Plan additional teaching sessions to address issues that come up as treatment gets under way—for example, concerns about addiction or how to deal with unpleasant side effects.

> What's the difference between a health care provider and an educator? You'll find there isn't one!

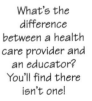

Opioid analgesics

Opioid analgesics are safe and effective in relieving many types of pain experienced by elderly patients. Although there are risks involved, they tend to be less threatening than most patients anticipate. Proper dosage and careful monitoring keeps the risk factor low. Still, therapy can cause cognitive impairment and, due to pharmokinetic changes associated with aging, the half-life of opioids in elderly patients is longer, so proper dosage is especially critical. Older patients tend to require a smaller dosage than younger patients to achieve pain relief. Also, a concurrent medical condition or its treatment regimen may increase patients' sensitivity to opioid analgesics.

Ah, that's much better

Steps to take to ensure safe, effective therapy include:
• around-the-clock dosing to maintain a stable blood level
• avoiding adverse reactions by starting therapy with shorter-acting opioids to determine the required level of pain relief before moving to longer-acting opioids
• determining the most effective administration method (oral is preferred)
• recognizing opioid metabolites (some are toxic)
• establishing a bowel regimen and increasing fluids if necessary (constipation is an adverse effect of therapy)
• avoiding concurrent use of sedatives
• recognizing and treating adverse reactions
• continuous assessment and proper documentation.
    You'll know opioid therapy is going well when the patient's functional ability increases, his sleeping patterns improve, and he reports little or no pain.

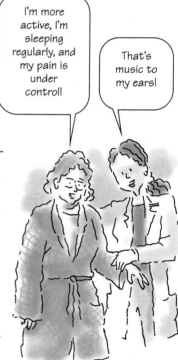

I'm more active, I'm sleeping regularly, and my pain is under control!

That's music to my ears!

When to avoid an opioid

While opioids can be a boon to pain management, several should be avoided if at all possible. These include:
• meperidine (Demerol; can cause renal neurotoxicity, delirium)
• pentazocine (Talwin; can cause delirium, agitation)
• propoxyphene (Darvon; minimal analgesic effect, potential for renal injury)
• methadone (Dolophine; a short-acting analgesic with a long half-life).

Patient-controlled analgesia

Patient-controlled analgesia (PCA) is helpful, safe, and can be administered I.V. or epidurally. When considering this option, first assess the elderly patient for a physical or cognitive impairment that might interfere with his ability to use PCA. Also, prepare patient education sessions to explain PCA equipment and proper use. An elderly patient can be intimidated by the technology.

Nonopioid analgesics

The nonopioid analgesics most commonly used in treating pain in elderly patients include acetaminophen, nonsteroidal anti-inflammatory drugs (NSAIDs), and a variety of adjuvant analgesics.

Acetaminophen

Acetaminophen relieves mild pain and reduces fever. It's commonly the drug of choice when aspirin and NSAIDs are contraindicated. Unlike these drugs, acetaminophen isn't anti-inflammatory. It doesn't alter platelet function and rarely causes GI problems.

Acetaminophen may slightly increase the effects of oral anticoagulants and thrombolytics and may increase the risk of liver toxicity if combined with phenytoin (Dilantin), barbiturates, carbamazepine (Tegretol), or isoniazid (Nydrazid).

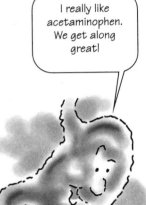

I really like acetaminophen. We get along great!

NSAIDs

In general, NSAIDs provide temporary relief from mild to moderate pain and may be used as adjunctive treatment in the management of cancer pain. Also, NSAIDs may be prescribed for pain associated with osteoarthritis and rheumatoid arthritis. In elderly patients, NSAIDs should be prescribed with caution and in lower dosages. Short-acting NSAIDs are a better choice because they minimize accumulation in tissues. NSAIDs shouldn't be prescribed if the patient has abnormal renal function, a history of peptic ulcer disease, or bleeding tendencies.

What's new? COX-2!

Elderly patients undergo more invasive procedures (for example, surgery for hip fracture or GI bleeding) than younger patients. COX-2 inhibitors, which don't affect platelet aggregation or increase bleeding time, are a better choice for this population. Research indicates that age has little if any affect on the safety or effectiveness of COX-2 inhibitors.

Although the dosage needs no adjustment because of the patient's age, treatment is routinely started at the lowest recommended dose. When using COX-2 inhibitors, it's important to monitor the patient for renal insufficiency and other side effects.

Salicylates

Caution is needed when prescribing salicylates to elderly patients, as they can be more susceptible to the toxic effects. The effects of aspirin on renal prostaglandins may cause fluid retention and edema, a significant drawback for elderly patients, especially those with heart failure.

Adjuvant analgesics

Adjuvant analgesics are drugs with other primary functions, but that provide analgesia in specific circumstances. The most effective pharmacologic treatment strategies for managing pain in elderly patients combine opioid, nonopioid, and adjuvant analgesics. Tricyclic antidepressants and anticonvulsants have been effective in relieving neuropathic pain; however, this combination carries a high risk of adverse reactions. Patients receiving adjuvant analgesics should be monitored frequently for incidental and continuous pain and for adverse reactions.

Local anesthetics

I.V. infusion of local anesthetics, such as lidocaine, is helpful in managing pain associated with neuropathies, musculoskeletal disorders, arthritis, and stroke. Common adverse effects include myocardial depression (reduced heart rate), paresthesia, dizziness, and tremors. Capsaicin (Zostrix) and lidocaine patch (Lidoderm), topical anesthetics, are used in the treatment of various neuropathies and herpes zoster.

Nonpharmacologic pain management

Although analgesics are the mainstay of pain management in elderly patients, nonpharmacologic interventions help reduce the psychological components of pain, thereby enhancing comfort and improving quality of life.

Nonpharmacologic interventions range from the conventional (whirlpools, massage, hot packs, electrical nerve stimulation) to the esoteric (aromatherapy, meditation, yoga, biofeedback); however, all can be grouped into three main categories: cognitive and behavioral therapies, physical therapies, and alternative and complementary therapies.

Nonpharmacologic interventions help reduce pain, stress, and anxiety and give the patient a sense of control over pain. Managing pain in the elderly patient usually involves a combination of interventions.

This may not be a masterpiece, but it sure took my mind off my aching back!

Cognitive and behavioral therapies

Cognitive therapies focus on influencing the patient's interpretation of pain. Behavioral therapies focus on helping him build the skills he needs to manage pain and change his reaction to it when it occurs. Examples of cognitive and behavioral therapies include distraction, meditation, biofeedback, and hypnosis. (For more information, see chapter 4, Nonpharmacologic pain management.) These techniques improve the patient's sense of control by encouraging his active participation in pain management.

Pain subtraction through distraction

In distraction, the patient is encouraged to focus on a stimuli other than his pain and the associated negative emotions. Reading, watching television, listening to music, painting or crafting, and humor are examples of distraction therapies. Focusing on the humorous side of life is beneficial because doing so reduces tension and stimulates endorphin production in the brain. Endorphins are the body's natural painkillers.

Just... reeeelaxxxxx...

Countless studies have illustrated that muscular and mental tension exacerbate pain. Relaxation techniques, such as meditation, guided imagery, and passive relaxation, are easy for older patients to learn and require no exertion. In fact, they require just the opposite — stillness, quiet, and focused thought.

All relaxation techniques have a common goal — to clear the mind and release pent-up muscular tension. By focusing attention on one peaceful thought, sound, or rhythm, the patient sets aside, at least for a time, any negative thoughts, worries, or concerns that he's harboring. At the same time, he focuses on relaxing tense muscles throughout the body. In guided imagery, a leader describes a peaceful mental journey to relaxation. If the patient is new to meditation, he may prefer this technique. Also, you can augment more structured relaxation sessions with patient teaching about the simple techniques he can use anytime to relax — for example, deep breathing.

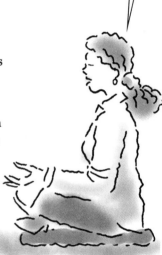

I am free from tension. I am free from distraction. I am free from all pain. I am free...

Physical therapies

Physical therapies use physical agents and methods to aid pain reduction. They are relatively inexpensive and easy to use. With appropriate teaching, patients and their families can use them on their own. Thermotherapy, biofeedback, transcutaneous electrical nerve stimulation (TENS), and massage are commonly used in managing pain in elderly patients.

Should I bring my thermal underwear?

Thermotherapy is the application of dry or moist heat to reduce muscular aches and pains, relieve stiff joints, improve circulation, and increase the pain threshold. Dry heat can be applied with a hot water bottle, a K-pad, or an electric heating pad. Moist heat can be applied with a hot pack, a warm compress, or a specialized heating pad.

Cold can also relieve pain by numbing nerve endings and reducing inflammation. In most cases, alternating heat and then cold is a more effective strategy for relieving pain than either method used alone.

I need some feedback

Biofeedback teaches the patient how to exert control over various autonomic functions. In a typical session, the patient watches or listens to a signal that coincides with a specific autonomic function—for example, his breathing, heart rate, or blood pressure. Working with a trained member of the health care team, the patient learns how to adjust his thoughts, breathing pattern, posture, and muscle tension to influence the chosen function. As his control improves, he applies what he has learned to controlling painful sensations.

Biofeedback can be useful for reducing chronic pain, such as headache, backache, stress-related pain, and GI pain. It's popular with patients because it gives them a sense of control over their pain.

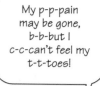

My p-p-pain may be gone, b-b-but I c-c-can't feel my t-t-toes!

A shock to the system

In TENS therapy, a portable, battery-powered device transmits painless alternating electrical current to a painful area. When used successfully, TENS can help an elderly patient with chronic pain reduce his need for analgesics and develop a sense of control over his pain. TENS therapy, which must be prescribed by a doctor, usually lasts 3 to 5 days, and sessions may run from minutes to hours to continuously, depending on the patient's ailment. Chronic nonmalignant pain, cancer pain, and pain associated with fractures, arthritis, and lower back strain are some of the conditions that respond well to TENS.

TENS is based on the gate control theory, which proposes that painful impulses pass through a "gate" in the brain. The painless electrical current delivered by the TENS unit blocks the painful stimuli, thereby altering the patient's perception of the pain.

TENS is contraindicated in the patient with a cardiac pacemaker because it can interfere with pacemaker function, and it should be used with caution in any patient with a cardiac disorder. It's also contraindicated in the patient with a cognitive impairment. TENS electrodes shouldn't be placed on the head or neck of the patient with a vascular or seizure disorder.

Massage therapy promotes relaxation and reduces stress. Hey, I should do this more often!

Ohhhhh, that feels so gooood...

Massage therapy helps relieve pain and fatigue, reduces swelling, promotes relaxation, reduces stress, and promotes sound sleep. In elderly patients, massage is particularly effective in relieving pain in the back, shoulders, hands, and feet. Massage can help communicate concern to cognitively impaired patients and to those faced with a language barrier.

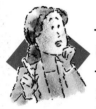

Quick quiz

1. Which of the following statements is *not* a misconception regarding pain in elderly patients?

A. Pain is a normal part of aging.
B. Elderly patients are more sensitive to pain.
C. Elderly patients routinely report pain when they feel it.
D. The adverse reactions associated with opioids make them too dangerous to use with elderly patients.

Answer: B. The misconception exists that elderly patients are *less* sensitive to pain.

2. Which of the following is *not* a benefit of massage therapy?

A. Relaxation
B. Sleeplessness
C. Relief from fatigue
D. Decreased pain

Answer: B. Massage promotes sleep.

3. Which of the following statements is true concerning the use of heat and cold for pain relief in elderly patients?

A. Alternating heat and cold is more effective than either method alone.
B. Heat is effective because it causes vasoconstriction.
C. Cold reduces inflammation by causing vasodilation.
D. The effects of heat last longer than the effects of cold.

Answer: A. The most effective way to use heat and cold is to alternate them.

Scoring

☆☆☆ If you answered all three questions correctly, congrats! You've overcome all barriers to managing pain in the elderly!

☆☆ If you answered two questions correctly, jump up and shout! You know what pain management is all about!

☆ If you answered only one question correctly, don't take a pain pill! Just review the chapter again, and you'll be better in no time!

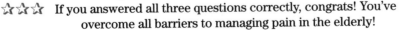

Addictive disease

Just the facts

In this chapter, you'll learn:

♦ definitions of terms related to substance abuse and dependency

♦ the current understanding of the neurobiologic basis of addiction

♦ pharmacologic and nonpharmacologic treatments for addiction

♦ approaches to pain management in addicted patients.

A look at addictive disease

All too often, the care of patients suffering from pain is complicated by misconceptions about pain, the medications used to manage it, and the nature of addiction. These misconceptions may create exaggerated or unfounded fears, prevent appropriate pain management, and cause patients to be stigmatized.

Off-kilter estimates

For one thing, many health care professionals overestimate the risk of patients becoming addicted to opioid analgesics. Some are reluctant to prescribe adequate dosages of opioids for pain, fearing the drugs may cause (or worsen) addiction.

Undertreated pain

Patients with undertreated pain who seek appropriate pain medication are sometimes mistakenly labeled as addicts by health care professionals. However, many more patients are undertreated for pain than are addicted to pain medications. Large surveys show that fewer than 1% of patients who receive prescribed opioids to treat acute pain become addicted.

Health care professionals may label a patient an addict just because he seeks pain medication.

In fact, patients with no history of addiction rarely become addicted to opioids when these drugs are prescribed for legitimate purposes.

Resigned to pain

Patients themselves may be reluctant to ask for analgesics out of fear they'll become addicted or be branded as addicts. They simply resign themselves to living with pain. (See *When your patient fears addiction.*)

Addressing addiction

What should you do if the patient reports a history of addiction or if you suspect he's addicted? In general, caregivers should try to address the patient's addiction and his pain management needs at the same time.

As appropriate, the patient should be referred to an outpatient treatment program. In the meantime, he may be prescribed a limit-

Myth busters

When your patient fears addiction

Many patients don't want to ask for analgesics (or refuse them) despite their pain due to misconceptions about addiction to painkillers. If you think this is the case with your patient, use the following information to dispel myths about these medications.

Myth: Many people become addicted to pain medication.

Fact: Patients rarely become addicted when pain medication is used appropriately. Many need pain medication only for a brief time—until the cause of pain goes away. When they're ready to stop taking the medication, the dose is reduced so that by the time they stop using it completely, the body has had time to adjust.

Myth: Someone who asks for pain relief is a complainer.

Fact: Patients have the right to ask for pain relief and should tell caregivers when they're in pain. The sooner they do so, the better—it's easier to control pain before it becomes severe.

Myth: Painkillers can make you "lose control."

Fact: Few people "lose control" when they take pain medication as prescribed. They may get sleepy, dizzy, or confused when they first start certain medications, but this feeling usually goes away after a few days.

Myth: Strong pain relievers should be saved for later.

Fact: Pain medications don't lose their effectiveness over time. Although drug tolerance can occur, it can be addressed effectively by increasing the dose.

ed amount of pain medication—preferably a drug that's less likely to be abused or sold on the street.

Barriers to pain management

If the patient has a history of substance abuse and is feeling pain, he may encounter tremendous barriers to receiving adequate pain management. Remember—he's entitled to the same quality of health care as another patient.

Providing care for a patient who has pain and addiction is challenging, but it can be rewarding as well.

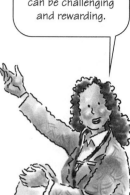

Caring for a patient who has pain and addiction can be challenging and rewarding.

Understanding addiction

In the past, addiction was seen as a personal or moral weakness or as a direct effect of the particular substance to which the person was addicted. Although these beliefs aren't supported by medical research, they've helped to shape society's attitudes toward people with addictive disease.

Important terms

To provide appropriate care, you need to understand the terminology of addiction.

• *Psychological dependence* refers to a person's belief that he must take a drug to cause or stop a particular effect.

• *Addiction* refers to a primary, chronic, neurobiologic disease with genetic, psychosocial, and environmental factors influencing its development and manifestations. It involves using the drug for nonmedical purposes, and it's characterized by such behaviors as impaired control over drug use, compulsive drug use, continued use despite adverse consequences, and drug craving.

• *Substance abuse* is a less severe form of—and commonly a precursor to—addiction or substance dependence. Compared to addiction, it usually has a shorter duration of impairment and cause fewer neurophysiologic symptoms.

• *Chemical coping* refers to behavior that appears to be addiction. For example, a patient who takes pills inappropriately to cope with stress.

Other key terms include pseudoaddiction, tolerance, physical dependence, and withdrawal or abstinence syndrome. (See *Defining key terms*, page 284.)

Defining key terms

Are you up-to-date on the definition of pseudoaddiction? Can you distinguish physical dependence from drug tolerance?

Many people use these and related terms inaccurately or inappropriately—and this can have consequences for patient care.

Pseudoaddiction

Pseudoaddiction is characterized by patient behaviors such as anger and escalating demands for more or different medications and results in suspicion or avoidance by the staff. It may be mistaken for addiction in patients with pain who don't receive adequate pain management.

Pseudoaddiction may be caused by under-treatment of pain. Unlike true addiction, it resolves when pain is treated effectively.

Tolerance

Tolerance is a state of adaptation in which exposure to a drug causes changes that diminish drug effects over time. The person then needs higher doses to obtain the same effects.

Physical dependence

Physical dependence is a state of adaptation manifested by withdrawal syndrome when the drug is stopped abruptly, the dose is reduced rapidly, or a drug antagonist is administered.

Withdrawal or abstinence syndrome

Withdrawal or abstinence syndrome refers to signs and symptoms that occur when a person suddenly stops taking a drug to which he has become physically dependent. Specific signs and symptoms depend on the particular substance. The presence of withdrawal doesn't mean that the patient is addicted.

Is it addiction, dependence, or tolerance?

Physical dependence and tolerance are normal physiologic consequences of extended opioid therapy for pain. Don't confuse these states for addiction.

Patients who take opioids on a regular basis for 1 to 4 weeks, such as after surgery, frequently experience symptoms of tolerance or physical dependence. Gradual dosage increases can overcome tolerance. Slowly tapering the dosage when pain diminishes can prevent withdrawal syndrome.

Addiction by the numbers

According to the federal Substance Abuse and Mental Health Services Administration, nearly 17 million Americans (7% of the U.S. population) were addicted to or abused alcohol or illicit drugs in 2001. Of these Americans:

• approximately 2 million were addicted to or abused both alcohol and illicit drugs.

• roughly 3 million were addicted to or abused illicit drugs but not alcohol.

• more than 11 million were addicted to or abused alcohol but didn't use illicit drugs.

Nearly 17 million Americans were addicted to or abused substances in 2001.

Addicts undercounted?

These figures may underestimate the true incidence of addiction because they come from self-reports. Earlier studies estimated the prevalence of alcohol and drug addiction at 14% and 7%, respectively.

Casual use doesn't count

If the substance itself, such as morphine or alcohol, were the primary cause of addiction, the number of drug and alcohol addicts would be much higher.

But many people smoke an occasional cigarette, have a few drinks, inhale marijuana at a rock concert, or experiment with illicit drugs without becoming addicted. The same is true of patients who receive controlled substances to treat pain; only a tiny number become addicted.

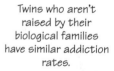

Many people can drink alcohol and use other drugs casually without becoming addicted.

Biological aspects of addiction

Addiction is a complex disease with a neurobiologic basis. Genetic makeup and environmental factors play important roles in its development.

Tale of the twins

Studies of twins and adopted persons suggest that genetic factors are the most powerful influences in addiction. Twins and adoptees who weren't raised by their biological families had similar addiction rates, suggesting that family environment was less important than shared genetic makeup.

Stress increases risk

Stress also has important links to substance use. Animal studies show that rats under stress learn to give themselves cocaine more quickly than nonstressed rats.

Also, studies of recovering addicts have found that their nervous systems are hypersensitive to chemically induced stress. The studies suggest the same may be true of emotionally induced stress.

Twins who aren't raised by their biological families have similar addiction rates.

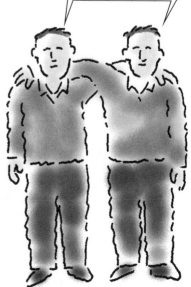

Addiction and mental illness

Many people who abuse substances also suffer from major psychiatric illnesses. Data suggest that up to 72% of persons who experience alcohol or drug addiction disorders at some time in their lives also meet the criteria for a psychiatric disorder.

Some people self-medicate with legal or illegal substances to relieve symptoms of anxiety, depression, or thought disorders. This temporary relief reinforces repeated use. If the substance they're using has the potential to cause physical dependence, they may experience unpleasant withdrawal symptoms. So to stop experiencing these symptoms, they continue using the substance.

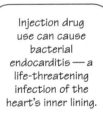

> Addiction often goes hand in hand with psychiatric illness.

And the survey shows...

The 2001 National Survey on Drug Abuse found a strong relationship between addiction and mental problems. Among adults reporting serious mental illness, 20% were addicted to or abused alcohol or illicit drugs. But among adults with no serious mental illness, only 6.3% were addicted to or abused alcohol or illicit drugs. An estimated 3 million adults had serious mental illness and addiction or abuse problems during the year.

Links between addiction and physical illness or injury

Persons with addictive disease are more likely than others to develop certain medical conditions.

Physical consequences

Addiction is associated with many medical conditions.

Alcohol aftermath

Chronic alcohol use may lead to:
- liver disease
- renal failure
- pancreatitis
- cardiomyopathy
- avascular joint necrosis
- neurologic disorders.

High stakes of smoking

Smoking is associated with:
- chronic obstructive pulmonary disease
- hypertension
- heart disease
- many types of cancer—especially lung cancer and head and neck cancers.

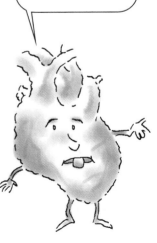

> Injection drug use can cause bacterial endocarditis—a life-threatening infection of the heart's inner lining.

Injection drug dangers

Injection drug use can lead to:
• hepatitis C
• human immunodeficiency virus (HIV)
• bacterial endocarditis
• soft-tissue infections.

Stimulant sorrows

Using stimulants, such as methamphetamine, can lead to stroke and other neurologic impairments.

Pregnancy perils

Pregnant substance abusers are less likely to receive adequate prenatal care than other pregnant women and more likely to have poor perinatal outcomes.

Increased injuries

Addicted persons also run a higher risk of traumatic injury. Impaired judgment while under the influence contributes to accidents and assaults.

Studies show alcohol use as a factor in roughly 39% to 50% of spinal cord injuries and 44% of traffic accident deaths. Obtaining substances illegally also puts a person at increased risk for violence.

Managing addiction

Like any complex chronic illness, addiction is best treated by professionals with specialized education and appropriate experience. As with diabetes or hypertension, addiction treatment is more likely to succeed when a multipronged approach is used and when treatment is tailored to the patient.

No simple answers

Because addiction has so many dimensions and disrupts so many aspects of a person's life, treatment isn't simple. Goals include helping the patient to:
• maintain a drug-free lifestyle
• achieve healthy functioning in family relationships, at work, and in society.

Effective approaches

Three decades of scientific research and clinical practice have yielded many effective approaches to drug treatment.

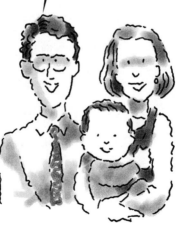

Helping the patient achieve healthy relationships with family members is one treatment goal.

Treating addiction effectively

According to the National Institute of Drug Abuse, successful drug addiction treatment hinges on the following principles.

Address all ills
• Treatment must address the patient's multiple needs—not just drug abuse.
• If the patient has a coexisting mental disorder, the addiction and mental disorder should be treated in an integrated way.
• The treatment program should include assessment for human immunodeficiency virus, acquired immunodeficiency syndrome, hepatitis B and C, tuberculosis and other infectious diseases, and counseling to help the patient change behaviors that place him at risk for infection.
• Individual or group counseling and other behavioral therapies are critical components of effective treatment.

One size doesn't fit all
• No single treatment approach is appropriate for every patient.

Monitoring is a must
• The treatment plan should be assessed continually and modified as needed to ensure that it meets the patient's changing needs.
• The patient must be monitored continuously for possible drug use during treatment.

Medicate as needed
• For many patients, prescribed medications are an important part of treatment—especially when combined with counseling and other behavioral therapies.

Expect a long haul
• Detoxification is only the first stage in addiction treatment and, by itself, does little to change long-term drug use.
• Recovery from addiction can be a long-term process and usually requires multiple treatment episodes.
• The patient must stay in treatment for an adequate time for the program to be effective.

Other principles
• Treatment must be readily available for those who need it.
• Treatment need not be voluntary to be effective.

Extensive data show that drug addiction treatments are as effective as treatments for most other chronic medical conditions.

Of course, not all treatment programs are equally effective. The National Institute of Drug Abuse has identified some basic principles that characterize the most effective drug abuse and addiction treatments. (See *Treating addiction effectively*.)

Shore up social supports

Because of the chaos that addiction creates in one's life, a patient being treated for addiction may need intensive social support and help in negotiating the health care system and other institutional systems.

Expect relapses

Keep in mind that a key feature of addictive disease is its chronic and relapsing nature. Few people achieve sobriety with a single course of treatment, and many must make repeated attempts before achieving sustained sobriety.

In other words, expect the patient to relapse. When he does, don't convey to him the notion that he has failed the caregiver, the treatment program, his family, or society.

> To treat addiction, the patient may receive a longer-acting substitute for the drug he's been abusing.

Pharmacotherapy for drug addiction

Drug therapy for addiction can help prevent withdrawal symptoms and normalize the patient's physiologic status. To reverse or prevent withdrawal symptoms without triggering reward mechanisms, treatment usually involves replacing the short-acting substance that the patient has been abusing with a longer-acting one that produces similar central nervous system effects.

In smoking-cessation programs, for example, nicotine patches and gum are commonly combined with nonpharmacologic treatments. This approach helps reduce the irritability and anxiety that commonly emerge as a smoker tries to quit—allowing him to concentrate on learning other skills.

Pharmacologic treatments for opioid and alcohol addiction also are well-established.

Pharmacologic treatment of opioid addiction

Medical detoxification—systematic withdrawal from the drug—usually is the first step in treating opioid addiction. Detoxification, which should be done under medical care, treats the acute physiologic effects of stopping drug use. Medications are available to aid detoxification from opioids.

Beyond detox

However, detoxification alone isn't adequate in treating addiction. Because it fails to address the psychological, social, and behavioral problems associated with addiction, it doesn't promote the long-lasting behavioral changes necessary for recovery. Long-term counseling and education are crucial as well.

Opioid detoxification

Opioid detoxification should take place in a licensed drug treatment program or under the direction of a doctor certified in addiction medicine. In outpatient settings, detoxification usually takes place over 21 days.

Drug switch

Opioid detoxification usually involves substitution therapy. The abused drug is replaced with a longer-acting opioid agonist, such as methadone (Dolophine) or levo-alpha-acetylmethadol (LAMM).

To start, the replacement drug is given in a small oral dose. Methadone, for instance, is given as a syrup. Its long half-life allows once-daily dosing for withdrawal prevention. LAMM, even longer-acting, can be given every 72 hours. Gradually, the dose is titrated upward in small increments to eliminate physical withdrawal symptoms.

More help on the horizon

Clonidine (Catapres) may be added as an effective and easy-to-use medication that increases patient compliance. It's given orally until the maximum dose is achieved, then the patient is switched to a patch.

If the patient is experiencing acute intoxication, naloxone (Narcan) is given.

A slew of symptoms

Symptoms of opioid withdrawal include an increase in pain, insomnia, fear, agitation, tremors, and autonomic nervous system hyperexcitability, which can cause sweating or chills, runny nose, changes in heart rate and blood pressure, abdominal pain and cramping, nausea, vomiting, and diarrhea.

Maintaining on methadone

Maintenance doses of methadone may be much higher than the doses used for preventing withdrawal symptoms. Additionally, some patients may need the drug longer—for months or even years—as a maintenance medication. (See *How methadone works*.)

For many patients, methadone has proven indispensable. Its stabilizing influence allows them to regain their physical and mental health, achieve educational and vocational goals, reunite with family, and enter or stay in the workforce.

Methadone-less detox

But some patients choose not to use methadone or LAMM when stopping drug use. Instead, they may receive only medications to lessen withdrawal symptoms—for instance, antihistamines to

> Methadone is commonly given as a syrup for opioid detoxification.

Now I get it!

How methadone works

An opiate analgesic, methadone hydrochloride (Dolophine) is used to detoxify and maintain patients with opiate dependence as well as to treat severe pain. The drug causes only mild euphoria and doesn't produce sedation.

Changes in perception
Methadone binds with opiate receptors at many sites in the central nervous system, including the brain, brainstem, and spinal cord. It alters the perception of and emotional response to pain.

Safety, stability, less stress
Methadone has numerous benefits over illicit opiates:
• It's much longer-acting than heroin and needs to be taken only once a day. A single dose is effective for preventing opiate withdrawal for about 24 hours, compared to just a few hours for heroin. When methadone is used for pain relief, however, it needs to be given more than once a day.
• It's taken orally, so it's safer than injecting drugs. The patient doesn't risk sharing needles and becoming infected with blood-borne viruses, such as hepatitis B or C or human immunodeficiency virus.
• The routine involved in methadone treatment encourages the patient to lead a stable lifestyle, improve his diet, and adopt a regular sleep pattern.
• The patient doesn't have to worry where his next "hit" will come from. Also, he can cut his ties to the illegal drug scene.
• When prescribed medically, methadone is much cheaper than illicit drugs.

ease anxiety and insomnia, antiemetics and antidiarrheals for GI symptoms, and nonopioid analgesics for generalized muscle and joint pain.

Opioid antagonist therapy
After detoxification, some patients may decide to use opioid antagonists, such as naltrexone (Trexan), instead of opioid agonists. Oral naltrexone, a long-acting synthetic antagonist, is given three or four times a week for a sustained period. To prevent withdrawal symptoms, patients must be detoxified and opiate-free for several days before starting naltrexone.

Blocking the high

Because naltrexone therapy blocks all opioid effects—including euphoria—noncompliance is common. For this reason, patients on naltrexone or another opioid antagonist must have a strong therapeutic relationship with caregivers, receive effective counseling, and undergo close monitoring for compliance. Naltrexone therapy has had only limited success.

Nonetheless, naltrexone is useful for patients who desire total abstinence because of their circumstances—for instance, impaired professionals and people being supervised by the criminal justice system.

Stable and functioning

Maintenance opioid agonist or antagonist therapy can stabilize recovering addicts so they can function normally. Many are able to hold jobs, avoid the crime and violence of the street culture, and reduce their exposure to hepatitis B and C and HIV by stopping injection drug use and drug-related high-risk sexual behavior.

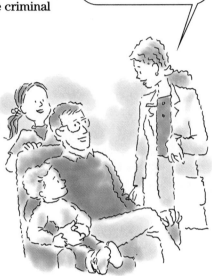

A patient receiving naltrexone must be monitored closely for compliance.

Pharmacologic treatment of alcohol addiction

The patient who wishes to stop abusing alcohol may receive disulfiram (Antabuse) to deter him from drinking. This drug causes nausea and vomiting, flushing, a severe throbbing headache, sweating, chest pain, tachycardia, confusion, and agitation if the patient consumes alcohol.

Disulfiram + Drinking = Danger

Be aware that disulfiram occasionally causes respiratory depression and cardiac collapse in the patient who's still drinking.

Smaller reward

To reduce the reinforcing effects of alcohol, a patient may receive naltrexone. This drug blocks opiate receptors in the brain and is thought to decrease the psychological reward brought by drinking alcohol.

Alcohol detoxification
Although detoxification alone isn't an effective treatment for alcohol addiction, it may be a useful first step in stabilizing the patient. As he detoxifies, caregivers can assess his overall physical and mental health and plan a more comprehensive approach to treatment that begins when he's more stable.

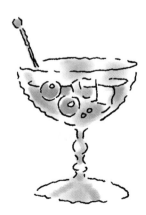

Detecting withdrawal syndrome

Alcohol withdrawal can be life-threatening if it progresses to delirium tremens. The patient's risk of withdrawal must be evaluated.

Usually, high-risk patients receive benzodiazepines, based on protocols tied to symptom severity and frequent reassessment. Patients with impaired liver or renal function need closer monitoring because of the danger of drug accumulation.

During alcohol withdrawal, such symptoms as nausea, tremors, paroxysmal sweating, anxiety, hallucinations, and disorientation may occur. However, the earliest withdrawal symptoms may be subtle and subjective with no outward manifestations.

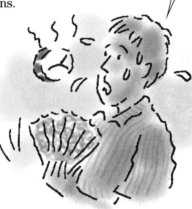

A patient going through alcohol withdrawal may experience sweating and other signs and symptoms.

Help is on the way

Maintenance therapy for the recovering alcoholic includes the use of disulfiram. The patient must abstain from alcohol for 12 hours before administration. The dose is 500 mg once per day for 2 weeks, then decreased to 250 mg once per day. However, be aware that the use of this drug has a low compliance rate if the patient self-administers.

Symptom scale

One tool used to detect withdrawal is the Clinical Institute Withdrawal Assessment of Alcohol Scale (revised)—CIWA-Ar for short. This scale provides a comprehensive symptom checklist for quantifying and monitoring the presence and severity of alcohol withdrawal symptoms. It yields a numerical score that helps the health care team recognize alcohol withdrawal in the early stages so they can begin pharmacologic treatment before withdrawal symptoms become severe. (See *Assessing alcohol withdrawal symptoms*, pages 294 and 295.)

Nonpharmacologic approaches

Most addiction specialists combine pharmacologic treatment with nonpharmacologic approaches, such as self-help groups and cognitive or behavioral therapy.

Twelve-step treatment programs

Self-help groups complement and enhance the efforts of professional substance abuse treatment. Well-known self-help groups include those affiliated with Alcoholics Anonymous, Narcotics Anonymous, and Cocaine Anonymous. These groups are based on the 12-step model. (See *Twelve steps to recovery*, page 296.)

(Text continues on page 296.)

Assessing alcohol withdrawal symptoms

You may want to use the tool below to assess the patient for alcohol withdrawal symptoms. Called the Clinical Institute Withdrawal Assessment for Alcohol (revised) (CIWA-Ar), it was developed by the Addiction Research Foundation. This assessment for monitoring withdrawal symptoms requires approximately 5 minutes to administer. The maximum score is 67. Patients scoring less than 10 usually don't need additional medication for withdrawal.

Nausea and vomiting

Ask "Do you feel sick to your stomach? Have you vomited?"

Observation:

0   no nausea and no vomiting

①   mild nausea with no vomiting

2

3

4   intermittent nausea with dry heaves

5

6

7   constant nausea, frequent dry heaves, and vomiting

Tremor

Arms extended and fingers spread apart. *Observation.*

0   no tremor

1   not visible, but can be felt fingertip to fingertip

2

3

④   moderate, with patient's arms extended

5

6

7   severe, even with arms not extended

Paroxysmal sweats

Observation:

0   no sweat visible

1   barely perceptible sweating, palms moist

2

③

4   beads of sweat obvious on forehead

5

6

7   drenching sweats

Patient: *John Krutz*

Date: *4/15/03*   Time: *1400*

Pulse or heart rate, taken for one minute: *92*

Blood pressure: *138/72*

Anxiety

Ask "Do you feel nervous?"

Observation:

0   no anxiety, at ease

1   mildly anxious

2

③

4   moderately anxious, or guarded, so anxiety is inferred

5

6

7   equivalent to acute panic states as seen in severe delirium or acute schizophrenic reactions

Agitation

Observation:

0   normal activity

1   somewhat more than normal activity

2

3

④   moderately fidgety and restless

5

6

7   paces back and forth during most of the interview or constantly thrashes about

Assessing alcohol withdrawal symptoms *(continued)*

Tactile disturbances

Ask "Have you any itching, pins and needles sensations, any burning, any numbness, or do you feel bugs crawling on or under your skin?"

Observation:

0 none

1 very mild itching, pins and needles, burning, or numbness

2 mild itching, pins and needles, burning, or numbness

③ moderate itching, pins and needles, burning, or numbness

4 moderately severe hallucinations

5 severe hallucinations

6 extremely severe hallucinations

7 continuous hallucinations

Auditory disturbances

Ask "Are you more aware of sounds around you? Are they harsh? Do they frighten you? Are you hearing anything that's disturbing to you? Are you hearing things you know aren't there?"

Observation:

0 not present

1 very mild harshness or ability to frighten

② mild harshness or ability to frighten

3 moderate harshness or ability to frighten

4 moderately severe hallucinations

5 severe hallucinations

6 extremely severe hallucinations

7 continuous hallucinations

Visual disturbances

Ask "Does the light appear to be too bright? Is its color different? Does it hurt your eyes? Are you seeing anything that's disturbing to you? Are you seeing things you know aren't there?"

Observation:

0 not present

1 very mild sensitivity

② mild sensitivity

3 moderate sensitivity

4 moderately severe hallucinations

5 severe hallucinations

6 extremely severe hallucinations

7 continuous hallucinations

Headache, fullness in head

Ask "Does your head feel different? Does it feel like there's a band around your head?" Don't rate for dizziness or light-headedness. Otherwise, rate severity.

0 not present

1 very mild

② mild

3 moderate

4 moderately severe

5 severe

6 very severe

7 extremely severe

Orientation and clouding of sensorium

Ask "What day is this? Where are you? Who am I?"

0 oriented and can do serial additions

① can't do serial additions or is uncertain about date

2 disoriented for date by no more than 2 calendar days

3 disoriented for date by more than 2 calendar days

4 disoriented for place or person

Total CIWA-Ar Score: _25_   Rater's initials: _EJ_   Maximum possible score: 67

Twelve steps to recovery

Twelve-step programs are support groups for people who live addictive lifestyles but want to make a change for the better. Members provide emotional and spiritual support to each another.

The first 12-step program, Alcoholics Anonymous (AA), was founded in 1935 and now has more than 2 million members.

Mission: Recovery

The main goal of 12-step programs is to find solutions to common problems and help others find recovery. To accomplish this goal, members share their stories, experiences, strengths, and hopes. Each new member is assigned a sponsor—someone who has "been there" and can help the newcomer recover from addiction.

Twelve-step programs bring together groups of people with the same or similar types of addictive diseases to study the principles of and steps to recovery.

A sober sponsor

Sponsorship is a key element in 12-step programs. Each new member is assigned a sponsor—a person who has achieved extended sobriety and is knowledgeable in the recovery program. The sponsor becomes the cornerstone of the new member's support system, helping him achieve and maintain a substance-free lifestyle.

The effectiveness of 12-step programs hasn't been rigorously studied. Although these programs are effective for many patients, others need additional treatment modalities. Many treatment models include 12-step meetings to augment or reinforce other approaches.

> In a 12-step program, a new member is assigned a sponsor to help him achieve a substance-free lifestyle.

Cognitive and behavioral therapies

Cognitive and behavioral therapies help the patient develop the skills they need to deal with the emotional states, social pressures, and interpersonal conflicts that may trigger a relapse of drug use. These therapies teach the patient how to make lifestyle changes, acquire healthy stress-management skills, and develop stronger social support networks. (See chapter 4, Nonpharmacologic pain management, for information about cognitive and behavioral therapies.)

Assessing the addicted patient with pain

If the patient is addicted, perform a pain assessment just as you would in another patient. Ask about the location, intensity, and quality of pain and its effects on his activities of daily living, mood, sleep, and relationships. Be sure to have him rate his pain intensity on a pain rating scale. (See chapter 2, Assessing pain.)

Sensitive subject

In addition to your pain assessment of the patient, look for behavior that raises suspicion of possible drug abuse. You may have difficulty soliciting information about the abuse of drugs. Be sure you ask him about it in a nonthreatening, nonjudgmental manner. If you suspect that the patient may use drugs, encourage him to discuss it honestly, emphasizing that drugs have profound effects that may result in serious drug interactions. If the patient admits to using an illegal drug, you should document the drug used, the amount and frequency of use, and the route of administration.

Other information to gather

In a nonjudgmental way, gather information about the patient's substance use. Find out:
• which drug or drugs he uses
• the amount he uses daily
• the administration route
• the time of last use
• his history of withdrawal symptoms
• his history of treatment for substance abuse.

An issue of trust

No data support the notion that an addicted patient reports exaggerated pain scores. Yet many people assume that anyone with addictive disease is dishonest. Caregivers may distrust an addict's report of pain and pain treatment effectiveness.

Unlike heart rate or blood pressure, pain can't be measured directly. Neither you nor the patient can prove or disprove that he's in pain, so you have to trust that he's telling the truth about his experience. Accept—and act on—his report of pain.

Remember, too, that certain outward signs, such as affect, behavior, and vital signs, may indicate pain—but that *absence* of these signs doesn't mean the patient isn't experiencing pain.

Patient-clinician relationship

If the patient is currently enrolled in a drug or alcohol treatment program, ask his permission for you to contact his counselor for information—including the medications used in his treatment plan and their current doses.

Don't withhold

If the patient is receiving methadone, LAMM, or another medication as part of his treatment program, know that it is *not* acceptable for caregivers to withhold this drug.

If a patient on naltrexone experiences pain or is expected to experience it (for example, if he's scheduled for a medical procedure that normally calls for opioids), suspend naltrexone therapy as ordered—ideally, 3 days before his anticipated need for opioids.

> Stop naltrexone therapy before the patient's anticipated need for analgesic opioids.

Managing pain in patients with addiction

Pain management for an addicted patient varies with the setting.

Inpatient management

If the patient is hospitalized, assume that he's suffering a relatively serious illness or injury and that inadequate pain management can jeopardize successful treatment for that condition. For reasons discussed earlier, the patient with addictive disease is at high risk for undertreatment of pain.

Multiple goals

A treatment plan should include a multidisciplinary team. The plan should include setting concrete and attainable goals, evaluating for psychiatric disorders, preventing withdrawal symptoms, considering tolerance when prescribing drugs, considering nonopioids or opioids with a lower abuse potential, frequently reassessing the adequacy of treatment, and recognizing drug abuse behaviors.

Stick to standards

Addicted patients should receive the same standard pain management measures—for instance, patient-controlled analgesia or epidural analgesia—when appropriate. The well-established principles of regularly scheduled (around-the-clock) analgesics and oral analgesic administration have added advantages for addicted patients.

Optimal analgesic schedule

A powerful stressor, pain can dramatically magnify drug craving. If the patient receives drugs strictly on an as-needed (PRN) basis, a significant delay may occur between his request for medication and analgesic administration. Or he may not even ask for pain medication for fear his request will be misunderstood.

During this delay, his pain may worsen. If he grows anxious and frustrated with the delay, this may create conflict between the patient and caregivers.

Stay regular

To minimize this problem, administer analgesics on a regular schedule rather than PRN whenever possible. This helps build the patient's trust and confidence in the pain management plan and can reduce his stress and drug craving.

Minimizing cues for craving

For a patient with a history of injection drug use, the hospital environment teems with cues that can trigger intense anxiety and drug craving. Needles and constrictive equipment, such as tourniquets and blood pressure cuffs, are powerful reminders of past injection use and may stimulate a strong desire to use drugs.

Cut down on cues

To reduce these cues, minimize blood withdrawals and use nonparenteral administration routes whenever possible. If exposure to needles can't be avoided, have the patient look away during the procedure or shield the equipment from his view.

Medications to avoid

Many addicted patients have overlapping medical conditions, such as cirrhosis, hepatitis, and renal complications of substance use. For this reason, avoid giving nonsteroidal anti-inflammatory drugs (NSAIDs) or acetaminophen for pain management. These drugs carry a higher risk of toxicity or adverse effects due to impaired drug metabolism or elimination.

Have the patient look away when you draw blood so the sight of the equipment won't trigger drug cravings.

Dealing with opioid tolerance

An addicted patient may have a markedly high tolerance for opioids. To achieve satisfactory pain relief, he may need analgesic doses that are several times higher than those given to nonaddicted patients.

Don't focus on doses

To determine if the analgesic regimen is appropriate, perform regular evaluations of the patient's pain level, sedation, and functional status. Use these criteria — not the number of milligrams given — to determine the effectiveness of the pain management plan.

Outpatient management

In outpatient settings, the steps outlined in inpatient management also apply. Pain management for patients with addictive disease presents unique challenges. Whereas health care providers control access to medication in inpatient settings, the outpatient setting puts medications in the patient's hands.

Taking medications as directed may pose a problem for someone whose underlying disease is characterized by compulsive drug use and lack of control. To manage this problem, the patient may need frequent outpatient follow-up. Also, smaller amounts of medication may need to be dispensed to discourage him from misusing analgesics.

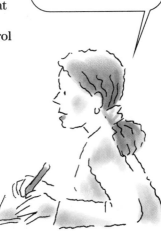

You may need to draw up a written agreement to clarify patient and provider responsibilities for analgesic use.

Sign here

If the patient's pain persists, a routine analgesic dosing schedule provides structure and may help decrease compulsive use. Having a trusted family member or friend dispense the analgesic may help as well.

If necessary, draw up a written agreement about expectations to help clarify the patient's and provider's responsibilities.

Pain and relapse

Be aware that periods of increased stress increase the risk of relapse in patients who've undergone addiction treatment. Pain is a powerful stressor. If the patient is experiencing pain, encourage him to increase his contact with his sponsor or other healthy social supports and to intensify his involvement in his treatment program.

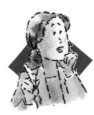

Quick quiz

1. Addiction is thought to result largely from which of the following?
    A.   Personal weakness
    B.   Moral weakness
    C.   Direct effects of the abused substance
    D.   Genetic factors

Answer: D. Addiction is a complex disease with a neurobiologic basis. Genetic makeup and environmental factors play an important role in its development. Studies of twins and adoptees who weren't raised by their biological families show similar incidences of addiction, suggesting that genetics have a powerful influence.

2. Goals of cognitive and behavioral therapy for addicted patients include all of the following *except*:
    A.   developing skills to deal with negative emotional states.
    B.   making lifestyle changes.
    C.   learning to go it alone.
    D.   developing stress management skills.

Answer: C. To overcome addiction, the patient must develop strong social support networks. One way to do this is through a 12-step recovery program, which typically assigns a sponsor to new members.

3. Which statement about opioid agonist detoxification is *false*?
    A.   It should take place in a licensed treatment program.
    B.   It starts with a high dose.
    C.   It can help the patient function normally.
    D.   It may be required for a prolonged period.

Answer: B. Methadone and other opioid agonists used for detoxification usually are given in small doses to start and then titrated upward in increments.

4. Which of the following is most likely to occur when analgesics are given on an as-needed basis to patients with addictive disease?
    A.   Conflict between the patient and staff decreases.
    B.   The patient's craving for drugs increases.
    C.   The patient loses trust in the staff.
    D.   The patient is less afraid to ask for pain medication.

Answer: C. Giving analgesics on an as-needed schedule causes delays in pain relief, which may lead the patient to distrust the staff.

Scoring

☆☆☆ If you answered all four questions correctly, great job! Your knowledge of addictive disease is a cut above!

☆☆ If you answered three questions correctly, nice job! You're well on your way to understanding what addictive disease is all about!

☆ If you answered fewer than three questions correctly, don't despair. A quick review of this chapter will put you back on the cutting edge of superior knowledge.

Lifestyle management

Just the facts

In this chapter, you'll learn:

◆ how chronic pain can affect a patient's lifestyle

◆ self-management skills that can improve the patient's functioning

◆ ways to promote positive life changes

◆ how to help the patient set appropriate goals, create new relationships, and restore joy to his life.

A look at lifestyle management

Patients with chronic pain face many challenges. The pain may interfere with nearly every aspect of life, forcing them to adjust physically, emotionally, and socially. It may prevent them from living their normal lifestyle, keeping a job, maintaining valued relationships, or even getting the medical help they need.

Chronic pain (commonly defined as pain lasting 3 or more months) is a complex phenomenon. Recently, scientists discovered genetic, anatomic, and pathophysiologic mechanisms within the nervous system that may explain chronic pain.

But until medical science produces effective treatments — or a cure — patients may be unable to fulfill their usual role functions. Forced to abandon long-held goals and dreams, many become frustrated and deeply depressed.

This chapter discusses the challenges encountered by patients with chronic pain and provides strategies to help them make positive life changes.

> The burden of chronic pain can make the patient feel that the weight of the world is on his shoulders.

Responses to pain

By its nature, pain tends to stop a person in his tracks, compelling him to take action to ease the pain. In acute pain, this response is protective—sometimes even crucial for survival. It prevents someone from trying to walk on a broken leg or ignoring a potentially life-threatening disorder.

Pain with no purpose

Unlike acute pain, chronic pain serves no useful purpose. It doesn't provide a warning or help ensure survival.

Even so, chronic pain may cause the patient to stop, or dramatically alter, his usual daily activities. This response only worsens his overall condition. Eventually, inactivity may lead to disability, social isolation, and despair so profound that the patient wonders if life is worth living.

Besides interfering with work, home, and recreational activities, chronic pain may severely limit any activity that requires sitting, standing, driving, or walking. It can turn even the simplest daily chore into a near-impossible task.

Ripple effects

The stress response to pain, combined with inactivity and medication effects, may cause secondary problems ranging from insomnia, obesity, and constipation to hypertension and depression. Social isolation and self-doubt may contribute to these problems.

In most cases, though, these effects can be minimized by increasing the patient's self-management skills, helping him make life changes, improving his role functioning, and enhancing his communication skills.

Self-management skills

Developing self-management and self-efficacy skills can dramatically improve the patient's functional and coping abilities. *Self-efficacy* refers to a person's estimate or personal judgment of his own ability to succeed in reaching a specific goal.

Studies suggest that for a patient with chronic pain, self-doubts about one's ability to manage pain, cope with pain, and function contribute to depression and disability. As the patient gains skills in these areas, he may find his pain decreases and he's able to increase his activity level. These gains can help restore some of the joy and hope he might have lost.

Building self-efficacy

Think of self-efficacy skills as tools in the patient's toolbox. Too often, caregivers offer only passive forms of therapy, such as taking medication or submitting to medical procedures.

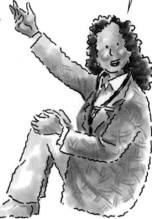

Taking medication is a passive form of therapy that doesn't require self-efficacy.

Pill-taking skill

In many cases, taking medication is the only skill that the patient is asked to master. His toolbox contains just one tool—the skill of taking pills.

But many patients with chronic pain feel they've already overused this tool and grow even more frustrated if nothing else is offered. To make matters worse (and perhaps set the stage for conflict), prescribers may deny or limit their access to medication. In essence, they're taking away the patient's only tool.

Passive treatments, such as pill-taking, reinforce the notion that the patient is powerless to deal with pain. It's no wonder that he may develop feelings of helplessness and self-doubt—feelings almost certain to lead to further disability and depression.

More tools for the box

To help the patient overcome learned helplessness and self-doubts, teach active self-management techniques—skills he can master and initiate himself.

Ways to enhance the patient's self-efficacy include:
• promoting skill mastery, such as pain management and coping skills
• persuading him to do things on his own behalf
• teaching him about his condition
• helping him reinterpret pain sensations
• encouraging him to connect with others with chronic pain who are coping well.

Promoting skill development

Skill development can be taught on an individual basis or as part of an integrated cognitive-behavioral education program. Core skills useful to the patient with chronic pain include:
• keeping a pain diary
• pacing activities
• mastering relaxation techniques
• using imagery
• using hypnosis
• restructuring thoughts
• communicating effectively.

Building my skills will help me cope with chronic pain.

I CAN COPE

I CAN DO BETTER

IT'S NOT THE END OF THE WORLD

I CAN GET THROUGH THIS

Self-exploration activities — engaging in activities, such as drawing self-portraits and setting personal goals — also can help. Even if these activities don't directly control pain, they can add to the insight and motivation the patient needs to improve his quality of life.

Keeping a pain diary

By keeping a diary that documents pain from day to day, the patient can observe his pain more closely, identify subtle changes in its nature, and evaluate the effectiveness of pain-relief interventions. As the patient reviews his diary entries, he can gain insight into the intricacies of his pain and response patterns.

Dear Diary

Advise the patient to make three daily entries in his pain diary, at the same times every day. Entries should include:

- the date and time
- the situation
- a self-rating of pain intensity on a scale of 0 to 10, where 0 represents no pain and 10 represents the worst possible pain
- a description of the physical characteristics of the pain
- a self-rating of emotional distress on a scale of 0 to 10
- the patient's response to pain or emotional distress. (See *A personal record of pain.*)

Pain watch

After a few weeks of keeping a pain diary and evaluating it regularly, the patient should begin to notice the relationship between his pain and:

- factors he can control such as activities that ease or worsen his pain
- factors outside his control such as the weather
- factors he might be able to control, such as irrational thought patterns, if he gained the skills.

Writer's block

Many patients struggle with writing diary entries. Perhaps they can't get past the natural response of denial and see the pain as their own responsibility rather than others'. Some simply wish to ignore the unpleasant topic of pain, trying instead to "push through" the pain and concentrate on other things.

Win the battle; lose the war

If the patient would rather "push through" pain than write about it, point out that this choice may help him win the battle against pain by getting through the day. But after fighting pain

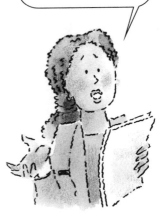

It won't read like Mother Goose's Nursery Rhymes, but a pain diary can help the patient identify pain patterns.

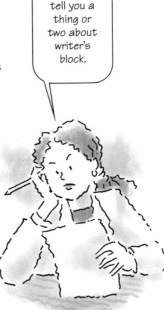

I can tell you a thing or two about writer's block.

Rein in the pain

A personal record of pain

A pain diary can help the patient self-manage chronic pain by shedding light on his pain and response patterns. Here's a sample pain diary entry:

> 3/25/03 8:00 a.m.
>
> Situation: Just finished breakfast.
>
> Description of pain: Experiencing burning pain in left shoulder. Pain rates a 5 on a scale of 0 to 10.
>
> Description of emotional distress: 6. I'm frustrated that I'm still having this much pain in my shoulder.
>
> Patient response: I took an additional pain pill and wrote for 10 minutes about my frustration.

A patient who tries to win the battle against pain could end up losing the war.

for hours, he may collapse from the energy drain — and his pain may get even worse. Ultimately, he could lose the war with pain.

Pacing activities

Pacing activities wisely can help the patient reduce pain and prevent exacerbations. Principles of pacing include:
• working smarter, not harder
• managing time effectively
• alternating pain-producing and pain-relieving activities
• using adaptive devices, such as reachers and over-sized eating utensils
• asking for and accepting help when needed. (See *Pacing for less pain*, page 308.)

Relaxation techniques

Chronic pain and its impact clearly qualify as stressors — conditions that trigger the stress response. The stress response causes

Rein in the pain

Pacing for less pain

Proper pacing of activities can go a long way toward easing a patient's pain or preventing flare-ups. Here's an example.

Dishwashing dilemma

Maribeth found that washing dishes increased her pain. In fact, she had to lay down for several hours afterward to recover.

Seeking a solution, the nurse advised her to analyze each stage of the activity to find out if she could link particular movements to increased pain. The analysis revealed that the most painful movements were carrying heavy pots to the sink, standing for more than 2 minutes at a time, and bending over to place dishes in the dishwasher.

Discoveries galore

Armed with this knowledge, the nurse helped Maribeth explore possible solutions. During this troubleshooting exercise, they found that:
• she could carry pots weighing less than 5 lb (2.3 kg) without increased pain
• if she rested one foot on a stepstool, she could stand for 10 minutes at a time before her pain worsened
• she experienced less pain if she crouched rather than bent over when placing dishes in the dishwasher.

Play-by-play ratings

Maribeth then rated her pain intensity during each segment of dishwashing. She discovered that if she sat down and rested for 5 minutes when her pain intensity rating increased to 7 (on a scale of 0 to 10), her pain intensity quickly dropped to her baseline rating of 5. But if she waited until her pain reached an intensity of 8 before sitting down, she needed more time to recuperate.

Pots, pans, and pacing

With the nurse's help, Maribeth used the principles of pacing to adapt to dishwashing.
• She switched from iron pots and pans to lighter-weight aluminum versions.
• She emptied the contents of pots before moving them and carried no more than four dishes at a time.
• She used adaptive equipment (obtained from an occupational therapist) to move items from the countertop to the lower rack of the dishwasher without bending.
• She set a timer for 10 minutes when starting to wash dishes. When the timer went off, she sat down for at least 5 minutes before returning to the task.
• Whenever possible, she delegated the task of loading and unloading the dishwasher to family members.

automatic body reactions, including increases in blood pressure, heart rate, and respiratory rate.

The patient with chronic pain commonly displays signs of acute and chronic stress and may attribute stress-related problems to his chronic pain. In fact, stress can impair physical, cognitive, and emotional functioning and rob the patient of the resources needed to cope.

Relaxation response

By practicing relaxation techniques, the patient can learn to achieve the *relaxation response*—a protective mechanism that helps to offset some of the negative physiologic effects of stress.

Beyond relaxing

Inform the patient that meditation and certain other techniques activate the relaxation response. (See chapter 4, Nonpharmacologic pain management.) Point out, however, that the relaxation response isn't just a matter of relaxing. It requires a focused mind and a passive attitude.

Ideally, the patient should use the chosen relaxation technique for 20 to 30 minutes in quiet, comfortable surroundings. Tell him he'll need to practice the technique daily for at least a month before he masters it. If appropriate, provide an audiotaped guide as a learning tool.

Bumps on Relaxation Road

The patient may need guidance and assistance to incorporate relaxation techniques into his daily routine. Although these techniques rarely cause discomfort directly, he may notice pain or other discomforts during practice until he has mastered the skill.

Some patients fall asleep when practicing relaxation techniques—perhaps because they're sleep deprived. A few have trouble eliciting the relaxation response because of intrusive memories of frightening past experiences. To overcome these obstacles, they may need guidance from a trained professional. As necessary, provide appropriate referrals.

Imagery

Using an imagery technique may help the patient alter his perception of pain. Imagery allows even the patient with severely limited mobility to visit his favorite places mentally without leaving home.

To start, the patient learns how to perform *pleasant* imagery techniques (such as picturing himself in a pleasant situation) to promote feelings of safety.

After he gains this basic skill, he may benefit from practicing *guided* imagery. In this technique, he learns to create pain-related images that he progressively alters in positive ways.

Taming the spikes and bolts

Imagine, for instance, that a patient visualizes his pain as a large steel ball with spikes that discharge lightning bolts. Using guided imagery, he can change that frightening image in various ways— by turning off the power source for the electricity, filing down the

> Meditation doesn't require incense and New Age music. A quiet, comfortable corner will do.

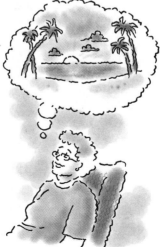

spikes, coating the ball with rubber, or shrinking it. These changes may allow him to perceive his pain as smaller, duller, and less intense.

Also, the image of turning off the power source and coating the ball may bring temporary relief from the electrical, shooting component of pain—the aspect of pain some patients find most bothersome.

Hypnosis

Hypnosis also helps the patient change his perception of pain. The first step in hypnosis is to achieve a state of deep relaxation. Next, the hypnotist makes suggestions designed to alter the patient's sensory and affective experience of pain. These suggestions may focus on:

• blocking the pain such as by having the patient picture a state of anesthesia
• making the pain less bothersome such as by telling the patient to feel the pain as a pleasant numbness.

Then the hypnotist turns the patient's attention away from the pain, makes posthypnotic suggestions to help him cope with the pain, and guides him back to an alert, refreshed state.

With adequate training, many patients can learn to hypnotize themselves. Hypnosis then becomes another tool in their toolbox of self-initiated skills.

Mindfulness techniques

If even simple movements or basic body positions cause pain, the patient may cut back severely on his activities. Some patients, however, go to the opposite extreme, ignoring the pain and overexerting themselves.

To help the patient find a happy medium between avoiding activity and overdoing it, teach him to be mindful of physical sensations and to avoid labeling all physical sensations as pain.

Name that sensation

A technique called labeling sensations involves guiding the patient through active range-of-motion exercises while he describes and analyzes his physical sensations.

To start, the patient is held in certain positions against gravity and asked to move a particular body part to a comfortable position. Then he's

Intrepreting pain descriptions

Sensations of burning, stabbing, or shooting pain may deter a patient from engaging in exercise or other activities. Yet these sensations don't necessarily mean that harm is being done. Point out that they may be errant signals from previously damaged nerves—not signs that the activity is causing further damage.

Painful clothing?

In allodynia, for instance, ordinarily painless stimuli evoke pain. The patient may experience pain flare-ups just from clothes rubbing against his skin—but mistakenly attribute the flare-ups to the activity he was doing at the time. Instead of stopping the activity, he'd be better off increasing it.

asked to verbalize the sensations he experiences—without using the word "pain."

The practitioner listens for such words as "sharp," "shooting," "catching," and "stabbing." These descriptions suggest that a particular movement is causing nerve impingement and thus should be modified or limited.

On the other hand, such words as "warmth," "tightness," "aching," and "throbbing" suggest muscle fatigue, which may result from muscle weakness. (See *Interpreting pain descriptions.*)

Next, the patient is asked to list five activities that normally increase his pain and five things he does in response.

Pain watch

Mindfulness techniques emphasize the value of paying attention to changes in pain triggered by particular movements or activities. Advise the patient to make a written note any time a movement or activity increases his pain. Tell him to document the character and intensity of his pain before he started the activity and then frequently during the activity.

Then, as appropriate, teach him how to modify activities to prevent pain exacerbations. For example, advise him to change activities if his pain intensity increases by more than one or two points.

Dealing with pain flare-ups and relapses

Chronic pain may occur in phases, with times of relative stability alternating with minor exacerbations and major flare-ups. For some patients, these fluctuations make it especially hard to sustain positive lifestyle changes.

Pain exacerbations and flare-ups can occur even if the patient does everything right. To help the patient cope with them, review the typical patterns of his pain and evaluate his skill in dealing with them.

Technique boutique

Next, hold a brainstorming session with the patient to come up with techniques he can use to:

- prevent pain exacerbations
- manage mild exacerbations to prevent major pain flare-ups
- deal with major flare-ups.

Then help the patient evaluate the ideas that emerge during the session, eliminating those that aren't practical and suggesting that he try those that seem worthwhile. Advise him to list the worthwhile techniques in writing and to keep the list available so he can refer to it whenever he feels hopeless in dealing with escalating pain.

I'm having more than just a mild exacerbation. I'm having a major flare-up! @#*!

Cognitive restructuring

Self-efficacy skills can go a long way in helping a patient cope with chronic pain. But when used alone, they're not enough. The patient also needs to learn ways to improve his mental health.

Thoughts can have a profound effect on mood and physical states, including the perception of pain. In patients with chronic pain, certain thought patterns — learned helplessness, catastrophic thinking, and self-doubts — are associated with high pain levels and may contribute to disability and depression.

Rethink that thought

Through a technique called cognitive restructuring, which originated in cognitive therapy, the patient can learn to change his thought patterns and content. Cognitive restructuring helps the patient identify irrational, negative beliefs and replace them with rational, truthful statements.

Cognitive restructuring can help the patient with chronic pain learn to:

- interpret pain signals in a less threatening way
- take a more active role in self-managing pain
- see the value of adopting healthier lifestyle practices
- remove self-doubts that are preventing him from participating in activities.

A penny for your thoughts

In cognitive restructuring, the goal is to make the patient aware of the content of his thoughts ("self-talk"). He learns to trace nega-

The right time to challenge

You can promote cognitive restructuring by challenging certain statements the patient makes about his pain. Consider challenging him, for example, when he expresses:

- half-truths about his chronic pain
- self-defeating thoughts
- exaggerated or catastrophic thinking
- pessimistic, hopeless, or helpless thoughts
- blame for a single person or event
- self-pitying thoughts ("Why me?!")
- "if only" thoughts ("Things could be the same as they were before my pain began, if only...").

tive thoughts to unpleasant physical and emotional feelings and undesirable behavioral responses to pain.

Techniques used to attain this skill include keeping a journal and paying attention to automatic thoughts and self-talk. Once the patient identifies his automatic thoughts and self-talk, a trained counselor challenges the truthfulness and helpfulness of negative ideas and asks him to restate them in more truthful and helpful terms.

Q & A

During this self-discovery process, the patient must repeatedly ask himself such questions as:

- What am I thinking?
- What do I need?
- What do I want?
- What can I do?

Validate or challenge?

To aid the patient with cognitive restructuring, provide support and encouragement while validating or challenging (as appropriate) statements he makes regarding his pain.

For instance, validate such statements as:

- "My pain is real. It isn't in my head. I'm not making it up."
- "I'm not responsible *for* my pain, but I am responsible *to* it."
- "I can cope. I may not want to, but I can."
- "I did the best I could at the time. What have I learned that may help me do better in the future?"

On the other hand, challenge the patient when he engages in negative mental habits. such as mind-reading ("They think I...") or

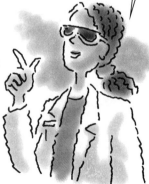

Cognitive restructuring helps the patient replace negative ideas with more truthful ones. Pretty cool, huh?

fortune telling (predicting dire events that may never happen). (See *The right time to challenge*, page 313.)

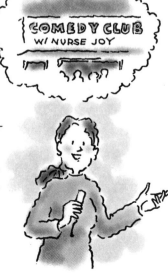

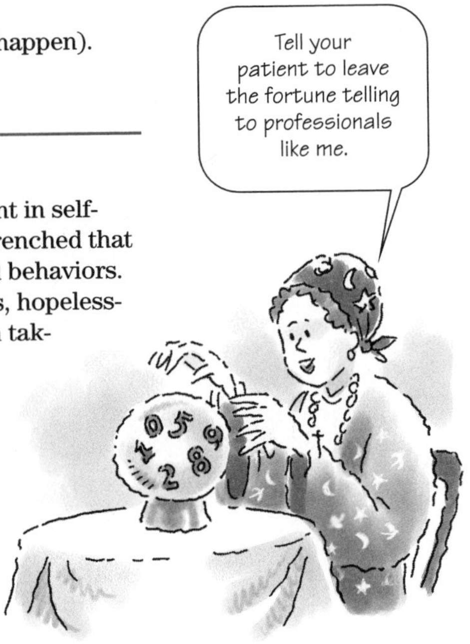

Tell your patient to leave the fortune telling to professionals like me.

Adopting a healthier attitude

Adopting a healthier attitude is another crucial element in self-management. Certain thought patterns may be so entrenched that they become a part of one's personality, thoughts, and behaviors. Distressing attitudes, such as pessimism, helplessness, hopelessness, and worthlessness, can prevent the patient from taking steps toward improving the quality of his life.

Hope mongering

To help turn a negative attitude around, have the patient identify his good qualities. Urge him to develop an interest in pursuits he's capable of doing despite his pain.

Try to instill hope, using humor as appropriate. Encourage him to get involved in altruistic endeavors, such as helping others, to take his mind off himself and improve his outlook.

Pursuing healthy pleasures

More than 2,000 years ago, Aristotle observed that pain is an emotional state. Emotions were viewed as points on a continuum, with ecstasy and pleasure on one end and pain and suffering on the other. People with chronic pain were seen as incapable of experiencing pleasure.

Sad spiral

Even today, many patients with chronic pain share that antiquated view. As a result, they may find themselves sliding down a spiral of despair:
• Pain causes the patient to discontinue meaningful or pleasurable activities.
• As a result, he becomes less active, more disabled, more socially isolated, and even more depressed.
• These changes further erode the quality of his life.

To help offset negative feelings and attitudes, encourage your patient to seek pleasure in healthy ways whenever possible. (See *Chasing beauty*.)

Chasing beauty

Chronic pain can strip all the pleasure from life. If the patient seems miserable, encourage him to balance the negativity by actively pursuing pleasure, seeking beauty in the environment, and creating opportunities to be with loved ones.

At every encounter, ask him what enjoyable things he has done since you last saw him or what experience of joy, beauty, or satisfaction has he had recently.

Happiness prescription

If necessary, consider writing the patient a "prescription" for the pursuit of happiness, to be taken Q.D. and PRN. This will remind him that he can choose to add enjoyment to his life.

Improving communication skills

The patient with chronic pain commonly finds himself in tenuous, conflict-filled relationships with the people he depends on — doctors and other health care workers, family members, friends, coworkers, or employers. For healthier relationships, he must gain skills in effective communication — the basic building block of relationships.

Communicating well requires clarity, assertiveness, and the ability to consider the other person's viewpoint. To communicate clearly, the patient must be consciously aware of how he feels and what he wants or needs from the other person. He must express himself assertively and listen closely to others' responses.

Role-playing, rephrasing

If necessary, role-play with the patient to help him rephrase his statements so they more clearly express his thoughts and feelings. If, for instance, he's seeking understanding, analysis, advice, or reassurance, help him analyze his statements to determine if they're phrased in a way that's likely to achieve these goals. Also guide his attempts to express himself in an assertive — but not aggressive — manner.

Let's pretend that I'm your wife. How would you describe your pain to me?

Practicing wellness behaviors

If chronic pain limits the patient's mobility, he's at risk for weight gain, excessive stress, and various chronic ailments. For instance, he may develop painful muscle spasms or contractures, headaches, pathologic bone fractures, poor healing, high blood pressure, and heart disease.

Chronic pain exacts a high psychological toll as well. The patient may develop anxiety disorders (such as panic attacks or post-traumatic stress disorder), mood disorders (such as depression), and even suicidal ideation.

Being "responsible to pain"

To help compensate for this vulnerability, the patient must adopt wellness behaviors and healthy lifestyle patterns. Explain to him that he's *responsible to his pain*. This means he must initiate steps that help manage his pain and reduce his risk of long-term complications.

Point out that—like a diabetic patient who must self-manage his diabetes—a patient with chronic pain must control his diet, exercise regularly, monitor the severity of his condition (such as by keeping a pain diary), and take medications as directed.

Getting regular exercise

Regular exercise is vital in achieving and maintaining good health. Research shows that people should do at least 30 minutes of moderate physical activity most days of the week.

Stretch and strengthen

Encourage a patient with chronic pain to do stretching, strengthening, and stamina-building exercises most days of the week, as tolerated. Strengthening exercises help prevent loss of muscle mass (a key factor in weight gain). Weight-bearing exercises help prevent bone density loss. (See *Exercise guidelines.*)

Overcoming barriers to exercise

Some patients with chronic pain resist exercise, believing it will hurt them and worsen their pain. Others simply have difficulty overcoming a sedentary lifestyle.

Exercise phobia

Fear that exercise will hurt and make the pain worse may lead to a pattern of learned helplessness, which has been linked to lower

Hey, let's do this for at least 30 minutes 5 days a week.

Exercise guidelines

The patient with chronic pain should do stretching, strengthening, and stamina-building exercises every day, if possible.

Stretching exercises

Experts recommend performing range-of-motion (ROM) exercises to all muscle groups every day. Of course, the patient may need to limit some movements to prevent harm. Besides ROM exercises, other options for stretching movements include physical therapy, yoga, and tai chi.

Strengthening exercises

Strengthening exercises may involve weight work (using body weight against gravity, to start) or pool-based exercises. Pool-based exercises are particularly well tolerated. Many patients with chronic pain feel good in a pool because of the warm, buoyant water.

However, they may not realize that water is heavy — it weighs 8 lb per gallon. Even simple movements in a pool can really work the mus-

cles. Someone who's deconditioned can easily overdo pool-based exercises, suffering muscle stiffness and soreness for hours or even days afterward.

To promote long-term success, advise the patient to start with 5 minutes of strengthening exercises and then increase by 1 to 2 minutes per session every week.

Stamina-building exercises

Give similar instructions about stamina-building exercises: Start with low amounts and progress slowly, using the patient's current activity level as a baseline. For example, if the patient's only exercise is walking 1 minute to his mailbox, encourage him to walk 2 minutes a day during the next week and then to increase walking by 1 additional minute a day each week thereafter.

---

endorphin levels and depression in a patient with chronic pain. As appropriate, challenge the patient's notion of the types and amounts of exercise he's capable of doing. Encourage him to increase his activity level as appropriate. However, be sure to review precautions he should take to prevent exercise-induced harm.

Sedentary lifestyle

If the patient is sedentary, remind him of the principle of inertia and momentum — bodies at rest tend to stay at rest, whereas bodies in motion tend to stay in motion.

The "use it or lose it" principle may apply as well. Tell the patient that if he doesn't use his ability to, say, walk a mile, he may eventually lose his ability to walk altogether.

Eating a healthy diet

Dietary recommendations for the patient with chronic pain fall into three main categories:
• adhering to principles of good nutrition

Painful links to food

Some patients with chronic pain report that high-sodium foods and food additives, such as aspartame and monosodium glutamate, can trigger their pain. For others, drinking caffeine or alcohol makes pain worse.

If you suspect that the patient's pain is linked to certain foods, advise him to note whether pain onset seems to follow ingestion of these foods. As necessary, instruct him to gradually eliminate pain-causing foods from his diet.

A patient with chronic pain should use me as a guide to choosing foods.

• using effective weight-loss strategies, as needed
• avoiding dietary supplements that may interact negatively with their disease state or medications.

Principles of good nutrition
Review such nutritional principles as:
• using the food pyramid to select foods and plan meals
• preparing and preserving foods for optimal nutritional value
• avoiding alternating cycles of meal-skipping and overeating.

Trigger control

If the patient has a condition with a specific pain trigger (such as migraine, rheumatoid arthritis, or interstitial cystitis), review these triggers with him. If he has Crohn's disease, pancreatitis, or a cachexia-causing disorder, teach him how to maintain good nutrition without exacerbating his pain. (See *Painful links to food.*)

Effective weight-loss strategies
If the patient must lose weight, refer him to a dietitian, who can develop an individualized diet plan.

Using supplements wisely
As appropriate, review the uses and recommended dosages of dietary supplements, such as daily multivitamins and minerals. If the patient has arthritis, he may want to learn about glucosamine, a supplement that may reduce arthritic pain.

However, point out that some supplements such as St. John's wort can interact with prescribed medications. Also mention that dietary supplements aren't regulated, so product quality and purity may be a problem.

Steer your patient away from dietary supplements that can interact with us.

Creating life changes

Many chronic pain sufferers have exhausted all medical treatments. Neither surgery nor other invasive procedures nor medications bring adequate pain relief.

The next step may be a referral to a psychiatrist or psychologist. However, these professionals commonly convey the notion that the problem is all in the patient's head.

Of sane mind?

Not surprisingly, the patient may end up questioning his sanity. He may feel trapped by circumstance, hopeless and helpless to do anything on his own. If friends or family members also express skepticism — such as implying that he's exaggerating his discomfort to gain sympathy or favors — only adds salt to the wound.

Owning pain

To reconstruct a fulfilling life demands creativity and fortitude. As a first step, the patient must take ownership of the pain. He must acknowledge that although he can't control the pain itself, he *can* control his response to it — and this can improve his quality of life.

Little c, big C

We all face countless choices every day — what to wear, what to eat for lunch, whether to look for a new job, or how much money to invest in the stock market.

A patient with chronic pain may feel overwhelmed when faced with choices — even trivial ones. To help him cope with decision-making, teach him to distinguish the "little c" choices from the "big C" choices.

• "Little c" choices are those that require little thought and have few, if any, consequences — for example, what to wear.

• "Big C" choices demand more thought and can have major long-term consequences. They include such issues as where to live and whether to quit (or return to) work.

Helping the patient explore his options can empower him to make necessary changes — especially the "big C" changes that can improve his life. Teaching him decision-making skills will also make him accountable for the consequences of refusing to make changes.

Help your patient explore his options when faced with major choices.

Grief and acceptance

Frustrated by multiple referrals and treatment failures, many chronic pain sufferers find themselves doing things that don't help their pain—all the while missing opportunities for more satisfying and productive functioning. As their attempts to control pain grow stronger and bolder, their frustration will increase if their pain persists.

Grieving over losses, and ultimately accepting them, can help the patient break this cycle. Research shows that the patient who accepts pain as part of his life is less distraught and functions better than one who persists in unproductive attempts to control pain.

Pie chart approach

To help the patient conceptualize and accept pain-related changes in his life, instruct him to draw a circle and then divide it into sections, like slices in a pie.

Next, have him assign each slice to a major area of his life—such as work, self-care, exercise, hobbies, and family time. The size of each slice should represent how much time he devoted to that area before his pain problem arose.

Slices of life

Next, have him darken the "slices of life" that have been affected by pain. Tell him to partially darken the slices (areas of life) where he has had to cut back and to totally darken the areas he has had to eliminate completely. For example, if he's able to work part-time, he should color 50% of the work slice. If he's unable to work at all, he should blacken the work slice.

Reclamation plan

After the patient completes the pie chart, review it with him. What does it say about pain's impact on his life? How would he change it if he could? If he's like many patients, he'd choose to reclaim lost portions of his life.

Without discouraging him from trying to regain what he's lost, point out another path: Rather than spend time and energy trying to get back what he's lost, he can grieve over and accept his losses, cherish his memories, and grow into new interests and activities.

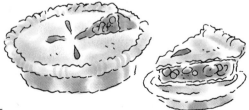

Life after hiking

Here's an example. Suppose the patient is an avid hiker—until a car accident leaves her with persistent pain and left-sided weakness. Even after she recovers from the accident, she's unable to hike.

She then grows deeply depressed. Every time she thinks of the mountains or hears someone talk about hiking, she becomes angry about her accident and despondent over her disability. She can't even bear to look at photographs taken on previous hikes.

Good grief

To help her grieve for her losses, you guide her through the pie chart exercise. With its stark black slices, her chart shows her exactly how much she has lost by being unable to hike.

She realizes she has lost not just her main hobby, but her major stimulus for staying in shape and her connection with nature and long-time friends. For the first time, she's able to understand the magnitude of her losses and grieve for them.

When whitening won't work

When you ask her what she would change about her pie chart if she could, she says she'd find a way to whiten the hiking slice. Yet she knows that isn't possible.

You point out that although she may never be able to hike again, there are other ways she can express her reverence for the mountains and stay connected with nature and friends. For instance, she can invite her former hiking partners to her house for monthly gatherings, organize albums of hiking photos, take scenic drives in the mountains, and write about her hiking experiences.

Out of the ashes...

After this exercise, the patient is finally able to look at photographs taken on previous hikes and discuss her hiking accomplishments with others. Grieving for her losses has allowed her to make choices about the future instead of doing nothing and continuing to feel miserable.

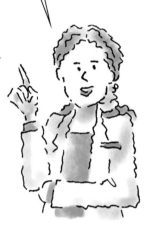

Point out that regaining what he's lost isn't the patient's only option. Accepting his losses might serve him better.

Changing the environment

For some patients with chronic pain, the external or internal living environment adds significant physical, emotional, and social stressors. For instance, stormy weather exacerbates pain in some patients. For others, maintaining a large house is physically exhausting.

Climate control

To escape pain-exacerbating weather, some patients may decide to move to a different climate. For those who can no longer keep up a large house, moving to a smaller space or into an assisted living facility can reduce stressors.

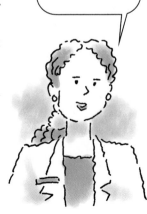

Looking at old photographs can help the patient grieve over and accept her losses.

Obviously, decisions about whether and where to move are "big C" choices with major consequences. Yet some people never even consider changing their living environment as an option.

If appropriate, broach this topic with the patient. Help him analyze his current needs and capabilities in light of the anticipated progress of his health problems.

Right place, right time

For instance, if death is imminent (expected within 6 months), suggest moving into a hospice. On the other hand, if the patient's likely to remain independent in daily activities for the foreseeable future, help him research assisted living facilities. If he's fully independent, suggest condominium living as a way to reduce the burdens of home maintenance, yard work, and costly upkeep.

Mood boosters

Of course, many patients whose pain is affected by climate can't (or won't) move to a more amenable region. In this case, encourage the patient to consider measures that may improve his psychological state.

The pampered patient

Say, for instance, a patient with fibromyalgia experiences pain flare-ups when the barometric pressure drops. To improve her mood on those days, advise her to pamper herself — say, by taking an especially long, hot bath that morning or doing an extra relaxation technique that day. Although these things won't change the weather or prevent pain flare-ups, they could give her a psychological lift and make the day less dreary.

Improving the home setting

Changes in the current home setting can help as well. For a wheelchair-bound patient, adding ramps and arranging the living space on one level of the home can make a big difference.

Reducing clutter and moving furniture can improve the traffic flow through the house and prevent injuries. Advise the patient to place chairs, stools, stepstools, and other furnishings where they're convenient and easy to use.

Less wash-day drama

Appliance location, style, and height also are important considerations. Having a laundry room on the same level as the bedroom eliminates the need to carry heavy loads up and down the stairs. Here are some other points the patient should consider:

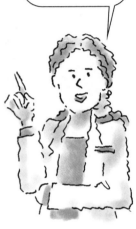

Moving to a smaller, more manageable space can reduce stress in a patient with chronic pain.

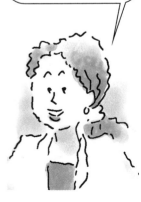

Suggest that a wheelchair-bound patient add ramps and rearrange his living space.

- A front-loading washer is easier to load and unload than a top-loading model.
- Putting the washer and dryer up on blocks minimizes the amount of bending required on laundry days.
- Having a convenient surface on which to fold clothes while sitting can help if the patient's pain increases when standing.

Making workplace changes

Roughly 30% to 50% of Americans suffer from chronically painful conditions. About 50 million of them experience pain-related disability.

Chronic pain accounts for nearly one-half million lost workdays in the United States, with more than $100 billion spent annually on health care, disability payments, and related costs. What's more, despite modified work and work-hardening programs introduced over the past few decades, return-to-work and full-duty capacity rates haven't improved appreciably.

Evaluating the options

Some patients with chronic pain try their best to maintain (or return to) full-duty work. Unfortunately, many find that the cycles of work and recovery from work become the focus of their lives, pushing out other interests. Others patients decide not to return to work for physical, mental, or social reasons.

Ad-reading advice

Whether your patient must change jobs because of chronic pain, wishes to keep his current job, or wants to return to work despite his condition, he needs help in evaluating his options.

To start, guide him in taking stock of his physical capacities, interests, marketable skills, and professional network. Encourage him to keep an open mind when reading the help wanted ads — and not to automatically assume he doesn't meet job requirements.

If the patient must make a career change, point out that he may need to regard this as a long-term goal, especially if it requires a special academic degree or a new skills set.

If he's unemployed but wants to return to work, point out alternatives to working full-time. For instance, he could look for part-time or volunteer work, with hopes of resuming full-time employment if workplace accommodations are satisfactory and his physical condition allows.

> Encourage your patient to keep an open mind when reading the Help Wanted ads.

Light vs. heavy duty

The nature of a job can affect a patient's decision to keep working, quit working, or change jobs. For a patient with chronic pain, jobs that require heavy labor are out of the question, whereas desk jobs or managerial or administrative positions may be feasible options.

Yet someone with light-duty work may be more likely to push himself beyond his capabilities in response to pressures from supervisors or coworkers—or his own guilt feelings. If you suspect your patient is pushing himself too far, discuss this with him.

> Jobs involving heavy labor may be out of the question for a patient with chronic pain.

Workers' compensation and disability claims

Studies show that such factors as anger, depression, self-doubt, and sociocultural issues (for instance, access to specific medical services) contribute to the number of people claiming to be disabled by pain.

However, if the patient is considering filing for workers' compensation or Social Security disability, point out that these systems are complex legal structures that don't always provide the services that chronic pain sufferers need. (See *Pursuing a disability claim.*)

Pursuing a disability claim

If the patient can't or won't return to work, point out that pursuing a Social Security disability claim can be problematic. Proving disability related to a pain problem may entail up to a 5-year legal battle, and the odds of winning are only about 50%. Ironically, some of the winners live to regret the confines of the "permanent, total disability" status they've been awarded.

Part-time work

If the patient already gets disability income, make sure he knows all the facts before taking a part-time job. Inform him that some people with disability income can lose their indemnities if they work even part-time. In other words, they're sacrificing $1,000 or so per month for a job that may pay as little as $200 per month.

Setting appropriate goals

Patients with chronic pain may be so focused on finding pain relief that they neglect other concerns. They may put long-term goals on hold or hang onto goals they had before pain onset — which are now unrealistic. Many grow discouraged, thinking their pain makes any effort futile.

But helping the patient set short-term and mid-range goals can motivate him to take steps on his behalf and set the stage for accomplishments he can be proud of.

Goal criteria

When helping the patient set goals, inform him that a goal should meet all of these criteria:
- objective (behavioral)
- measurable
- realistic
- desirable
- "I"-centered.

Goal honing

If the patient chooses a nebulous goal, such as "I will have less pain," point out that this goal doesn't meet the criteria. Help him define exactly what "less pain" means to him, and work with him to build his new goal around that.

Then ask him to choose a pain intensity rating (objective and measurable) that would let him comfortably perform activities of daily living (realistic and desirable). Finally, make sure the goal is something he can accomplish on his own ("I"-centered).

Thus, the patient's new goal might be: "I will get 30 minutes of exercise every day and comply with my medication regimen so my pain doesn't exceed an intensity rating of 4."

> Help your patient develop an action plan that addresses obstacles to reaching his goals.

and... action

Act against obstacles

After the patient has established appropriate goals, help him identify physical, cognitive, emotional, or social factors that might prevent him from achieving these goals. Then help him develop an action plan that addresses the obstacles.

Creating new relationships

Creating new relationships can be crucial for patients with chronic pain. For many, breathing new life into relationships or finding a new partner or friend helps them transcend the limits imposed by pain and create even better lives than they had before.

Relationships that may need work include those with intimate partners, family members, friends, coworkers, and even casual acquaintances. The patient also may need to evaluate his relationship with himself, his spirituality, and the meaning of life to create a new and more fulfilling life.

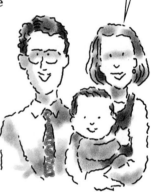

My husband is going to try to work on relationships with us, his coworkers, and others.

Enhancing intimacy

Intimate relationships may suffer from a partner's well-intentioned attempts to help. Instead of relying on others to do things for them, patients with chronic pain need to find activities they can do independently.

A cascade of concern

If the partner is overly solicitous, the patient may become even more inactive and dependent, and the relationship may become strained.

If you suspect this is the patient's situation, encourage his partner to find the right balance between staying supportive but not promoting dependence or reinforcing excessive disability. At the same time, urge the patient to delegate only those activities and responsibilities he finds really difficult. (See *Promoting intimacy.*)

Links between chronic pain and abuse

Although intimate relationships commonly need rebuilding, in some cases abandoning them may be a better choice. Research shows a strong link between chronic pain and a history of abuse. Chronic headaches, myofascial pain, and low back pain have been linked to abusive relationships.

According to some studies, as many as half of women with chronic pelvic or abdominal pain have been sexually abused. This supports the need to take a careful history about abusive relationships when assessing patients with chronic pain.

Promoting intimacy

Intimate relationships commonly benefit from adjustments in the sexual realm. A patient's painful condition or pain medications may impair his libido and sexual responsiveness. He may worry that he's unable to satisfy his partner sexually. Meanwhile, the partner's main concern may be to avoid exacerbating the patient's pain.

Solutions for sex
To help restore a mutually satisfying relationship, investigate those issues with the patient and his partner, as appropriate. To help them deal with physical and emotional obstacles and explore feasible solutions, follow these guidelines:
• Mention that pain-relieving endorphins are produced and released during orgasm.
• Suggest that the couple time their sexual activity to coincide with the peak effect of pain medications.
• Urge the couple to explore various sexual positions to find those that are best tolerated. Also suggest that they explore different ways of expressing sexuality.
• If the patient is on antidepressants or opioids (which can affect sexual functioning), recommend that he take the dose after, rather than before, sexual activity.

Finding peer support

Relying solely on family members and friends for support can be problematic because they may be unable to provide pain-specific support for the patient.

Peer support, in contrast, can be a saving grace for the patient with chronic pain, helping him feel less alone. Connecting directly with other chronic pain sufferers can help the patient better understand the incomprehensible, cope with the intolerable, and find the inner strength to transcend the apparent limits imposed by chronic pain.

Web of support

Ways to make connections with peers range from joining supportive Web sites and online chat groups to attending support groups. The best forms of peer support encourage self-expression in a supportive environment

Joining a support group can help the patient feel less alone.

without allowing members to dwell on pain. Validating and accepting pain are necessary, but should be accompanied by information-sharing and role-modeling effective coping strategies.

Model organization

The American Chronic Pain Association (ACPA) serves as a good support group model. The ACPA is structured to keep the focus on helping people improve their situations. It also provides training materials for group leaders. To contact the ACPA, call 1-800-533-3231 or visit *www.theacpa.org*.

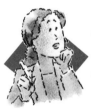

Quick quiz

1. Which statement about chronic pain is *true*?
   A. It's a chronic, relapsing, treatable disease linked to addiction.
   B. It may be explained by certain genetic, anatomic, and pathophysiologic mechanisms within the nervous system.
   C. It's a biopsychosocial disorder caused by ineffective coping.
   D. It's a mental disorder resulting from anxiety and depression.

Answer: B. Researchers have discovered genetic, anatomic, and pathophysiologic mechanisms within the nervous system that may explain chronic pain.

2. In patients with chronic pain, helplessness, catastrophic thinking, and self-doubts are associated with:
   A. low levels of disability.
   B. high levels of pain.
   C. low levels of depression.
   D. high levels of endorphins.

Answer: B. In patients with chronic pain, certain thought patterns — learned helplessness, catastrophic thinking, and self-doubt — are associated with high pain levels and contribute to disability and depression.

3. Which of the following interventions is *not* likely to enhance a patient's self-efficacy?
   A. Teaching the patient about his condition
   B. Teaching relaxation techniques
   C. Numbing the pain with nerve blocks
   D. Urging the patient to do things for himself

Answer: C. Numbing the pain with nerve blocks is a pharmacologic intervention. Although it may ease the patient's pain, it isn't a self-efficacy skill that the patient can initiate to manage his pain.

4. Which technique promotes the process of grief and acceptance?
- A. Pushing through pain
- B. Trying to reclaim what's been lost
- C. Reducing activities
- D. Evaluating losses

Answer: D. The patient must evaluate losses caused by chronic pain before he can grieve over and accept them.

Scoring

☆☆☆ If you answered all four questions correctly, fantastic! Your insight into lifestyle management is the best!

☆☆ If you answered three questions correctly, you've done a very credible job! And you can handle lifestyle management with ease.

☆ If you answered fewer than three questions correctly, take heart. A quick review of this chapter will be painless.

Appendices and index

Herbs used in pain management

With herbal remedies gaining wider acceptance among the general population, you may find that some of your patients are using these remedies for pain relief. This chart lists herbs that may used to eliminate, minimize, or prevent various types of pain.

Abdominal pain
- bitter orange
- Chinese cucumber
- Chinese rhubarb
- ground ivy
- khella

Analgesia
- aconite
- allspice
- arnica
- bethroot
- borage
- butterbur
- capsicum
- celandine
- devil's claw
- horse chestnut
- indigo
- lemongrass
- meadowsweet
- nettle
- parsley
- passion flower
- peach
- poplar
- red poppy
- safflower
- scented geranium
- turmeric
- wild lettuce
- willow
- wintergreen
- yerba maté

Antispasmodic effects
- American hellebore
- anise

- black haw
- bloodroot
- blue cohosh
- boldo
- butterbur
- cardamom
- celery
- clary
- cowslip
- dill
- fennel
- galangal
- ginger
- goldenrod
- hops
- jambolan
- lady's slipper
- lemongrass
- lovage
- madder
- parsley
- passion flower
- peppermint
- skunk cabbage
- tree unicorn root

Arthritis
- autumn crocus
- bearberry
- black pepper
- bogbean
- burdock
- capsicum
- celery
- chaparral
- chaulmoogra oil
- couch grass

- evening primrose oil
- feverfew
- fumitory
- ginger
- guggul
- kelpware
- male fern
- mayapple
- meadowsweet
- methylsulfonyl-methane
- morinda
- nettle
- nutmeg
- oregano
- pau d'arco
- rose hip
- safflower
- sassafras
- shark cartilage
- squill
- thuja
- thunder god vine
- vervain
- willow
- wintergreen

Backache
- butterbur
- rue

Cluster headaches
- melatonin
- benzoin
- bloodroot
- mullein

Dental pain

- allspice
- arnica
- asparagus
- bloodroot
- Chinese rhubarb
- clove oil
- coriander
- elderberry
- male fern
- mallow
- marigold
- meadowsweet
- prickly ash
- rosemary
- tansy

Diabetic neuropathy

- capsicum
- evening primrose oil

Dysmenorrhea

- black cohosh
- black haw
- black pepper
- butterbur
- caraway
- catnip
- chaparral
- daisy
- dong quai
- false unicorn root
- feverfew
- guarana
- Jamaican dogwood
- lady's mantle
- marigold
- night-blooming cereus
- parsley
- passion flower
- peach
- peppermint
- ragwort
- shepherd's purse
- squaw vine
- squill
- tree of heaven

- tree unicorn root
- valerian
- wild lettuce
- wild yam
- willow
- wintergreen

Earache

- male fern
- mullein
- peach

Fractures

- butcher's broom
- royal jelly
- shark cartilage

Headache

- black pepper
- blue flag
- butterbur
- castor bean
- catnip
- Chinese rhubarb
- clary
- cola
- cowslip
- daisy
- damiana
- dehydroepian-drosterone
- dong quai
- elderberry
- ephedra
- feverfew
- ginkgo
- green tea
- guarana
- Jamaican dogwood
- kava-kava
- lady's slipper
- lemon balm
- marjoram
- meadowsweet
- melatonin
- morinda
- passion flower
- peach
- peppermint

- pulsatilla
- ragwort
- rosemary
- rue
- saffron
- shepherd's purse
- stone root
- tansy
- turmeric
- valerian
- wild ginger
- willow
- yerba maté

Inflammation

- arnica
- blue cohosh
- boldo
- borage
- butcher's broom
- castor bean
- chaulmoogra oil
- Chinese rhubarb
- clary
- coffee
- comfrey
- daisy
- devil's claw
- fenugreek
- ginger
- goldenrod
- ground ivy
- indigo
- marigold
- meadowsweet
- methylsulfonyl-methane
- nettle
- pau d'arco
- peach
- prickly ash
- pulsatilla
- rue
- skullcap
- St. John's wort
- turmeric
- willow

Joint symptoms
- daisy
- juniper
- Queen Anne's lace
- ragwort
- rosemary
- thuja
- wild lettuce
- willow

Labor pain
- blue cohosh

Leg pain/swelling/edema
- horse chestnut

Migraine
- butterbur
- castor bean
- catnip
- clary
- cola
- daisy
- dehydroepian-drosterone
- dong quai
- feverfew
- Jamaican dog-wood
- lemon balm
- passion flower
- peppermint
- pulsatilla
- tansy
- wild ginger
- willow

Muscle pain
- allspice
- eucalyptus
- fenugreek
- horseradish
- juniper
- male fern
- marjoram
- methylsulfonyl-methane
- peppermint
- prickly ash

- rosemary
- St. John's wort
- wild lettuce
- wintergreen

Muscle spasms
- bay
- blue cohosh
- rue
- tonka bean

Muscle strains
- daffodil

Neuralgia
- aconite
- angelica
- betony
- black pepper
- capsicum
- cowslip
- daisy
- devil's claw
- dong quai
- elderberry
- hops
- Jamaican dog-wood
- lemon balm
- male fern
- passion flower
- peppermint
- pulsatilla
- rosemary
- wintergreen

Oral pain
- acidophilus

Osteoarthritis
- bogbean
- capsicum
- glucosamine sul-fate
- nettle
- S-adenosylme-thionine
- shark cartilage

Phantom limb pain
- capsicum

Postherpetic neuralgia
- capsicum

Premenstrual symptoms
- black cohosh
- bugleweed
- chaste tree
- clary
- couch grass
- dong quai
- ginkgo
- morinda
- nettle
- shepherd's purse
- wild yam
- willow

Reflex sympathetic dystrophy
- capsicum

Rheumatic diseases/rheumatism
- aconite
- angelica
- arnica
- asparagus
- autumn crocus
- birch
- blessed thistle
- bloodroot
- blue cohosh
- bogbean
- boldo
- boneset
- borage
- broom
- capsicum
- cat's claw
- celery
- chaparral
- chaulmoogra oil
- chickweed
- daisy
- elderberry
- eucalyptus
- evening primrose oil
- feverfew

- fumitory
- galangal
- horsetail
- juniper
- kava-kava
- kelpware
- lemon balm
- mayapple
- meadowsweet
- mullein
- nettle
- night-blooming cereus
- nutmeg
- parsley
- pau d'arco
- pokeweed
- poplar
- prickly ash
- ragwort
- rue
- sarsaparilla
- shark cartilage
- St. John's wort
- sweet flag
- thuja
- thunder god vine
- thyme
- tree unicorn root
- wild yam
- wintergreen

Sciatica
- aconite
- broom
- male fern
- nettle
- ragwort
- rose hip
- rosemary
- St. John's wort

Sprains
- arnica
- chaulmoogra oil
- comfrey
- daisy
- meadowsweet
- ragwort

- rue
- tansy
- yerba santa

Teething pain
- mallow

Toothache
- allspice
- asparagus
- Chinese rhubarb
- coriander
- elderberry
- male fern
- marigold
- meadowsweet
- prickly ash
- rosemary
- tansy

Glossary

addiction: physical or psychological dependence on a substance or activity, characterized by a craving beyond the individual's voluntary control

adjuvant analgesic: a drug typically administered for an indication other than pain relief (for instance, an anticonvulsant or an antidepressant) that's given to relieve pain in certain conditions

agonist: a drug that enhances or stimulates a receptor

analgesia: absence of pain in a conscious person, resulting from therapeutic intervention (such as with medication)

antagonist: a drug that nullifies the action of an agonist drug at a receptor site

balanced analgesia: absence of pain that's achieved by administering drugs from several classes of analgesics (such as nonsteroidal anti-inflammatory drugs, opioids, and local anesthetics) via one or more administration routes

biofeedback: a technique in which an individual receives visual or auditory information from monitoring devices about certain physiologic functions, such as blood pressure, muscle tension, and brain wave activity, and then learns to control these functions

breakthrough pain: worsening of pain that occurs either intermittently and spontaneously or in association with a particular kind of activity

dermatome: the area of the skin that's supplied with afferent (sensory) nerve fibers by a single posterior spinal root

efficacy: the ability of a drug or treatment to produce the desired therapeutic effect

epidural: located on or outside the dura mater of the spinal cord

half-life: the amount of time required for a drug's plasma concentration to decrease by 50%

lancinating: darting, tearing, sharp, knifelike (as pain)

metabolite: any product (such as food or waste product) of metabolism

modulation: inhibition of the cells that are responsible for transmitting pain impulses

narcotic: an obsolete term for what are now called opioids; current usage of the term is primarily in a legal context to refer to various substances of potential abuse

neuralgia: severe stabbing pain caused by several disorders that affect the nervous system

neuropathic pain: pain associated with inflammation or degeneration of the peripheral nerves

nociceptive pain: pain associated with activation of primary afferent neurons by a noxious stimulus

nociceptor: a sensory receptor that conveys nociceptive information about a noxious stimulus

nonopioid: a class of drugs once called "nonnarcotic" that includes acetaminophen and nonsteroidal anti-inflammatory drugs

nonsteroidal anti-inflammatory drug: aspirinlike drug that reduces inflammation and pain resulting from injured tissue

noxious stimulus: any stimulus (such as a cut, a pinch, or a burn) that's damaging to normal tissue

opioid: natural, semisynthetic, or synthetic drug that relieves pain by binding to opioid receptors in the nervous system

opioid agonist-antagonist: a drug that acts as an agonist at one type of opioid receptor site and as an antagonist at another opioid receptor site

pain: an unpleasant sensory or emotional experience associated with actual or potential tissue damage; any experience described in terms of such injury

parenteral route: an I.M., subcutaneous, or I.V. route of drug administration

paresthesia: abnormal or heightened touch sensations, such as burning, numbness, prickling, and tingling, that commonly occur without external stimuli

patient-controlled analgesia: treatment that allows the patient to control I.V. delivery of an analgesic (usually morphine) via a programmable device to maintain therapeutic serum levels

pharmacodynamics: the biochemical and physical effects of drugs and the mechanisms of drug actions

pharmacokinetics: the action of a drug within the body, including its absorption, distribution, metabolism, and excretion

pharmacotherapeutics: the use of drugs to prevent or treat disease

physical dependence: physical reliance on an opioid as evidenced by withdrawal symptoms if the opioid is abruptly stopped or an antagonist is administered

preemptive analgesia: treatment to prevent or minimize pain before an injury occurs (such as administration of epidural analgesia before a surgical procedure)

pseudoaddiction: behaviors (such as anger and escalating demands for more or different medications) that are associated with patients who aren't receiving adequate pain relief

rescue dose: a bolus or extra dose of medication given as needed to relieve pain that persists despite a regimen of pain medication given at regularly scheduled intervals

somatic pain: pain involving the musculoskeletal system

substance abuse: drug or alcohol use that can lead to social, occupational, psychological, or physical problems

titration: adjustment of a dose until a desired endpoint is reached

tolerance: decreasing response to a constant dose of a drug or the need for an increased dose to maintain a constant response

transduction: conversion of one form of energy to another

visceral pain: pain involving the body's internal organs

Web sites for pain management

- Agency for Healthcare Research and Quality
www.ahrq.gov

- American Academy of Hospice and Palliative Medicine
www.aahpm.org

- American Academy of Pain Management
www.aapainmanage.org

- American Cancer Society
www.cancer.org

- American Council for Headache
www.achenet.org

- American Journal of Nursing
www.nursingcenter.com

- American Nurses Association
www.nursingworld.org

- American Pain Society
www.ampainsoc.org

- Arthritis Foundation
www.arthritis.org

- Centers for Disease Control
www.cdc.gov

- Food and Drug Administration
www.fda.gov

- Gerontological Society of America
www.geron.org

- Hospice Foundation of America
www.hospicefoundation.org

- Internet Alcohol Recovery Center
www.med.upenn.edu/~recovery

- Medline
www.medline.com

- Medscape
www.medscape.com

- National Clearinghouse for Alcohol and Drug Information
www.health.org

- National Council on Alcoholism and Drug Dependence
www.ncadd.org

- National Hospice and Palliative Care Organization
www.nhpco.org

- National Institute of Nursing Research
www.nih.gov/ninr

- National Library of Medicine
www.nlm.nih.gov

- National Rehabilitation Information Center
www.naric.com

- Oncology Nursing Society
www.ons.org

- Reflex Sympathetic Dystrophy Syndrome Association of America
www.rsds.org

Selected references

American Academy of Pain Medicine, American Pain Society, American Society of Addiction Medicine: *Definitions Related to the Use of Opioids for the Treatment of Pain.* Glenview, Ill.: American Academy of Pain Medicine, American Pain Society, American Society of Addiction Medicine, 2001.

American Pain Society. *Guideline for the Management of Pain in Osteoarthritis, Rheumatoid Arthritis, and Juvenile Chronic Arthritis,* 2nd ed. Glenview, Ill.: American Pain Society, 2002.

Braunwald, E., et al., eds. *Harrison's Principles of Internal Medicine,* 15th edition. New York: McGraw-Hill Book Co., 2001.

Del Borgo C., et al. "Multidimensional Aspects of Pain in HIV-infected Individuals," *AIDS Patient Care and STDs* 15(2):95-102, February 2001.

Dijkstra, A., et al. "Readiness to Adopt the Self-management Approach to Cope with Chronic Pain in Fibromyalgic Patients," *Pain* 90(1-2):37-45, February 2001.

Dodd, M., et al. "Advancing the Science of Symptom Management," *Journal of Advanced Nursing* 33(5):668-76, March 2001.

Loeser, J.D., et al., eds. *Bonica's Management of Pain,* 3rd ed. Philadelphia: Lippincott Williams & Wilkins, 2001.

Main, C.J., and Spanswick, C.C. *Pain Management: An Interdisciplinary Approach.* Edited by Parker, H., and Watson, P. New York: Churchill Livingstone, Inc., 2000.

Marnetoft, S.U., and Selander, J. "Multidisciplinary Vocational Rehabilitation Focusing on Work Training and Case Management for Unemployed Sick-listed People," *International Journal of Rehabilitation Research* 23(4):271-79, December 2000.

McCaffery M., and Pasero, C. *Pain: Clinical Manual,* 2nd ed. St. Louis: Mosby–Year Book, Inc., 1999.

Miaskowski, C. "Different Kinds of Pain," *Pain Management Nursing* 2(4):119-20, December 2001.

Mior, S. "Exercise in the Treatment of Chronic Pain," *The Clinical Journal of Pain* 17(4 Suppl): S77-85, December 2001.

Oncology Nursing Society (November 2000). "Oncology Nursing Society Position on Cancer Pain Management" [Online]. *www. ons.org/xp6/ONS/Information. xml/Journals_and_Positions. xml/ONS_Positions.xml/ Cancer_Pain_Management.xml/* [2003, January 17].

Osterweil, D., et al. *Comprehensive Geriatric Assessment.* New York: McGraw-Hill Book Co., 2000.

Physician's Desk Reference, 56th ed. Montvale, N.J.: Medical Economics Co., 2002.

Powderly, W.G., ed. *Manual of HIV Therapeutics,* 2nd ed. Philadelphia: Lippincott Williams & Wilkins, 2001.

Raj, P.P., ed. *Practical Management of Pain,* 3rd ed. St. Louis: Mosby–Year Book, Inc., 2000.

Rees, V.W., et al. "Injury Among Detoxification Patients: Alcohol Users' Greatest Risk," *Alcoholism: Clinical and Experimental Research* 26(2):212-17, February 2002.

St. Marie, B., ed. *Core Curriculum for Pain Management Nursing.* Philadelphia: W.B. Saunders Co., 2002.

Stuifbergen, A.K., et al. "An Explanatory Model of Health Promotion and Quality of Life in Chronic Disabling Conditions," *Nursing Research* 49(3):122-29, May-June 2000.

U.S. Department of Health and Human Services (January 30, 2001). "Healthy People 2010: Leading Health Indicators" [Online]. *www.healthypeople.gov/ document/html/uih/uih_4.htm/* [2002, July 9].

World Health Organization (2002, May). "WHO Policy Perspectives on Medicines: Traditional Medicine — Growing Needs and Potential" [Online]. *www.who.int/ medicines/library/trm/trm_ polpers_eng.pdf/* [2003, January 17].

Index

A

Abdominal pain
  acute, 145-148, 147t
  HIV-AIDS and, 237, 238
Abstinence syndrome, 284
Acetaminophen, 56-57, 86,134
  in cancer pain, 210
  in chronic nonmalignant pain, 166
  in elderly patients, 276
  in HIV-AIDS pain, 227
  in pediatric pain, 259
Acquired immunodeficiency syndrome.
    See HIV-AIDS pain.
Actiq, 83
Acupressure, 121
Acupuncture, 120-122, 172
  in cancer pain, 220
Acute pain, 11, 131-156
  assessment of, 132-133
  chronic nonmalignant pain versus,
    31-32, 158
  dosing schedules for, 144-145, 156
  in children, 262
  management plan for, 133-134
  medication administration routes in,
    140-143
  nonpharmacologic interventions for, 145
  pharmacologic management of, 134-140
Acute pain disorders, 145-155
Addiction. *See* Addictive disease.
Addictive disease, 133, 281-302
  biologic aspects of, 285
  dosing schedule for, 299, 301
  management of, 287-298
  mental illness and, 285-286
  myths about, 282
  nonpharmacologic approaches to,
    293-296
  outpatient management of, 300
  pain assessment in, 297-298
  pain management in, 298-300

Addictive disease *(continued)*
  patient management in, 298-300
  pharmacotherapy for, 289-293
  physical illness and, 286-287
  statistics for, 284-285
  understanding, 283-287
A-delta fibers, 7
Adjustment, 9
Adjuvant analgesics, 67-81, 86
  in acute pain, 136-137
  anticonvulsants as, 67-69
  benzodiazepines as, 76-77
  in cancer pain, 214
  cholinergic blockers as, 79-80
  corticosteroids as, 80-81
  in elderly patients, 277
  ergotamine alkaloids as, 75-76
  in HIV-AIDS pain, 230
  local anesthetics as, 69
  muscle relaxants as, 71-72
  in pediatric pain, 260
  psychostimulants as, 77-78
  selective serotonin reuptake inhibitors
    as, 74-75
  serotonin 5-HT1 receptor agonists as,
    73-74
  topical anesthetics as, 70-71
  tricyclic antidepressants as, 72-73
Adverse reactions, in elderly patients, 273
Aerocaine, 70
Aging. *See also* Elderly patients.
  pharmacodynamics and, 273-274
  pharmacokinetics and, 271-273
AIDS pain. *See* HIV-AIDS pain.
Alcohol addiction, 292
Alcoholics Anonymous, 293
Alcohol withdrawal, 293
Allodynia, 5, 9
Almotriptan, 73
Alprazolam, 76

Alternative and complementary therapies,
    106-122
  acupuncture as, 120-122
  aromatherapy as, 108-109
  chiropractic treatment as, 118-120
  defining terms in, 106
  in pediatric pain, 261
  massage as, 116-118
  music therapy as, 109-111
  Therapeutic Touch as, 111-114, 113i
  yoga as, 114-116
American Chronic Pain Association, 328
Amides, 69, 70
Amitriptyline, 72
Amoxapine, 72
Analgesia. *See also specific type.*
  in acute pain, 134-140
  balanced, 135
  in cancer pain, 209-217
  in chronic nonmalignant pain, 165-170
  in elderly patients, 274-277
  in infants and children, 248
  preemptive, 135, 155
Analgesic drug interactions, 232, 234-236t
Analgesic infusion flow sheet, 43, 45i
Analgesics, adjuvant. *See* Adjuvant anal-
    gesics.
Anesthetics. *See* Local anesthetics *and*
    Topical anesthetics.
Angina, 6
Antabuse, 292
Anticonvulsants, 67-69, 185
  in cancer pain, 215
  in chronic nonmalignant pain, 169, 201
  in HIV-AIDS pain, 231
  and human immunodeficiency virus drug
    interactions, 236t
Antidepressants, in cancer pain, 215
Antiemetics, 184
Antiretroviral drug interactions, 232,
    234-236t
Antispasmodic agents, 71
Appendicitis, 6

i refers to an illustration; t refers to a table.

i refers to an illustration; t refers to a table.

refers to an illustration; t refers to a table.

i refers to an illustration; t refers to a table.